# Psychotherapy with African American Women

# PSYCHOTHERAPY WITH AFRICAN AMERICAN WOMEN

## Innovations in Psychodynamic Perspectives and Practice

Edited by

**Leslie C. Jackson**
**Beverly Greene**

*Foreword by Pamela Trotman Reid*

The Guilford Press
New York   London

© 2000 The Guilford Press
A Division of Guilford Publications, Inc.
72 Spring Street, New York, NY 10012
www.guilford.com

Printed in the United States of America

**Library of Congress Cataloging-in-Publication Data**

Psychotherapy with African American women : innovations in psychodynamic perspectives and practice / edited by Leslie C. Jackson and Beverly Greene.
    p. cm
    Includes bibliographical references and index.
    ISBN 1-57230-585-1 (cloth)
    1. Afro-American women—Mental health.   2. Psychodynamic psychotherapy.
  3. Afro-American women—Psychology.   I. Jackson, Leslie C.   II. Greene, Beverly.
RC451.4.M58 P795 2000
616.89'14'08996073—dc21                                    00-030870

*This book is the culmination of the survival, observations, and creativity of all the women who came before and after me and who enriched my life. This book was made possible because of my great-grandmother, Annie, my grandmother, Mary, and my mother, Theresa, who gave me strength. The friends, students, and clients whom I have been fortunate to have over the years planted a seed for this book. I hope they are pleased.*

*–Leslie C. Jackson*

*For my father,*
*For your time and attention to the essential details of our lives,*
*For taking any and many jobs, working endless hours,*
*And bearing indignities with dignity,*
*To give your children a better life. . . .*

*–Beverly Greene*

# About the Editors

**Leslie C. Jackson, PhD, ABPP (Clinical Psychology)**, is a professor in the Psychology Department at Georgia State University and a licensed psychologist in private practice in Atlanta, Georgia. Dr. Jackson spent most of her professional career in Los Angeles, where she worked as a staff psychologist at the UCLA Counseling Center and as a consultation education specialist at USC's Counseling Centers, and was an associate professor in the Multicultural Community/Clinical Proficiency Program at the California School of Professional Psychology, Los Angeles. As a licensed psychologist in California in private practice for 10 years, she consulted with community organizations, educational institutions, and mental health agencies on issues of diversity in clinical practice with African Americans. Dr. Jackson is an active presenter at professional workshops and conferences. She has also served as an associate professor in the School of Professional Psychology at Wright State University in Ohio. A member of the Association of Black Psychologists and the American Psychological Association (APA), she received an APA Minority Fellowship for graduate studies in clinical psychology, became a Fellow of the American Orthopsychiatric Association, and a Fellow of the Academy of Clinical Psychology in 1997. Dr. Jackson has advanced postdoctoral training in psychoanalytic psychotherapy from the Wright Postgraduate Training Center in Los Angeles. Additionally, she holds a Diplomate in Clinical Psychology from the American Board of Professional Psychology. She has served on many local, state, and national boards of directors in California, Ohio, and now Georgia, and is an editorial and consulting reviewer for two APA journals: *Cultural Diversity and Ethnic Minority Psychology* and *Professional Psychology: Research and Practice.* Her research and publications focus on diversity issues in training and service delivery. Dr. Jackson has received several awards and commendations within the field: a Distinguished Humanitarian Contribution from the APA in 1992 and the California Psychological Association in 1993; Kellogg Women of Color Leadership Fellow in 1988; and a Distinguished Faculty Contribution Award from the California School of Professional Psychology in 1993.

**Beverly Greene, PhD, ABPP (Clinical Psychology)**, is a professor of psychology at St. John's University and a certified clinical psychologist in private practice in Brooklyn, New York. A Fellow of the American Psychological Association (APA), the Academy of Clinical Psychology, and the American Orthopsychiatric Association, she holds a Diplomate in Clinical Psychology from the American Board of Professional Psychology. Prior to joining the faculty of St. John's University in 1991, Dr. Greene worked in public mental health with the New York City Board of Education, Inpatient Child and Adolescent Psychiatry at Kings County Hospital, and Outpatient Community Mental Health at the University of Medicine and Dentistry of New Jersey in Newark. Dr. Greene is the recipient of numerous national awards for distinguished scholarly and professional contributions, including the 1992 Award for Distinguished Professional Contributions to Ethnic Minority Issues (APA Division 44) for her development of lesbian-affirmative theoretical perspectives and clinical applications with African American women; 1995 and 1996 Psychotherapy with Women Research Awards from the Division of the Psychology of Women of the APA for substantial and outstanding contributions to the theory, practice, and research of psychotherapy with women; and the 1991 Women of Color Psychologies Publication Award from the Association for Women in Psychology for publications deemed significant contributions to the development of greater understanding of the psychologies of women of color. She is coeditor of *Women of Color: Integrating Ethnic and Gender Identities in Psychotherapy* (Guilford Press, 1994), which received a 1995 Distinguished Publication Award and a 1995 Women of Color Psychologies Award. Dr. Greene is also the recipient of the 1996 Outstanding Achievement Award from the APA's Committee on Lesbian, Gay, and Bisexual Concerns for pioneering scholarship and training efforts on the interaction of gender, ethnicity, and sexual orientation in mainstream professional psychological publications and practice. She was the founding coeditor of *Psychological Perspectives on Lesbian, Gay, and Bisexual Issues* (Sage), a series of annual publications sponsored by the Society for the Psychological Study of Lesbian, Gay, and Bisexual Issues of the APA (Division 44), and is a consulting editor and editorial board member of numerous scholarly journals. She is the coauthor of the undergraduate text *Abnormal Psychology in a Changing World* (Prentice Hall, 2000), editor of *Ethnic and Cultural Diversity among Lesbians and Gay Men* (Sage, 1997), and coeditor of the recently published *Education, Research, and Practice in Lesbian, Gay, Bisexual, and Transgendered Psychology: A Resource Manual* (Sage, 2000).

# Contributors

**Joan M. Adams MSW,** is director of clinical quality and inservice training at the Postgraduate Center for Mental Health in New York City, where she is also a senior supervisor and training analyst in the Adult Analytic Training Program and a supervisor in the Analytic Group Therapy Training Program. A clinical social worker, she was trained and certified in individual and group analytic psychotherapy at the Postgraduate Center. She is also in private practice in individual and group psychotherapy in New York City. Ms. Adams's training, teaching, and consultation focus on issues of diversity in mental health and higher education.

**Jessica Henderson Daniel, PhD, ABPP,** is an assistant professor in the Department of Psychiatry at Harvard Medical School, a codirector of training in psychology and an associate director of leadership education in the Adolescent Health Training Program at Children's Hospital, and a senior research associate at the Judge Baker Children's Center. In private practice for 22 years, she has a particular interest in the development of African American females. From 1989 to 1993 she chaired the Board of Registration of Psychologists in the Commonwealth of Massachusetts. Under her leadership, Massachusetts became the first and remains the only state, to require both instruction and training about people of color in order to be licensed as a psychologist. She is the recipient of the A. Clifford Barger Excellence in Mentoring Award at Harvard Medical School and the 1999 Kenneth and Mamie Clark Award from the American Psychological Association of Graduate Students in recognition of her mentoring graduate students of color.

**Beverly Greene, PhD, ABPP** (*see* "About the Editors")

**Leslie C. Jackson, PhD, ABPP** (*see* "About the Editors")

**Yvonne M. Jenkins, PhD,** is a staff psychologist at the University Counseling Services, Boston College, and a psychologist in private practice in Brookline, Massachusetts. She has served on the staff of the Harvard University Mental Health Service and on the faculty of the Jean Baker Miller Institute at Wellesley College. Dr. Jenkins's professional publications and training interests include mental health issues associated with cultural diversity, college mental health, and women's mental health issues. Recent publications include *Diversity in College Settings: Directives for Mental Health Professionals* (Routledge, 1999).

**Michele Owens-Patterson, PhD,** is a clinical psychologist in private practice for 17 years. She is a clinical supervisor at New Hope Guild's East New York Children's Clinic, an adjunct clinical supervisor at City College's Doctoral Program in Clinical Psychology, and an assistant clinical professor at the Derner Institute of Advanced Psychological Studies of Adelphi University. Dr. Owens-Patterson has advanced training in psychotherapy and psychoanalysis. She has spent much of her career focusing on African American children's and adolescents' issues as well as on the issues and concerns of women of color. She designed and conducts a conflict resolution project for elementary school children and their parents. Her other interests include multiculturalism in the delivery of mental health services, depression in Black women, parenting issues for African American children and adolescents, mental health programming for at-risk youth, and psychological issues of upward mobility in African American families.

**Regina E. Romero, PhD,** is in the private group practice of Psychological and Educational Associates, Inc., in the Washington, DC, area and is also an adjunct faculty member at Howard University. She has taught diversity classes at Loyola University in the Baltimore area and at the Trinity College Graduate Workshop Program in Washington, DC. Dr. Romero served as the director of inpatient clinical services at St. Luke Institute, and as a consultant to the National Leadership Institute, the University of Maryland, and Clinical Associates, Camp Springs, Maryland. Dr. Romero is a member of the Association of Black Psychologists, the American Psychological Association, and the Washington Area Council on Alcohol and Drug Abuse. She is also a National Institute of Mental Health Fellow.

**Kumea Shorter-Gooden, PhD,** is a professor in the Multicultural Community/ Clinical Proficiency Program at the California School of Professional Psychology, Los Angeles, and a licensed psychologist in Pasadena, California. Her courses include intercultural lab, multicultural mental health, community–clinical issues, and advanced psychodynamic interventions with multicultural populations. She has served as the director of the Student Counseling Center at the Claremont Colleges in Claremont, California; as clinical director at the Community Mental Health Council, a comprehensive community mental health center in Chicago; and as the director of the Umoja Extended Family Juvenile Program, a residential and counseling program for inner-city, African American adolescents in New Haven, Connecticut. Her research and publications focus on identity development of African American women.

**Cheryl L. Thompson, PhD,** is an associate professor of clinical psychology at Seton Hall University in South Orange, New Jersey, and a member of the faculties of the New York University Postdoctoral Program in Psychotherapy and Psychoanalysis and the Institute for Psychoanalysis and Psychotherapy of New Jersey. A certified clinical psychologist in private practice in Millburn, New Jersey, she has published several articles and book chapters on the impact of race on the development of psychopathology in African American patients, and is interested in juvenile delinquency and the variables that lead to serious antisocial behavior. She has served as an expert witness in juvenile waiver cases.

**Frances K. Trotman, PhD,** is the founder/director of the Contemporary Counseling and Psychotherapy Institute, with offices in Teaneck, Weehawken, and West Long Branch, New Jersey, where she has been in practice for over 25 years. An associate professor and director of the Graduate Program in Psychological Counseling at Monmouth University in West Long Branch, New Jersey, Dr. Trotman has served as president of the New Jersey Association of Black Psychologists and the Bergen County Association of Licensed Psychologists. She has also served as an officer and on several boards of the American Psychological Association and its divisions. A recipient of the Psychologist's Recognition Award, she has numerous professional publications. She is currently writing a textbook on the psychology of African American women and is editing a volume on alternative parenting.

**Judith C. White, MS, CSW, CGP,** is a psychotherapist and psychoanalyst in private practice in New York City. A faculty member and supervisor in the Advanced Training Program for Group Practice at the Jewish Board for Family and Children's Services, she is also a supervisor in the Psychoanalytic Training Institute of the Postgraduate Center for Mental Health and a member of their Analytic Group Workshop faculty. She has served as the director of counseling at Malcolm King Harlem College Extension in New York, where she received that institution's 1985 Award for Outstanding Service from the Friends of Malcolm King. Dr. White is a long-standing member of the Association of Black Social Workers, the Eastern and American Group Psychotherapy Associations, and the Black, Hispanic, and Asian Caucus of the Postgraduate Center for Mental Health. She has made numerous presentations and has published articles on the mental health of African Americans and the impact of race/ethnicity on individual and group psychotherapies with both Black and White women.

**Lisa Whitten, PhD,** is an associate professor of psychology at the College of Old Westbury, State University of New York. Active in the Association of Black Psychologists for over 20 years, she has served two terms as president of the New York chapter and as eastern regional representative. She has a private practice in Queens, New York, and is president of Maximizing Excellence, an educational and consulting firm. An early proponent of bringing race and culture to the center of undergraduate instruction, she presented a workshop on infusing Black psychology into the introduction to psychology course at the Teaching Undergraduate Psychology Conference, SUNY Farmingdale, in 1987. Dr. Whitten has contributed material related to race and culture to *Psychology: An Introduction* (Brown & Benchmark, 1994) and to the course planner to accompany *Psychology: The Contexts of Behavior* (Brown & Benchmark, 1992). In 1993 her article on race and culture became one of only three such articles ever published in the first 19 years of the journal *Teaching of Psychology*. Her professional interests and research focus on parent education, survival guilt, and survival conflict in African American college students.

# Foreword

There exist at least two myths of African American women; they are either "good" or "bad." The "good" African American woman is strong, maternal, hard-working, devoted to family, and quiet. (Note that quietness is traditionally considered a virtue in children, Blacks, and women.) The "bad" African American woman is ugly, lascivious, lazy, negligent, emasculating, and loud. Both views are based on stereotypes born of a need to justify public policies or societal treatment of African American women; they do not come from data or any close investigation of reality. Thus, when psychologists attempt to address therapeutic needs, obvious anxieties, or behavioral problems, they must ask, "What do we know about African American women?" Too often the answers have been couched in terms of these myths as well as other mistaken notions that may abound.

It also seems rare that the literature of psychology examines the difficulties that African American women face, unless their losses somehow affect the greater segments of society. The personal trauma and problems of coping have remained private and invisible, events that these women must cope with by themselves. We in psychology have looked past the illness and death, the loneliness and pain, the broken relationships and the crises of self-doubt that African American women experience. We have also ignored the cultural and the social situations that contribute to mental, emotional, and even physical problems.

The state of African American women requires much more lightheartedness and understanding. For psychologists, this group represents an understudied, overlooked, and distorted topic. In part, the dearth of knowledge about African American women has resulted from a bifurcation of their dual identity as ethnic group members and as women. For some decades, researchers who examined ethnicity or race often ignored the issues of gender and the impact of sexism, so that studies of the ethnic experience have been told from the male perspective. The feminist literature had a similar narrow focus, with a concentration on majority women, leaving women of color out of the discourse. Indeed, for African American women, the experience of having one segment or the other of one's identity overlooked is common as they are subsumed under other groups' categorizations.

Another reason for the ignorance about African American women is the unwillingness to recognize the differences that exist within Black communities; we have not chronicled the heterogeneity or the myriad factors that distinguish the subgroups and subcultures. African American women are Baptist and Catholic; they are descended from the Caribbean and from southern U.S. states; they work in varied occupations, from doctors, lawyers, and educators to factory workers and domestics; they identify themselves as heterosexuals and lesbians, married and single, mothers, lovers, sisters, and daughters.

While learning to realize our differences, we have also not acknowledged sufficiently our similarities with other ethnic groups, those who are people of color and those who are not. When there has been a failure to cope successfully, this has been noted, but we have not fully understood the stresses and the strains of establishing identity or the struggles in dealing with life in America as an African American woman. In addition to this essentialism that serves to ignore African American women, and other women of color, there has been an oversimplification, a belief in parsimony that discounted complicated explanations. Particularly in psychology, we try to select one domain, one trait, one characteristic—or, in this case, one category of persons to examine. Therefore, we conduct our analyses without fully demanding an understanding of the system and the contexts in which the trait or the person operates. We do this so regularly that our students and even we, as researchers, begin to believe that this is not only legitimate, but that it is indeed the best and maybe the only way to proceed toward understanding our complicated world. We want to understand "pure phenomena," as one colleague explained it to me. "I came into psychology," he said, "to learn about the rules and the principles of behavior." Obviously he, and many others, believe that behavior can exist in a vacuum.

We all really know that it is not possible to study one trait in isolation, whether it is intelligence or generosity, athletic skill or musical talent. Everything has an environment in which it is manifest. We know that everything must be considered in context even in the physical sciences—when chemists isolate an element, they proceed further to learn how it operates in conjunction with others, how it combines and interacts, and how it is influenced by temperature and other conditions. So, too, in the behavioral sciences we cannot study one trait without considering the person who possesses it; neither is it possible to study one category of persons in isolation, unless they truly live in isolation. Obviously, this is not the condition of African American women.

To best understand complicated lives and complicated people, such as African American women, we therefore will require analyses that consider them as they live within the context of families, communities, and societies. We cannot just examine them as though they alone control the key elements of their behavior, personality, and experiences. We must understand them and the important issues of their lives, including the influence of others, and their views of themselves across and within a variety of domains. If we do not look at the complexity of African American women, we will explain and understand only part of the picture.

Given an understanding of African American women in context, through this book, Leslie C. Jackson and Beverly Greene provide new knowledge and innovative perspectives for therapists and others interested in unpacking the stereotypes and uncovering some degree of complex reality. The topics and the contexts explored in this volume avoid the easy answers and confront the issues of daily life for African American women. Remarkable in their experience and insight, the editors and contributors replace stereotypes and myths to create a complicated view of women in relationships, women in a variety of contexts, and women facing themselves in society. Additionally, they deliver a set of strategies that have proven useful in treating the concerns of African American women in therapeutic situations.

In the chapters written by women of color about women of color, there is a blend of theory with application, psychoanalytic perspective with real-world experience. The offer is not a panacea; instead, we are given thoughtful suggestions and challenges to stereotypic approaches. This is the beginning of the light and it is hoped that it will spark useful treatment and clearer practice for African American women and guide those therapists who serve them.

PAMELA TROTMAN REID, PhD
*University of Michigan*

# Preface

## WHY A BOOK ON PSYCHODYNAMIC PSYCHOTHERAPY AND AFRICAN AMERICAN WOMEN?

As editors of this volume we decided to bring together a group of clinicians from around the country to give voice to the silence around psychodynamic psychotherapy with African American women. This process began with a focus group dialogue with a group of African American women attending the 1994 American Psychological Association conference in Los Angeles. The group discussed whether they thought an edited book on psychodynamic psychotherapy was needed that focused specifically on the issues of African American women. There was overwhelming support for this idea, and the women began sharing their experiences as students, clinicians, supervisors, and clients as evidence of the lack of literature to guide the training of future clinicians. We found in our collective experiences in graduate school, our training as clinicians, and our experiences as psychotherapy clients that there was almost no information available that addressed the complexity of our collective experiences as African American women. We wanted to address deficits in the psychological literature that ranged from offering limited information on theory and interventions to giving distorted and offensive information that leads to damaging interventions. While historically the literature on culture and ethnicity may have been descriptive, it lacked a psychological perspective. There was little or no focus on how factors based on culture and ethnicity would be played out in a therapy context and what appropriate interventions for them might be. Similarly, the emerging psychological literature on gender focused on gender as the primary locus of discrimination for all women. It overlooked the salience of ethnicity as a dimension that transforms the meaning and experience of gender, sexism, and heterosexism.

This volume specifically addresses these issues and explores psychotherapy with African American women and a wide range of their potential presentations in the psychotherapy hour from psychodynamic perspectives. The authors explore both the common and the distinct dilemmas that confront African American women in their attempts to negotiate a society that is hostile to them on multiple levels and that continually challenges their psychological functioning. The chapters show the wide range of ways of understanding these dilemmas and explain creative and innovative reformulations of psychodynamic theory as well as concrete techniques. Contributors provide information about issues that concern African American women that are common to their lives and experiences, but that are, from our perspective as African American women and clinicians, often missing from the theoretical paradigms that are prevalent in the field and conspicuously absent in the therapeutic inquiry.

The absence of the African American female perspective in the psychological literature and in clinical practice may be attributed in part to the ethnocentrism of the mental health profession. Most psychological theories were developed in the context of a dominant European American cultural perspective, more specifically by White males. The European American perspectives consistently fail to acknowledge other experiences that differ from their dominant cultural perspectives. Moreover, in these "traditional" theoretical frameworks, when differences cannot be denied, those outside the dominant culture are often stigmatized and/or pathologized. This stigmatization occurs because the meaning of these differences, stereotypes, and social constructions stimulates projections that have been internalized about African American women. These unconscious projections are remnants of a patriarchal, racist, classist, and heterosexist society. This creates a cognitive dissonance in the self-perception of dominant culture members, resulting in defensive responses. If these defensive responses fail, then the "traditional" theoretical framework and the dominant culture become the model that is used to understand the complex experiences of African American women. Often the theorists from the dominant culture, male or female, are writing from their positions as dominant cultural beings. They view African American women from a position of power, and are generally invested in maintaining this hierarchy without examination. The failure to examine oneself as a dominant cultural being, or as any other being, for biases inherent in one's theoretical position contradicts a fundamental ethical responsibility for self-examination, both in capacity and in behavior. The very core of this professional responsibility is one in which self-examination is intrinsic not only to psychodynamic thinking, but to the ethical functioning of mental health professionals. Why, one may ask, is this important?

While training programs today are more compelled to address the dimensions of gender, class, culture, sexual orientation, and so forth, they still rely primarily on perhaps one course in a curriculum and limited numbers of faculty of color to teach such courses. They also continue to rely on a mental health literature and many theoretical paradigms that remain, albeit better than they once were, still lacking in many ways. These experiences and our sense of what has been missing from the literature provided the impetus for our development of this book. We believe that the experiences we have discussed were also operative in the thinking of this book's contributors. Such experiences have clearly played an important role in compelling them to develop creative theoretical and practical psychotherapy approaches that build on and even challenge previous approaches in their clinical work with African American women.

The collective experience and knowledge of the contributors shows their desire to improve the delivery of psychological services to African American women and is reflected in their roles as senior faculty, supervisors, researchers, and trainers in mental health over many years. Their cumulative experiences as African American women and clinicians make this book a compilation of work on the development of theory and intervention strategies with African American women clients that is on the cutting edge. While the authors examine the common experiences and struggles in the lives of African American women, they also challenge the notion of universality, reminding us of the richness and complexity of difference within this group.

We assert that if mental health professionals are to have an authentic understanding of human behavior, they must be able to appreciate how differing dimensions of human identities inform and transform one another rather than dichotomizing them as if they either developed, are experienced, or are responded to in isolation from one another. We specifically address these issues in African American women. We view African American women as having multiple identities that shift in salience depending on the context, their personal history, self-perception, and experiences.

## WHAT IS THIS BOOK ABOUT?

These chapters offer reformulations of various psychodynamic theories. In addition, they show how these theories can be applied to specific dilemmas of African American women. The authors tried to point out the inherent bias of the original theories in their omission of considerations of culture, gender, class, sexual orientation, and other dimensions in a historical and sociopolitical context. This is reflected most concretely not only in their failure to consider the importance of these identities to African American women's experience of themselves but also in their tendency to stigmatize these identities. None of the traditional psychodynamic approaches integrated perspectives on class, gender, sexual orientation, and other identities in ways that reflect their true complexity. Without maintaining the perspective that all identities are interrelated one loses the ability to effectively intervene clinically and/or to develop research paradigms that accurately reflect the lives of African American women.

The contributors' analysis and reformulation of existing theory serve as the basis for the creative and innovative clinical applications discussed in their chapters. We are given an important synthesis of theoretical innovation and clinical application.

Another unique aspect of this book is that the authors' work is a result of their shared personal experiences as African American women as well as their empathic professional work with African American women across the country. Despite the varying locales and circumstances of their practices, there is a surprising consistency in this body of work. There are many important correspondences in African American women's experiences that cut across their differences and their presentations to therapists across the country that have been reflected in the content of the chapters in this book.

These chapters come from a uniquely African American female perspective. The authors represent the heterogeneity among African American women that mirrors the experience of the women we serve. The exploration of the material covered in this volume required more of these authors than distant intellectual analysis. The contributors are personally acquainted with many of the painful experiences that their clients bring to them. Their intimate knowledge of their clients' dilemmas makes the therapy more empathically complex and challenging, but potentially more rewarding. In practice this requires managing the unique countertransference feelings that surface during the course of the work. Writing about these issues required contributors to revisit these experiences both emotionally and intellectually. What is less articulated and acknowledged is that writing about the work requires managing painful feelings as well. Despite the challenges in the process, we believe the end product is richer.

## GIVING OUR VOICE TO THE SILENCE

Some of the challenges that have emerged in creating this book mirror the broader experience of African American women. The historical absence of affirmative theory and research about many of the issues discussed in this book represents a kind of silence about them. We know that silence is often another form of oppression. Breaking that silence threatens the dominant culture status quo as well as the status quo among African Americans. This, in turn, created an additional challenge for these authors. These challenges are organized around issues of power and control, competence, and rejection for airing "dirty cultural laundry" and violating the cultural taboo that requires homogeneity as proof of group and cultural loyalty. Traditionally, African American women are devalued and as such their thinking and intellect is devalued. For the authors, this book was an opportunity to give our clients and ourselves a voice in a climate in which we are used to having our experiences labeled and talked about rather than naming, claiming, and talking about them ourselves. We are used to being labeled and defined by others, both outside and inside the group, and have been treated as if our collective perceptions were historically, interpersonally, and intrapsychically inaccurate. Even when our perceptions as African American women have been presumed to be accurate, we have been treated as if we should not articulate them, such as we all witnessed with Anita Hill. We are aware that when we say that African American women must be understood as individuals as well as part of a group, we recognize that this may be seen as a perspective that threatens the survival of the community. However, we also recognize that we are contributing another level of knowledge for the intellectual and scientific community to grapple with. While there are many different perspectives represented on any one of the dimensions we have articulated, we believe that the diverse experiences of African American women warrant more than what any one worldview offers, and we make our contribution in that way.

LESLIE C. JACKSON
BEVERLY GREENE

# Contents

## CHAPTER 1

# The New Multiculturalism and Psychodynamic Theory

## Psychodynamic Psychotherapy and African American Women

### LESLIE C. JACKSON

This book explores doing psychodynamic therapy with African American women. We hope that our readers will develop a broader understanding of what is both useful and problematic when applying psychodynamic theories to their African American female clients. We created this book because we want to help mental health professionals identify the differences among intrapsychic, cultural variables, and social constructions, so as to better understand how these interacting variables affect the coping and functioning of African American women.

Deconstructing the cultural underpinnings of psychoanalytic theory is not a new endeavor for therapists working with people of color. Communities of color have long been suspicious of psychoanalytic models because of their traditional focus on the individual, as well as their failure to acknowledge racist and sexist assumptions underlying the theory of personality development. Ironically, however, those same theories have also been used to study the effects of racism, sexism, and identity development by psychoanalysts who have transformed the psychodynamic theoretical understanding of African Americans and women to include the effects of cultural and social constructions on development and coping (Bulhan, 1985; Fanon, 1967; Greene, 1993; Grier & Cobbs, 1968; Mattei, 1996).

Yet advances in theory development within the psychodynamic domain, such as object relations, self psychology, relational models, and the efforts to

1

include social and cultural knowledge, offer a new opportunity for cultural competent treatment using these models. As with any one model, there continue to be limitations. The broader analytic community has yet to acknowledge that these theories are not universal theories, and that they reflect the political and social realities in which they developed. The European American ethnocentric point of view provided an opportunity for therapists to support and sustain cultural stereotypes and social constructions about African Americans in our society. Theorists developed these models without considering either the effects of "other" social and culture factors or the effects of being the "other" on personality functioning. Taylor (1999) pointed out how this theoretical inadequacy has resulted in two "solutions" used by mental health professionals trying to bridge the gap between theory and practice with people of color. The first is to make the client fit the particular theory, and the second is to "stretch the frame of reference to fit the client" (p. 175). The former solution is embedded in the etic, or universal, notions of theory and is a denial of difference; the latter solution assumes that the clients' unique differences would be the primary focus of treatment. This results in denying within-group differences and prevents the client from experiencing his or her individual uniqueness. Consequently, these models have been associated with the pathologizing of various groups, for example, ethnic minority populations, women, gay and lesbian populations, and in general all people who are not White, middle-to-upper class, and of European ancestry.

## THE MULTICULTURAL CONTEXT

Over the last 20 years multicultural training and research have shifted from examining client variables to concentrating on therapist variables. One of the elements of the multicultural concentration is the need for therapists to acknowledge an awareness of their own ethnocultural attitudes and beliefs. Specifically, therapists who are able to explore their own cultural and ethnic backgrounds are more likely to appreciate the nuances of cultural and ethnic identity and how they effect one's perceptions of self and the other in a sociopolitical context. The therapist's exploration of his or her family dynamics around issues of ethnicity, gender, culture, and power will provide therapists with the experience to help clients explore their own backgrounds and possible intrapsychic derivatives. A focus on the ethnocultural effects of the psychotherapy process and our ability to form empathic connections will broaden our understanding of how the therapeutic process can be effective with people of color in general and African Americans in particular.

Training students to work effectively with clients who are different from the therapist is especially important given the fact that fewer students of color are entering graduate training programs. Cultural competence training and research has also given us the necessary data to acknowledge the cultural and ethnic diversity within communities of color. Therefore, cultural competency training is needed for all clinicians working with people of color. Over the last 10 years there has been a proliferation of guidelines for cultural competency published by state licensing boards and professional organizations, such as the American Psychological Association. Researchers have identified issues for therapists—whatever their theoretical orientation—to consider when working with diverse clients, for example, issues of racial identity, cultural identity/acculturation, social class, language, and worldview. Additionally, theoreticians have added to the armamentarium of information available to therapists working with clients who are different—for example, feminist theory, African-centered models, and social construction theory have expanded our understanding of how issues of difference and power effect the therapeutic relationship.

The challenge for those of us trained in psychodynamic models is to expand our understanding of the therapeutic relationship in diverse dyads, and to elaborate upon the theories we use to become more inclusive. Contemporary psychodynamic models offer us an opportunity to examine cultural constructs within the client's social environment, as well as the ethnocultural experience that occurs between the therapist and the client. Dynamic therapists should consider the following questions when deciding to work with African American clients because these questions challenge the eurocentric bias built into theory:

1. How does the experience of early childhood development (if the nuclear family is not the model) effect the development of healthy or unhealthy personality?
2. When is the development of autonomy or separation an appropriate or inappropriate marker of healthy functioning?
3. How have the effects of slavery, marginalization, and discrimination affected the development of personality?
4. What is the importance of the effects of racial identity development, skin color, and hair (being either idealized or devalued) on the development of African American personality?

Presently, the traditional dynamic theories are not prepared adequately to address these issues in either their theories or in the relational issues that arise within the scope of practice.

Likewise, our knowledge of psychopathology today reflects the integration of biological, psychological, social, and cultural phenomena. The context in which we learn about psychopathology often affects our understanding of the unique contribution or balance among these four factors. Individual cultural experiences will effect both the therapist and the client, and this can result in the therapist and client disagreeing on the nature of the problem and treatment recommendations. Alarcon, Foulks, and Vakkur (1998) describe the role of culture in the therapeutic relationship as a constant variable that will influence how the client defines his or her problem, whether or not he or she will seek and comply with treatment, and how he or she will experience the relationship with the therapist. This experience is particularly consequential for African American women entering psychotherapy, for they bring with them a unique history in American culture that will effect the understanding of their lives in most dramatic ways in psychotherapy. The ethnic, gender, sexual, and social stereotypes projected onto African American women have been significantly different from those projected onto African American men, even though both groups share the historical experience of discrimination and powerlessness. For example, African American men do not share the historical sexism imposed on African American women. It is through these cultural lenses that the African American female will define her therapeutic issues and experience the psychotherapy relationship.

Recent changes in the mental health field, for example, the inclusion of cultural and biopsychosocial models, have affected our view of pathology, resulting in it being redefined by women, gay and lesbian groups, and people of color. Now that both cultural and social factors have been recognized as contributing to our understanding of pathology, many of us understand that sometimes psychopathology must be viewed through the lens of our unique cultural experiences. Nonetheless, most dynamic theories have yet to embrace the social reality of the nondominant groups in our society. Therefore, these theories still reflect the worldview of the more privileged in society who have the power to decide who is sick, what type of treatment they need, and how to provide it.

Some African American psychologists have challenged the culturalist belief of psychodynamic theories as eurocentric and inappropriate for African American populations. Most of the African culturalist constructs coming from the African American community are attempts to more fully capture the experience of African Americans in this country. But we believe that it is a false assumption that an African-centered paradigm is *always* more appropriate than any other theory for the African American community. The African American community in the 1990s represents a composite of racial and cultural diversity. For example, the Caribbean peoples who have recently emigrated to the United States in great numbers bring their own unique cultural history, and interracial pairings have resulted in a very heterogeneous Black U.S. community. Additionally, within the U.S. African American community, there are tremendous political, regional, social class, and educational differences. All of this diversity demands new ways to understand our clients. We suggest that no one theory can appropriately respond to every African American seeking or needing services. This reality requires a shift in understanding and training procedures. Alarcon and colleagues (1998) advocate a shift toward clinical applicability rather than theoretical appropriateness, allowing therapists more flexibility in deciding what a client may need given his or her particular circumstance. The experience of slavery, marginalization, and decades of ongoing discrimination requires mental health professionals to recognize that the "African American community" will also have assorted reactions to these experiences. It is a reasonable assumption to recognize that no one theory will be useful for every problem or for any particular group of Black people.

## PSYCHODYNAMIC THEORIES: THE MYTH OF UNIVERSALITY

Psychodynamic theories are culture-bound social constructions embedded in the particular worldview of their time. These theories have been espoused as universal theories of development of personality and pathology despite the evidence to the contrary. Communities of color have justifiably criticized dynamic theories from the beginning because these theories reinforced the various biases, stereotypes, and prejudices that were prevalent in our society.

In particular, Freud's drive theory focused on the contradictions and conflict that existed between biological drives (sexual and aggressive) and the sociocultural forces in his society. This theory was developed in the late 19th and early 20th centuries and identified issues that were the salient cultural issues of that era, for example, the suppression of women and sexuality. Freud offered a psychological explanation for the cultural value system of his own period. He concurrently espoused his theory of psychosexual development, a theory that initiated the psychological labeling of female inferiority to males as biologically derived and ignoring sociocultural influences; Freud later expanded his theory of personality with a structural model that supplemented drive theory. Structural theory proposed that one's intrapsychic (internal/unconscious) conflicts were the result of the interplay between the three psychic structures of the mind: id, ego, and superego. This theory introduced the beginnings of our understanding of ego functions and defenses. One important ego function is the regulation of self-esteem by evaluating perceptions of the self and the social environment. This level of theory development was supported by the evidence he collected from female patients with neurotic symptoms. These women were not living in a society where their development of self-esteem was supported by societal expectations for women; hence they were labeled neurotic.

Ego psychology, developed in the late 1940s and early 1950s, expanded our knowledge of ego functions. It focused on developing a framework for repairing developmental arrests. This theory continued to promote a universal theory of development and employed "normal" male development as the standard of health. If you look closely at the tenets of ego psychology, you see that its focus on personality development over the life span promotes the achievement of autonomy and individuation within the family and culture—not the prevailing view for many diverse cultures within the United States.

Object relations theory focuses on one's need to both attach and to be separate. Within this process the theory focuses on how we meet our needs within a relational context using a developmental model. Object relations theory promotes the notion of the universal nuclear family and the role of the powerful mother, who is all-giving and readily available, as necessary for the child's healthy personality development. This notion plants the seeds to pathologize other family constellations and primary caregivers—for example, grandparents. Additionally, it promotes an adherence to sex-role stereotyping of males and females in our society.

The latest theory to come from the dynamic school is self psychology with its exclusive focus on how the "self" develops and the techniques used to restore impaired development. Self psychology proposes that repeated empathic failures by caregivers result in an unhealthy development of the self. This theory does not focus exclusively on mothers or on the nuclear family for healthy development of a child. But even with its specialized focus on the "self" or the "individual," there is some flexibility in how personality development may be understood in other cultural contexts.

The newest relational model, created in response to analytic models that failed clearly to delineate healthy female development, has an exclusive focus on female development. This model was developed by European American feminists. It is flawed because it promotes their own experiences as the universal experience of women and fails to address the realities of race and ethnicity.

So what is there left to salvage? Well, some feminists have been successful in influencing how these theories could be useful with White women, in terms of how we understand their development and appropriate treatment strategies. Likewise, gay and lesbian groups have been successful in depathologizing gay and lesbian issues. Today, psychologists of color are challenging dynamic theories to be more inclusive.

The notion of what is meant by culture, how it influence one's view of health, and what would be considered a useful intervention is an appropriate start. Culture continues to be misunderstood and misapplied to various groups. Psychologists also selectively attend to the social, economic, and political realities of the people they treat for the maintenance of the status quo. To acknowledge the reality of racism, sexism, and heterosexism in American society would strengthen our ability to see the usefulness, and the damage, caused by theoretical misuse of these theories.

## HISTORICAL LEGACY AND COPING

### Slavery

The focus of psychodynamic theory on how one copes and defends in response to pain and trauma in early life is useful for understanding some unique experiences of African American women. How African American women deal with trauma is one issue that helps to illustrate the confluence of ethnicity and gender, and how that represents a unique cultural variable to consider. Jenkins (1993) discusses how under the U.S. slavery system the African American woman's "survival was dependent on this oppressive institution, which exploited her biological reproductive capacity, required her to work, care for, and live *through* others despite her own needs and constant subjection to social malevolence resulting in trauma" (pp. 119–120). A particularly poignant legacy of slavery and a continuing cultural constraint is the ideal of the "strong Black woman," who is selfless, nonsexual, all-giving, and protective of others in her family and community. The "Mammy" stereotype is the "strong Black woman" in its most pejorative form. During slave times, this role was adaptive for survival, but it also required a connection to the oppressor and a disconnection from the self (Abdullah, 1998). Many African Americans complain that this portrayal is often reinforced in the corporate world. This is not to imply that it is not reinforced in other work environments. To approximate the psychological emotional state that would assure a sense of survival in a continuous and unpredictable hostile environment demands a person who has a range of coping strategies available to her. Yet experiencing a continuous state of emotional trauma should disrupt the ability to develop effective coping strategies in response to constant trauma.

### Racism

For most African Americans the experience of racism is a traumatic experience. But because our society continues to deny racism as an everyday experience, some African Americans do not experience it as traumatic. Pierce (1988) discusses the daily insults that African Americans experience, calling them "microinsults" and "microaggressions." African American women are coping with the effects of racism and sexism through institutional and cultural practices. The subtle and indirect nature of these insults may result in feelings of powerlessness because of the incongruent experience between the individual's feeling state and her perception of the event. In their daily lives African American women either minimize these experiences to mask their anger and persistent feelings of powerlessness or internalize the experiences because the negative stereotypes and beliefs about African Americans in general and African

American women in particular are congruent with the perceptions of self and others within the African American population. Additionally, African Americans are placed in a double bind because to address a racial, ethnic, or sexist experience at work or in social situations often results in victim blaming or more aggressive action against the accuser.

Thompson (1998) explains that for many African American clients racial trauma is rarely brought up in therapy because the experience of racism is often so implicit that one is not completely sure whether it is racism or is not. Nevertheless, she notes in contrast "if Whites experienced some of these events they would be outraged, and these experiences would become therapeutic material" (p. 454). Psychodynamic theory helps the therapist and the client to understand the complex interplay between what is experienced intrapsychically and what is experienced outside in the world. Through this understanding the therapist can help the client to differentiate between the two and help the client to feel empowered and understood. Discussing experiences of discrimination both inside and outside the African American community is often a relief. But the therapist, particularly the African American therapist, should be mindful that he or she is not acting out his or her own issues with racism and sexism.

## Sexual Assault

Sexual assault is another very traumatic event, whether experienced as a child or as an adult. European American women have long fought the notion that childhood sexual assault was nothing more than the fantasized material of "neurotic" women, as Freud argued. Specialized treatments of sexually assaulted children and their families using dynamic and other theories have proliferated because of the political clout of feminists over the last 20 or more years. Nevertheless, sexual assault in the African American community continues to be endured by women and to be hidden. The neglect of the mental health profession adequately to protect and treat African American women and young women is tied to racial and gender stereotypes projected on the African American women by the larger society. Wyatt (1997) reports in her research on African American women and sexuality that over half the women in her study had not reported childhood sexual abuse to anyone. Often, instead of receiving professional counseling, a young African American woman who has been sexually assaulted receives a message from her family "that she should be strong and get on with her life" (p. 60). The message to young African American women to be strong is a common cultural message within the community. Specific cultural stereotypes often support this cultural constraint projected onto and internalized by African American women. Self-blame, isolation, and poor interpersonal relationships are common defensive reactions of many women who were sexually assaulted as children. Yet for some African American women these defensive responses may go untreated while concurrently they are encouraged to "be strong and get on with their lives."

## Stereotyping

African American women are still perceived as sexually permissive and readily available, two stereotypes perpetuated by White American society and internalized by some African Americans. These stereotypes were fashioned during slavery to rationalize the sexual exploitation of African American female slaves by their White masters. Today we clearly see the institutionalization of this image of sexual permissiveness in movie and television portrayals of African American women. Our society has therefore internalized these images. Wyatt (1997) illustrated this by sharing a personal experience. She stood in a hotel lobby waiting for her husband and children, dressed to attend a wedding. "Two young white men came out of the hotel bar and headed my way. When they got within earshot, one loudly exclaimed, 'She must cost at least $100!'" (p. 27). This experience left her shaken, angry, hurt, and humiliated. Hers was not an isolated experience. The price African American women pay for any such experience is far too high. My own experience as a clinician and supervisor has left me appalled at the number of psychological evaluations I have read where psychologists have documented client histories of sexual trauma and rape, but this information has been ignored in the formulation of diagnoses and treatment plans. Perhaps the general psychology community believes that African American women are neither traumatized nor affected by these events?

## Self-Image

Another source of trauma for African American women centers around the shame associated with beauty. Skin color, hair texture, body images, and facial features have all been distorted by projections from the European American culture's need to idealize themselves and to devalue the "other." This too has its historical roots in U.S. slavery. The rape of female slaves by slave owners created a cohort of people within the slave population who were biracial. Slave holders created a stratified community within a community based on skin color. This mirrored the boundaries that they had established in the larger society, where the way to identify a slave was primarily or exclusively based on color.

A complicated by-product of the multiracial history for African Americans has been the reality of dealing with multiple identities both within and outside the African American community. Biracial and bicultural differences are perhaps difficult for most people to negotiate in their life span, but for African Americans our society again "colors" these differences with both psychological and political reality. The global belief that America is a melting pot of various cultures, religions, and lifestyles never really applied to "Black folks," no matter what their color. Negotiating these differences is always stressful and often traumatic.

To understand the intrapsychic issues associated with traumatic events such as repeated exposure to racism, institutional discrimination, degrading stereotypes, and devalued self-images, one has to first look at how we understand trauma in the psychological literature. We generally think of trauma as psychological and stressful responses to life-threatening events (Herman, 1992). Another generally accepted understanding of trauma is related to the literature on posttraumatic stress disorder (PTSD). Marmar, Foy, Kagan, and Pynoos (1994) note that "psychological sequelae following traumatic life events are in part determined by the circumstantial factors of the trauma" (p. 240). They list various traumatic events and kinds of trauma victims: "combat trauma, repeated endangerment to the self, witnessing the death and dismemberment of buddies, . . . rape trauma victims, use of physical force, display of weapon, and injury, . . . [and] battered women" (p. 240). Curiously, they exclude racial trauma as a stressful event. It could be argued that racial trauma is not viewed as a traumatic event as a way to deny the existence of racism. Lewis (1996) posits that there is a built-in resistance to recognizing trauma because of individual defenses. Additionally, she points out that some people are immune to traumatic events while others are more vulnerable to experience even minor events as traumatic. While this is probably both theoretically accurate and empirically proven, using this logic would deny the effects of racism and the cumulative effects of racism's "microinsults" and "microaggressions" on African Americans.

Whether all African American women are traumatized or only some of them by the historical legacy of slavery, racism, sexual assault, and stereotyping, there is a high probability that many will be traumatized and yet remain silent. To help an African American woman gain the insight and inner strength needed to confront this coping strategy, the therapist must understand some culture-specific strategies. Richardson and Wade (1999) discuss seven coping strategies used by African American women that are the result of family and community attempts to hold onto their dignity in a hostile environment starting with slavery. These beliefs have resulted in maladaptive defensive reactions in the daily lives of African American women. These beliefs are often misunderstood by therapists. The seven emotional inherited beliefs are:

1. There will never be enough of anything I need, especially love.
2. I'm not good enough to be loved.
3. I'll lose anyone who gets close to me.
4. It's not safe for me to face my anger.
5. No matter what I do, it won't make a difference.

6. I have to control everyone and everything around me to protect myself from being hurt again.
7. My body is not my own. . . . (pp. 22–24)

Therapists working with African American women using dynamic models can help their clients differentiate those experiences that are societal-level experiences from intrapsychic issues. Clients can gain insight into their own functioning and the historical cultural imperative to be all-suffering for the community at the expense of the self. Helping African American women to feel empowered and in touch with their needs will only strengthen the African American community, not fracture the community—as some would fear. Dynamic theories and their accompanying techniques are useful because they provide therapists with tools to help clients explore the relationship between historical emotional learning and the affective defensive response of their experiences.

## PSYCHODYNAMIC TECHNIQUE AND THE USEFULNESS OF PSYCHOTHERAPY

The purpose of this book is not to endorse a particular dynamic theory or technique but to provide an overview of the usefulness of psychotherapy for African American women using the general principles and techniques of dynamic models. One of the most useful principles is the critical importance of the collaboration between the therapist and the client. The theories that focus on the curative nature of the therapeutic relationship are most helpful when working with African American women. For some women clients, this therapeutic relationship may be the only relationship in their lives in which they are not required to take care of someone else. This relationship should be nurturing, understanding, empathic, and appropriately confrontational. Various dynamic theories have specific requirements for the therapeutic relationship to be effective in working with clients. Dynamic theories may use techniques that are either more intensive, with in-depth focusing on the development of insight, or they may be supportive, helping clients with problem-solving needs without delving into the unconscious. Finally, dynamic theories allow the client and the therapist together to reawaken the humanness of the client's experience and to open doors to new ways of being that are healthy and satisfying for the African American woman.

## Useful Elements of Dynamic Models

Object relations theory focuses on the clinician's ability to help the client re-experience past and present difficult relationships by using the therapeutic relationship as a template for the client's displacements and projections. The clinician gives the client an opportunity to project onto the therapeutic relationship his or her fears regarding intimacy, dependence, separation, and individuation. These experiences will help the clinician understand how the client experiences him- or herself in both past relationships and the current therapeutic relationship. Through this encounter the client can explore both internal and external influences on the development of his or her identity and the self.

Ego psychologists using the therapeutic relationship can evaluate the strengths and weaknesses of the client's ego functioning both within and outside the therapeutic encounter. These functions are paramount to healthy adjustment to the social reality of the client. One important ego function, defensive functioning, protects the client from what he or she may perceive as potential danger and the development of anxiety or other symptoms. Schamess (1996) outlines four dangers that require adequate defensive functioning: "1) Conflict among the different agencies of the mind (id, ego, super-ego); 2) conflict in interpersonal relationships; 3) conflict in relation to social norms and institutions; and 4) the disruption of psychological equilibrium that occurs in response to trauma" (p. 79). These four dangers are more perilous when one is responding to a racist and sexist environment.

Self psychology focuses on the unique bond between the child and the child's caretaker. Specifically, the theory focuses on whether or not the child's empathic needs were met during development. The therapeutic relationship then becomes the vehicle to reenact these empathic failures through the transference. Through the transference relationship, the client can displace past conflicts and object relationships onto the therapist. The therapist then gives the client an empathic validating response through the interpretation of the transference that helps to undo past empathic failures. These failures relate to appropriate and genuine responses to childhood behavior that Kohut and Wolf (1978) called "mirroring." The child also requires empathic responses to his or her internal functions that in turn create a calming and comforting function that the child achieves through appropriate and genuine "idealizing" responses from the caregiver.

It is our belief that by understanding both client and therapist cultural perspectives we will create a way for African American women to have the freedom to choose a therapist and treatment modality that may best fit their needs. This will also create an environment where we can treat them with respect and they can more fully understand their experiences.

## SUMMARY

In this book we attempt to acknowledge both the strengths and limitations of psychodynamic models. The need to create a more culturally appropriate way to work with African American women is a challenge for the mental health field as a whole. While psychodynamic theories are guilty of selectively focusing on the individual, it does not have to be at the expense of the client's social and cultural environment. A treatment plan that includes empowering, empathy, understanding, and support will not be guilty of maintaining the status quo. With such treatment, "the individual is likely to become more effective in focusing on the insufficiencies of their social environment, and become increasingly effective in efforts to change their condition" (Jones, 1998, p. 472).

Faculty and clinical supervisors need to be aware of the importance of cultural competence as we train and supervise students to work with African Americans in general and African American women in particular. Without additional multicultural awareness and knowledge training, transference, resistance, and countertransference issues can and will be used to continue to pathologize African American women. We hope that this awareness will help therapists to acknowledge the power dynamics within the therapeutic dyad and to understand the various levels of difference or "otherness" within the therapeutic dyad. This awareness and knowledge will serve to prevent therapists from acting out their own issues around difference.

## REFERENCES

Abdullah, A. S. (1998). Mammy-ism: A diagnosis of psychological misorientation for women of African descent. *Journal of Black Psychology, 24*(2), 196–210.

Alarcon, R. D., Foulks, E. F., & Vakkur, M. (1998). *Personality disorders and culture: Clinical and conceptual interactions.* New York: Wiley.

Bulhan, H. A. (1985). *Franz Fanon and the psychology of oppression.* New York: Plenum Press.

Fanon, F. (1967). *Black skin, white masks.* New York: Grove Press.

Greene, B. (1993). Psychotherapy with African-American women: Integrating feminist and psychodynamic models. *Journal of Training and Practice in Professional Psychology, 7,* 49–66.

Grier, W. H., & Cobbs, P. M. (1968). *Black rage.* New York: Basic Books.

Herman, J. L. (1992). *Trauma and recovery.* New York: Basic Books.

Jenkins, Y. M. (1993). African-American women: Ethnocultural variables and dissonant expectations. In J. L. Chin, V. De La Cancela, & Y. M. Jenkins, *Diversity in psychotherapy: The politics of race, ethnicity, and gender* (pp. 117–135). Westport, CT: Praeger.

Jones, E. E. (1998). Psychoanalysis and African Americans. In R. L. Jones (Ed.), *African American mental health: Theory, research, and intervention* (pp. 471–477). Hampton, VA: Cobb & Henry.

Kohut, H., & Wolf, E. (1978). The disorders of the self and their treatment: An outline. *International Journal of Psycho-Analysis, 59,* 413–425.

Lewis, J. L. (1996). Two paradigmatic approaches to borderline patients with a history of trauma. *Journal of Psychotherapy Practice and Research, 5,* 1–19.

Marmar, C. R., Foy, D., Kagan, B., & Pynoos, R. S. (1994). An integrated approach for treating posttraumatic stress. In R. S. Pynoos (Ed.), *Posttraumatic stress disorder: A clinical review* (pp. 239–271). Lutherville, MD: Sidran Press.

Mattei, L. (1996). Coloring development: Race and culture in psychodynamic theories. In J. Berzoff, L. M. Flanagan, & P. Hertz, *Inside out and outside in: Psychodynamic clinical theory and practice in contemporary multicultural contexts* (pp. 221–245). Northvale, NJ: Jason Aronson.

Pierce, C. M. (1988). Stress in the workplace. In A. F. Conner-Edwards & J. Spurlock (Eds.), *Black families in crisis* (pp. 27–33). New York: Brunner/Mazel.

Richardson, B. L., & Wade, B. (1999). *What mama couldn't tell us about love.* New York: HarperCollins.

Schamess, G. (1996). Ego psychology. In J. Berzoff, L. M. Flanagan, & P. Hertz, *Inside out and outside in: Psychodynamic clinical theory and practice in contemporary multicultural contexts* (pp. 67–101). Northvale, NJ: Jason Aronson.

Taylor, M. (1999). Changing what has gone before: The enhancement of an inadequate psychology through the use of an Afrocentric–feminist perspective with African American women in therapy. *Psychotherapy, 36,* 170–179.

Thompson, C. J. (1998). Does insight serve a purpose? The value of psychoanalytic psychotherapy with diverse African American patients. In R. L. Jones (Ed.), *African American mental health: Theory, research, and intervention* (pp. 453–467). Hampton, VA: Cobb & Henry.

Wyatt, G. E. (1997). *Stolen women: Reclaiming our sexuality, taking back our lives.* New York: Wiley.

CHAPTER 2

# The Interweaving of Cultural and Intrapsychic Issues in the Therapeutic Relationship

## KUMEA SHORTER-GOODEN
## LESLIE C. JACKSON

Neither the burgeoning literature on psychotherapy with women nor the developing field of cross-cultural counseling and psychotherapy says much about the issues involved in doing psychotherapy with African American female clients. In general, the specific psychological issues of African American women are ignored, assumed to be the same as those for European American women, or grouped with those of African American men.

While African American women may share some of the same psychological and sociocultural realities with African American men, their gender informs and transforms their experience of culture and racism. Similarly, African American women may share some of the many realities of gender oppression with other women, but their race transforms and informs their gender identity in ways that are unique for them. The interactive effects of race and gender in the lives of African American women create special challenges that are unique to them, but are rarely discussed in the literature of women or of ethnic minorities (Greene, 1993; Smith & Stewart, 1983).

Our analysis of these unique challenges serves as the focus of this chapter. We explore the issues of race and gender in psychodynamic psychotherapy with African American female clients. We focus on the culture-specific issues that affect the therapeutic process with African American female clients, and we pay attention to the different issues that arise in connection with the therapist's race and gender. Using an object relations perspective, we examine the rela-

15

tionship between the client and the therapist and its psychic meaning for both. In sum, we hope to highlight for therapists of African American female clients the relational issues they need to be attuned to, as well as how they might respond to or intervene around these issues in an effective manner.

## THEORETICAL APPROACH

Our theoretical approach integrates a psychodynamic orientation with a culture-specific understanding of African American women. Many have questioned the appropriateness of psychodynamic psychotherapy for African American clients. Some therapists have criticized psychodynamic approaches as eurocentric and therefore inappropriate for people of African origin (Atwell & Azibo, 1991; Hamilton-Bennett, 1998; Phillips, 1990). While psychodynamic work may not be a good fit for *all* African American clients, just as it is not appropriate for *all* European American clients or for *all* clients of any race, its focus on exploration, uncovering, and insight is certainly valuable for many. In fact, psychodynamic psychotherapy can enable the client to free herself from an internal conflict that may have intrapsychic as well as external origins. Jones and Matsumoto (in Jones, 1998) indicate that

> psychotherapy that improves the functioning of an African American does not adapt the person to the existing social order or preempt a desire for social change. On the contrary, the individual is likely to become more effective in focusing on the insufficiencies of their social environment, and become increasingly effective in efforts to change their condition. . . . Psychotherapy may enhance an individual's capacity to assert what control he or she can over their personal existence . . . despite an often unfavorable social context. (p. 472)

In our view, psychodynamic therapy provides a process that enables African American women to understand internal and external oppressive influences in their lives and to be empowered to reduce both. In fact, these internal and external issues are almost always intertwined, can be difficult to differentiate, and as a result often lead to reductionist thinking. For example, some therapists limit their focus to intrapsychic issues and thus minimize environmental events as incidental or as mere reflections of what is going on intrapsychically. Others focus exclusively on the role of the environment in shaping personality and consequently ignore personal emotional issues. Part of our task here is to facilitate the differentiation and handling of these issues in the therapy of African American women.

Object relations theory focuses on the way in which significant interpersonal relationships are internalized and become central to the way the person interacts in the world (Hamilton, 1990; Horner, 1984). Interpersonal difficulty is conceived as the result of childhood disruptions in trying to separate and individuate the developing "self" from others, and consequently being unable to integrate both good and bad aspects of the self and others. These developmental disruptions are centered around childhood attachment experiences that shape the development of one's perceptions of both the internal self and the external world. The theory states that humans have a need for attachment. Therefore, childhood loss of significant others and negative attachment experiences will have an effect on one's ability to relate to significant others in one's life as an adult. In therapy, the theory posits that the quality and nature of the client–therapist interaction and relationship is ultimately therapeutic. For African American women, object relations theory presents an opportunity to explore how they developed a sense of self in the context of their familial relationships and also in the context of a racist and sexist society.

## CULTURAL ISSUES OF AFRICAN AMERICAN WOMEN

To work competently with any cultural group, therapists need to have some familiarity with the culture and lifestyles of that group. Thus, to do ethical and effective psychotherapy with African American women, clinicians need to be informed about who African American women are and what challenges they face in their lives. African American women wrestle with several common cultural issues as a result of being women of African descent in a racist and sexist society. We offer the caveat that we are not attempting here to describe the cultural concerns of *all* African American women. Moreover, we believe that it is important that therapists sensitively assess the degree to which these issues are salient for *any particular* African American female client with whom they are working. Nonetheless, we want to emphasize a couple of salient issues that therapists would be wise to look and listen for, because they are likely to affect the therapeutic relationship between an African American woman and her therapist. Specifically, we will focus on issues of identity and self-esteem, resiliency and vulnerability, and attachment and dependency. It is our belief that these developmental issues are affected by cultural norms as well as by sexism and racism in the larger society.

Therapists should be aware of the double jeopardy African American women experience by virtue of their membership in two devalued groups (Giddings, 1984; Reid, 1988). Racism and sexism, the legacy of slavery, continue to the present day (hooks, 1981; Reid, 1988). This "double whammy" impacts the African American woman's identity and self-esteem. Thus identity development and the development of a positive sense of self are affected by the internalization of racial and gender stereotypes, as well as by the experience of external racial or gender trauma.

Often the African American woman's struggles around identity and self-esteem are manifest in concerns about looks and beauty (Okazawa-Rey,

Robinson, & Ward, 1987). Reid (1988) points out that the African American woman represents the antithesis of what is considered American female beauty. In terms of skin color, hair texture and length, facial features, and body shape, most African American women do not approach the European American ideal of beauty.

It is important to note, however, that how African American women see themselves is not simply a function of how they are viewed in mainstream European American culture. There is evidence that the African American community serves as a buffer against the negative images and messages that are communicated by the mainstream culture (Barnes, 1980). Nonetheless, the negative messages often creep through in some form (Greene, 1994).

Sometimes the struggle around identity and self-esteem manifests itself in the African American woman's choice of a therapist: When she is free to choose her own therapist, whether she seeks out an African American therapist or a therapist of a different race, and whether she picks a woman or a man, may well say something about her identity and her sense of self. Object relations theory would expect these relational issues to be revealed in the choice of therapist. Jones (1998) points out that "psychoanalytic theories help [us] to understand how race and identity concerns can serve a variety of psychological purposes, and how they are most often interwoven with the patient's other important psychological conflicts" (p. 475).

Another significant cultural issue that African American women wrestle with is the message that it's important to be strong (Greene, 1994; Robinson, 1983; Shorter-Gooden & Washington, 1996). African American women are often socialized to be tough, resilient, and self-sufficient. Survival often depends on these qualities, as African American women are often single or single-parent heads of households, and, when married, are often substantial contributors to the family income. Many African American women have typically learned that their job is to take care of others, both emotionally and financially (Robinson, 1983). Acknowledging vulnerability becomes difficult and holding onto a sense of strength and sustaining resilience are paramount. Being in psychotherapy and acknowledging one's vulnerabilities runs counter to this cultural expectation.

As a result of the cultural emphasis on strength and self-sufficiency, attachment and dependence are sometimes seen as problematic, and oftentimes frightening. Strength and dependence are seen as conflictual. In romantic and sexual relationships, the difficulty with attachment and dependence can create conflicts. Sometimes this is manifested as a need to devalue one's strength in order to form an attachment. Conversely, at times feelings of attachment and dependency are experienced as a loss of personal strength. Of course, this conflict can easily get displaced onto the therapeutic relationship as well. What does it mean if feeling attached to one's therapist means feeling weak and incompetent? Therapists need to be aware of the enactment of this cultural dynamic, which may make it hard to engage the client or alternatively may contribute to a disempowered, passive, and compliant client.

In summary, it is important for therapists to be attuned to how the African American female client puts together a sense of identity and self-esteem and how she handles vulnerability and resilience, and attachment and dependency. These are a few of the core cultural issues that often affect the therapeutic relationship. Other examples of cultural conflicts are covered elsewhere in this book. The above issues will be highlighted in the discussions and case examples that follow.

## DEVELOPING A THERAPEUTIC ALLIANCE

The issues for any therapist in the early stages of psychotherapy revolve around establishing a relationship with the client and beginning to understand who the client is, what her difficulties are, and how the therapeutic relationship can be of help to her. Forming a *therapeutic alliance* is important in psychodynamic therapy because this working partnership between the client and the therapist provides the place in which the work of therapy gets done. As Paolino (1981, p. 103) points out, the therapeutic alliance involves, among other things, the client making "an identification with the real person of the therapist"; establishing "a real congruence between the patient's and therapist's concepts of mental health and psychic growth"; and developing a shared "confidence and hopefulness in the treatment" and an enthusiasm about working together. Greenson (1967, p. 192) defines the therapeutic alliance, or what he calls "the working alliance," as the "relatively nonneurotic, rational rapport which the patient has with his analyst."

The development of an effective therapeutic alliance is contingent on a number of factors. The client's *cultural transference* toward the therapist, the therapist's *cultural countertransference* toward the client, and the *real relationship* are all important ingredients in the development of the therapeutic alliance.

Our premise is that these issues are particularly important for African American female clients. It seems to us that the more marginal the client is in the society, or the more dissimilar she is from those in the mainstream culture, or alternatively, the more dissimilar the client and therapist are from one another, the more salient are the issues of cultural transference, cultural countertransference, and the real relationship. African American women are marginalized by virtue of their race and their gender, and they are very often in therapy with professionals who do not share their race and/or gender. The implication is that therapists must be prepared to deal with both their clients' and their own feelings, attitudes, and beliefs around race, ethnicity, and gender to avoid repeating this marginalization process.

## Cultural Transference

Comas-Díaz and Jacobsen (1991) emphasize that to do effective therapy, one must pay attention to "ethnocultural factors in transference and counter-transference reactions" (p. 392). Ridley (1989) defines *cultural transference* as the "emotional reactions of a client of one ethnic group transferred to a thera-pist of a different [ethnic] group" (p. 64). We define *cultural transference* even more broadly as the emotional reactions of a client to the therapist based on the client's sense of who the therapist is culturally with respect to race, ethnicity, religion, gender, age, social class, and other factors. This broader definition of "cultural transference" looks beyond race to acknowledge other obvious dif-ferences between the client and the therapist, and it also allows for "cultural" reactions by a client to a therapist who is similar with respect to race and gender. The cultural transference and how it is acknowledged and dealt with is an important element in forming the therapeutic alliance. We propose that object relations theory with its focus on the relational matrix between the therapist and the client offers an opportunity to understand early traumas and how they have influenced the client's internal representations of self and object relational needs. When the therapist helps the client begin to acknowledge and address the cultural transference, the client starts the process of gaining insight into her self and object representations, and the therapeutic alliance is strengthened.

A relevant example of this is the African American female client–African American therapist dyad. Many African American female clients find it rela-tively easy to identify with an African American therapist, to feel confident and hopeful about working with their therapist, and to experience a congruence between their concepts of mental health. The African American female client often has an initial positive feeling regarding her African American therapist (irrespective of gender), typically based on assumptions that the client makes about her similarity with the therapist or shared understandings or experience. Often the client feels that she can "let her hair down" with the African Ameri-can therapist, that she is "at home." In other words, there is an initial positive cultural transference. This feeling may be particularly strong for those African American clients who are feeling discriminated against, for African Americans who are feeling uncomfortable with spending much of their time in predomi-nantly European American settings, or, for those, conversely, who are isolated from contact with European Americans.

Let's look at a specific example of an initial positive cultural transference that facilitated the therapeutic alliance. The client was a 33-year-old married female who was treated by an African American male therapist. She was on disability because of stress from a large predominantly White corporation where she had worked for 12 years in increasingly responsible secretarial posi-tions. She was enraged at the company for mistreating her. She disclosed early on that she felt the company was systematically working on ridding itself of its

African American staff. The therapist believed that she had been mistreated by the company, perhaps because of her race; but he also noted that she had significant characterological features that clearly had exacerbated her problems on the job.

What is important here is her ability early on to connect with the African American therapist in a way that might have been difficult with a European American therapist, particularly if the European American therapist was not "tuned into" the client's cultural transference. Because the client was angry at European Americans at her place of employment, these feelings could have been transferred to a European American therapist, and, especially if the therapist was not aware (i.e., in denial) of this cultural transference, could have seriously jeopardized the development of a therapeutic alliance. Regarding this client and a European American therapist, it would be crucial for therapy success that the therapist convey, in the first couple of sessions, his interest in and willingness to explore the client's feelings about her job and about what it meant to the client to see a European American therapist. The client may or may not be willing to talk about these issues early on with a European American therapist whom she does not yet trust; what is really important, however, is that she hear the therapist's willingness to deal with these issues.

Sometimes initial positive cultural transference feelings will facilitate the beginnings of the therapeutic alliance. Yet these same positive feelings may blind the therapist to difficulties in establishing a more genuine, ongoing alliance. For example, take a well-educated African American middle-class client in her late 20s, who, in the first couple of sessions with an African American female therapist, seemed eager to start therapy and noted how grateful she was to have found an African American woman therapist. One indicator to the therapist that an effective therapeutic alliance had been formed was the client's willingness to talk openly about sexuality and sexual issues in her relationships. However, after several months of once-a-week therapy, the therapist realized that the client was not really engaged emotionally in the therapy process, and that she seemed to defend against feeling close to the therapist. Because of the client's strong initial positive cultural transference, the therapist was blinded to the client's rather superficial engagement and was slow to realize that there were significant problems in the client's capacity for relatedness. The client's positive cultural transference, as exemplified by her joining with the therapist around their shared African American identity and her ability to talk about sexuality, masked some of the client's difficulties with genuine intimacy.

As this last example indicates, it is important to look at the cultural transference not only in intergroup therapeutic relationships, for example, an African American female client with a non-African American male or female therapist, but also in intragroup therapeutic relationships, for example, an African American female client with an African American male or female therapist. Even when the African American female client is eager to work with an

African American female therapist, the therapist's understanding of and ability to deal with the cultural transference is still important in facilitating the therapeutic alliance.

Another intragroup example is the African American woman who remarked to her African American female therapist in the first session that she had expected to see "Angela Davis" sitting in the room. Her perception was based on how a friend and previous client had described the therapist when she urged this new client to call her. As the therapist explored what "Angela Davis" meant to her, it became clear that there was something about this client's sense of what it took to be a competent, successful African American woman that was conveyed in this cultural transference image. The client projected onto the therapist the qualities of strength and toughness she associated with Angela Davis, and this could have resulted in the client presenting her most compliant and passive side to the therapist. The therapist's ability to recognize this cultural transference helped to facilitate a discussion of these issues and, thanks to this discussion, the development of a therapeutic alliance. This example focuses attention on the importance of the issue of strength in African American women's lives. In the case of this client, it points to one internalized image that African American women use as a model of strength. The question to ask is "How would the cultural transference of a strong and powerful therapist promote or hinder the development of a therapeutic alliance if the cultural transference was not confronted?"

One of the challenges in the African American female client–African American female therapist dyad is that how the client feels about herself may be immediately projected onto the therapist. If the client, for example, has negative feelings about being Black and female, these feelings may be thrust onto the therapist through the process of projection or of projective identification. Helms (1985) talks about the therapeutic challenges when the client's negative ethnic identity is projected onto the therapist. Comas-Díaz and Jacobsen (1987) suggest that the client's ethnocultural identification can result in a negative reaction to a therapist she experiences as similar as well as to a therapist she experiences as different:

> Ethnocultural identification is a process whereby patients attribute ethnocultural characteristics to their therapists. It is similar to the concept of projective identification, where the patient projects parts of the self into the object (in this case the therapist). (p. 236)

The therapist who is not attuned to this process will have difficulty engaging the client and sustaining the therapeutic process.

Socioeconomic differences between the client and the therapist may lead to other sorts of cultural transferences. A client who is on public assistance may have a negative cultural transference toward a therapist whom she believes to be upper class—and for some African American female clients, being educated is equivalent to being upper class. On the other hand, another client, also on public assistance, might have a very positive cultural transference toward such a therapist, seeing this therapist as a successful representative of herself or as an example of what she can become.

Our aim is not to suggest that only certain race or class pairings of therapist and client are workable, but rather to draw attention to the myriad ways in which clients react to therapists. We want to emphasize that therapists need to be tuned into these varied possibilities in order to help clients deal with the initial feelings that, if ignored, might well prevent the development of a therapeutic alliance and might lead to a premature termination of the therapy. These cultural constructs are not limited to class issues, but include gender, skin color, hair, and how the therapist presents him-or herself initially to the client.

Premature termination is often a problem when cultural transference is not attended to. Let's look at the case of a 19-year-old African American female college student who was referred by her dean to the college counseling center after she made a suicidal gesture in reaction to being snubbed by a newly made European American male friend. The college dean was concerned about the student not only because of her scary suicidal gesture, but because the young woman had come to the attention of the resident advisors as an "angry, volatile person" whom the European American students in particular feared. The student seemed to keep people on this mostly European American campus at a distance, and she sometimes cursed and yelled at those around her with seemingly little provocation. The well-meaning European American male psychologist who saw her talked with her about the suicidal gesture, about her adjustment as a first-year student to college life, and about the student's family life, but the psychologist felt frustrated with the interaction and with the guardedness of the client and her limited engagement in the process. Not surprisingly, the student failed to attend the next appointment.

It is important to note that the psychologist had not explored with the client the racial element of the problems she was having, nor had he raised the issue of how the student felt about talking with a European American therapist about these issues. There are many possible reasons why this student chose not to return for a second therapy session. However, one reasonable hypothesis is that significant cultural transference issues enacted in this first session with the European American therapist blocked formation of a therapeutic alliance.

Because of premature termination, we cannot know what was going on with this young woman intrapsychically and culturally. But let's hypothesize based on what we do know. The extremity of her reported behavior—a suicidal gesture in response to being snubbed, and cursing and yelling with little provocation—suggests an intrapsychic relational component to her difficulties. But there also appears to be a strong cultural element: the young woman's behavior suggests that she may be acting out feelings of being culturally devalued. Moreover, being one of a few African American women at this college may have contributed to a sense of differentness and alienation that may have exacerbated this feeling. The young woman's cursing and yelling suggests that she devalues others—perhaps a reversal and a projection of her own feelings of being devalued *by* European Americans *onto* European Americans. She may have been involved in projective identification with her new European American male friend, where she projected onto him parts of herself that then contributed to him interacting with her in familiar (i.e., snubbing/devaluing), though destructive, ways. Her suicidal gesture in response to being snubbed certainly suggests a significant problem with self-valuation, which may be the result of a combination of intrapsychic and cultural issues. It seems likely that what was happening with this young woman on campus and in the therapy session reflected the interweaving of cultural and intrapsychic issues.

If the therapist had found a way to address these issues, or at least to acknowledge them, this effort might have paved the way for the client to begin to engage in the therapy process. The client had a strategy of relating to European Americans, based at least in part on her cultural transference, and unless this strategy, and the need for it, were examined, the therapy was likely doomed.

## Cultural Countertransference

We have focused thus far on the client's cultural transference and how that affects the development of a therapeutic alliance. A closely related issue is the therapist's cultural countertransference. Based on Ridley's (1989) definition, we define *cultural countertransference* as the therapist's emotional reactions to the client based on the client's race, ethnicity, religion, gender, age, social class, or the like. Clients, of course, are not alone in the consultation room. Therapists, too, have reactions that are based on experiences that occur outside the therapy hour. In fact, in a couple of the examples already given, the reader has perhaps wondered about the therapist's cultural countertransference to the client.

For example, in the case of the well-educated middle-class client in her 20s who shared openly about sexual issues, her African American female therapist was slow to realize that the client's initial superficial engagement around their shared Black identification masked some real difficulties in connecting with the therapist. We can hypothesize that there was something about the therapist's cultural countertransference that got in the way of her seeing the client more clearly. Perhaps the therapist tends to idealize African Americans who are well educated and from the middle class. This form of idealization may have led to an overidentification with the client (Comas-Díaz & Jacobsen, 1991), which then blinded her to their differences and to the client's problem areas. Perhaps the therapist felt so buoyed by the client's strong positive feelings about working with an African American female therapist that she found it difficult to see beyond her own need for validation.

Another example was the case of the European American counseling center psychologist who saw the "angry and volatile" African American female student after she made a suicidal gesture. The psychologist's cultural countertransference may have been to feel anxious, intimidated, and like he had to walk on eggshells around the client. This is a common reaction for non-African American therapists who have to deal with strong affect, particularly anger, emanating from African American clients. His emotions may have prevented the psychologist from dealing as directly as he should have with the issues at hand, including the salient issue of this young woman being Black but being surrounded by White students and staff. Or, on the other hand, it may be that this particular therapist experienced a cultural countertransference that involved feeling a need to rescue and protect a "poor, mistreated Black girl." In fact, in this case, through discussion with a colleague, the therapist became aware that he felt guilty as a White person about the racism directed toward African Americans in this society; that he was concerned about the small number of African American students enrolled at the college; and that, as a result, he often was inclined to assume the role of protector or rescuer vis-à-vis African American women. In an attempt to protect and rescue the client, and, perhaps, to hide his own "whiteness" (about which he felt some guilt), the clinician avoided dealing with the client in a direct manner around the racial aspects of what was transpiring on campus and with him.

Thus, it is important not only for therapists to consider their clients' cultural transference, but also their own cultural countertransference as a way of understanding what is happening in the therapy process and as a way of fostering the therapeutic alliance. For therapists to consider their cultural countertransference, they need to be able to get in touch with what it is. To do this, it helps to consult with colleagues and supervisors. In addition, therapists should seek both content-oriented and awareness-oriented training in working with diverse clients. Training experiences will help therapists identify their own biases and stereotypical beliefs about African American women and provide them with an opportunity to learn how their attitudes contribute to the development of cultural countertransference reactions.

## The Real Relationship

Cultural transference and cultural countertransference attitudes are brought by the client and therapist into the therapeutic encounter and may not have anything to do with the reality of the particular clinician or client seated in the room. However, the real relationship between the pair is another important element that can facilitate or get in the way of the development of a therapeutic alliance. The *real relationship* is defined by Greenson (1967) as the parts of the relationship between the therapist and the client that are realistic, in other words, not inappropriate or fantasized, and genuine. The client has objective perceptions and reactions to the therapist based on the therapist's appearance, office furnishings, dress, style of speech, personality, and other "real" aspects of the therapist (Paolino, 1981). Whereas the cultural transference and cultural countertransference cannot be directly observed, because they have to do with attitudes and feelings that are inside the client and the therapist, the real relationship is observable.

Greenson (1967) and Paolino (1981) believe that ignoring the reality elements of the therapy can undermine the client's self-esteem and reinforce the client's feeling of being abnormal. Additionally, inattention to the real relationship can hinder the client's capacity to differentiate between reality and fantasy.

Where there are significant differences, for example, in race, class, or gender, between the therapist and the client, it seems that issues of the real relationship may be particularly salient and may be particularly likely, if unaddressed, to impede the therapy. However, differences between the therapist and the client often lead to anxiety in the clinician and a resultant defensiveness (Bradshaw, 1978; Pinderhughes, 1989). The added danger in not dealing with the real relationship with a client of color is that this avoidance on the therapist's part "implicitly reinforces a denial of the client's sense of self" (Pinderhughes, 1989, p. 170). In other words, since part of the client's sense of self is based on being a Black person in a White-dominant society, to deny the reality of these issues and how they affect the actual or real relationship between the client and the therapist can undermine the client's sense of self. For African American females whose sense of self is already challenged by a racist and sexist society, the therapist's avoidance of differences between the therapist and the client is not healthy for the client.

Dealing with the real relationship means acknowledging and helping the client to acknowledge the actual differences between the client and the therapist—differences that may become barriers to the therapeutic relationship if left unacknowledged. As an example, let's look again at the case of the angry African American female college student who saw a European American male psychologist after feeling snubbed by a European American male friend. To facilitate the therapeutic alliance, the clinician needs to acknowledge the reality that the client and the therapist are different racially, and that the clinician is, in fact, of the same race and gender as the person by whom the young woman feels spurned. By bringing up this issue, or responding nondefensively to it if the client initiates this discussion, the therapist conveys to the client that he is willing to deal with the reality of her situation and the reality of the context in which her therapy is occurring. He is not focused solely on what is intrapsychic; for example, he does not assume that the client's reactions to him are entirely based on her feelings about the White friend who snubbed her or on her general cultural transference to European American males. The client's reactions to the White male therapist are assumed to be based, at least in part, on who the White therapist is and how he comes across in his interactions with the client. For example, the client and the therapist may have very different worldviews and cultural styles—styles of communication, of dress, and so on. Of course, the idiosyncratic meaning that the client attributes to this particular therapeutic relationship is important to explore at some point in the therapy. However, if the observable, obvious issues in the therapeutic relationship are not attended to, then it is likely the therapy will end prematurely, as it did in this case.

One of the challenges for the therapist is to work to try to distinguish between the client's cultural transference, the therapist's own cultural countertransference, and the real relationship. Of course, there is also the traditional transference (the noncultural components) as well as the traditional countertransference (the noncultural components) to wrestle with and sort out too. While we have talked about each of these constructs separately, the reality is that in the therapy moment it can be very difficult to differentiate them. One can only know over time, for example, how much of the client's reaction to the therapist is a function of the client's history with people whom she deems to be like the therapist culturally and ethnically (cultural transference) versus a function of who the therapist is and how the therapist presents herself (real relationship). Obviously, there is usually an interaction effect. And this effect is not static; rather it changes and evolves over time.

We know that it can be difficult to distinguish between the cultural transference and the real relationship; moreover, we also know that the cultural transference and the cultural countertransference are mutually influenced by each other. In the first minutes of the first therapy session, the therapist's initial cultural countertransference and how she or he begins to relate to the client impacts the client's initial cultural transference and how the client begins to relate to the therapist, which impacts the therapist's developing cultural countertransference, and so on. In other words, these are complex, interwoven processes that change and evolve over time. The astute therapist is tuned into this fluid and often ambiguous process and engages in an ongoing process of generating and testing hypotheses about what is going on. The danger, of course, is that the client will terminate before the therapist is able to help the client sort out what's getting in the way of the therapeutic alliance.

In sum, to build a therapeutic relationship, it is vitally important for therapists to pay attention to relationship issues—cultural transference, cultural countertransference, and the real relationship—that impact the developing therapeutic alliance. Attention to these issues and appropriate interventions in response to these issues can determine whether or not the nascent therapeutic relationship becomes an ongoing one.

## WORKING THROUGH THE THERAPEUTIC RELATIONSHIP

While the previous section focused on the issues of cultural transference, cultural countertransference, and the real relationship in the beginning of a therapeutic relationship with an African American woman, this section focuses on the relevance of these concepts in the middle and latter stages of psychotherapy. And we will do that by offering an extended case example.

A 45-year-old professional African American woman saw a European American female therapist to address her persistent long-standing feelings of depression. She was dissatisfied with her life: with a lack of intimacy with her husband, with the demands of parenting two children, and with the stress of her job as a manager in a predominantly White organization. In once-a-week psychodynamic psychotherapy, she focused on her presenting concerns as well as on her family history. She had grown up in a family of five children, where she was assigned the role of family achiever. She was the conforming, "goody-two-shoes" daughter who never rocked the boat or was cause for concern. And while she was the focus of parental expectations in terms of academic and future career performance, she was not accorded much nurturance and emotional support from her parents. Her parents considered her the independent, smart child, who did not need much from anyone.

The client seemed to connect well with the therapist from the beginning and the therapist had the sense of a solid therapeutic alliance. In the first year and a half, the client almost never missed a session, and she progressed in terms of becoming less demanding of herself and less perfectionistic. The client's theme had been "I have to be perfect in order to be okay," and this had softened. However, the therapist was aware that the client continued to wrestle with feelings of depression and to have significant difficulties with closeness and intimacy—in her relationship with her husband as well as in her relationship with the therapist.

The therapist conceptualized the client as operating at the level of whole-object relations; the client had fairly well-integrated self- and other-representations. In other words, internally the client experienced herself and others as having good and bad qualities. However, the client's persistent depression seemed connected to her difficulty in fully acknowledging her feelings. Unwanted affects were repressed. In the therapy, the client could express angry feelings about her husband and about her job, though not about the therapist, and the client seemed to have difficulty expressing any feelings of dependence. For example, though the client seemed very engaged with the therapist and the therapy, she had difficulty acknowledging what seemed to be the important role of this therapy experience in her life or in admitting any feelings of sadness or loss when there were vacation breaks. Moreover, the therapist was cognizant of the fact that the client almost never mentioned race or racial issues or anything about her feelings about the therapist being White.

The therapist regretted that she had not brought these issues up earlier in the treatment. The therapist had felt it unnecessary to bring up issues of race early in the therapy because her sense of the client was that the client had a healthy Black identity and that there were not significant conflicts around issues of race. Moreover, the therapist was unsure about how best to bring these issues up. She had some discomfort with addressing the racial difference between them. What may have heightened this uneasiness on the therapist's part was the relative similarity between the therapist and the client in many regards (e.g., gender, age, educational achievements, marital status, and number of children). The therapist's countertransference was "This client is a lot like me. We aren't very different." The cultural countertransference that contributed to this perception was an attitude, on the part of the therapist, that a well-educated professional African American is not really "Black," that is, that racial issues are not very salient in this population.

Through consultation with others about the case, the therapist came to the conclusion that it was important to encourage the client to explore issues around race and the race of the therapist. The therapist had begun to feel that these issues were getting in the way of the client's increased closeness and engagement in the therapeutic process, which paralleled the client's difficulties with intimacy with her spouse. Over a period of several months the therapist asked the client about her feelings about the therapist, and specifically about the Black/White difference between them. The therapist inquired about the client's relationships with Whites on her job, about the racial identification of various friends who had been discussed previously, and about the client's decision to see a White therapist. Slowly but surely, the client was able to disclose more and more about these issues, while admitting how difficult it was for her to talk about these things with the therapist.

The client revealed that she had very different relationships with European Americans than with African Americans. All of her family members and friends were African American. While, in many ways, she functioned very well in White settings, she had significant ambivalence about Whites. While this pattern of relationships seemed generally healthy and adaptive for the world in which she lived, it became clear that her ambivalence about Whites, which was coupled with substantial involvement with Whites on the job, in her church, and, of course, in her therapy, served a defensive function. This pattern enabled her to keep her distance and avoid intimacy and dependency—the pattern she had learned and was reinforced for as a child growing up.

Unconsciously, the client seemed to feel safer with a European American therapist with whom she felt she could maintain greater distance and protect herself from the danger of feeling close and getting little in return. The client's cultural transference seemed to involve seeing the White therapist as a potentially helpful person, but a person whom the client could not fully trust or rely on. Not surprisingly, after the therapist facilitated discussion of these issues, the affective tone of the therapy changed. The client's growing ability to access her ambivalent feelings about race helped her to better access her ambivalent feelings about attachment and dependence. The engagement of the client in the therapeutic process deepened, and the client began to feel less depressed and to feel closer to her husband and others in her life.

This case is an example of the interweaving of intrapsychic and cultural issues and the significance of the unfolding of these issues for the therapy of the client. In this case, cultural issues did not jeopardize the beginning of therapy; instead, they endangered the client's continued progress in a therapy that seemed to begin well with a good therapeutic alliance. For the client to continue to make progress through the therapeutic relationship, it was important for the therapist to consider and sort out with the client how race impacted the client's life and, importantly, the therapeutic relationship itself.

## SUMMARY

This chapter focused on the interweaving of cultural and intrapsychic issues in the therapeutic relationship with African American female clients. We paid attention to the impact of the relationship in the development of the therapeutic alliance as well as to relationship issues that can hinder the middle and latter stages of psychotherapy. The constructs of cultural transference, cultural countertransference, and the real relationship were defined and utilized as anchors for our discussion and for making sense of the case vignettes.

Because African American women are doubly marginalized in this society by virtue of their race and gender, it is especially important that therapists who work with African American women are mindful of the cultural issues that pervade the consultation room. Thus an exploration of and attention to the interplay of intrapsychic and cultural factors is important in understanding the African American woman's personality development and the unfolding interaction between the African American female client and her therapist. The goal of the culturally sensitive therapist, using a psychodynamic model, is to increase the African American female client's awareness of her needs, her motivation, and her identity as a Black woman, and thereby to strengthen her coping skills and her ability to live a reasonably satisfying life. This has been our goal in working with African American women.

## REFERENCES

Atwell, I., & Azibo, D. A. (1991). Diagnosing personality disorder in Africans (Blacks) using the Azibo nosology: Two case studies. *Journal of Black Psychology, 17*(2), 1–22.

Barnes, E. J. (1980). The Black community as the source of positive self-concept for Black children: A theoretical perspective. In R. L. Jones (Ed.), *Black psychology* (2nd ed., pp. 106–130). New York: Harper & Row.

Bradshaw, W. (1978). Training psychiatrists for working with Blacks in basic residency. *American Journal of Psychiatry, 135*(12), 1520–1524.

Comas-Díaz, L., & Jacobsen, F. M. (1987). Ethnocultural identification in psychotherapy. *Psychiatry, 50,* 232–241.

Comas-Díaz, L., & Jacobsen, F. M. (1991). Ethnocultural transference and countertransference in the therapeutic dyad. *American Journal of Orthopsychiatry, 61*(3), 392–402.

Giddings, P. (1984). *When and where I enter: The impact of Black women on race and sex in America.* New York: Bantam Books.

Greene, B. (1993). Psychotherapy with African-American women: Integrating feminist and psychodynamic models. *Journal of Training and Practice in Professional Psychology, 7,* 49–66.

Greene, B. (1994). African American women. In L. Comas-Díaz & B. Greene (Eds.), *Women of color: Integrating ethnic and gender identities in psychotherapy* (pp. 10–29). New York: Guilford Press.

Greenson, R. (1967). *The technique and practice of psychoanalysis.* New York: International Universities Press.

Hamilton, N. G. (1990). *Self and others: Object relations theory in practice.* Northvale, NJ: Jason Aronson.

Hamilton-Bennett, M. (1998). Healing the African American collective requires more than the psychoanalysis of individuals. In R. L. Jones (Ed.), *African American mental health: Theory, research, and intervention* (pp. 497–501). Hampton, VA: Cobb & Henry.

Helms, J. E. (1985). Cultural identity in the treatment process. In P. Pedersen (Ed.), *Handbook of cross-cultural counseling and therapy* (pp. 239–245). Westport, CT: Greenwood Press.

hooks, b. (1981). *Ain't I a woman? Black women and feminism.* Boston: South End Press.

Horner, A. J. (1984). *Object relations and the developing ego in therapy* (Rev. ed.). New York: Jason Aronson.

Jones, E. E. (1998). Psychoanalysis and African Americans. In R. L. Jones (Ed.), *African American mental health: Theory, research, and intervention* (pp. 471–477). Hampton, VA: Cobb & Henry.

Okazawa-Rey, M., Robinson, T., & Ward, J. V. (1987). Black women and the politics of skin color and hair. *Women and Therapy, 6,* 89–102.

Paolino, T. (1981). *Psychoanalytic psychotherapy: Theory, technique, therapeutic relationship, and treatability.* New York: Brunner/Mazel.

Phillips, F. B. (1990). NTU psychotherapy: An Afrocentric approach. *Journal of Black Psychology, 17*(1), 55–74.

Pinderhughes, E. (1989). *Understanding race, ethnicity, and power: The key to efficacy in clinical practice.* New York: Free Press.

Reid, P. T. (1988). Racism and sexism: Comparisons and conflicts. In P. A. Katz & D. Taylor (Eds.), *Eliminating racism: Profiles in controversy* (pp. 203–221). New York: Plenum Press.

Ridley, C. (1989). Racism in counseling as an aversive behavioral process. In P. B. Pedersen, J. G. Draguns, W. J. Lonner, & J. E. Trimble (Eds.), *Counseling across cultures* (pp. 55–77). Honolulu, HI: University of Hawaii Press.

Robinson, C. R. (1983). Black women: A tradition of self-reliant strength. *Women and Therapy, 2*(2–3), 135–144.

Shorter-Gooden, K., & Washington, N. C. (1996). Young, Black, and female: The challenge of weaving an identity. *Journal of Adolescence, 19,* 465–475.

Smith, A., & Stewart, A. J. (1983). Approaches to studying racism and sexism in Black women's lives. *Journal of Social Issues, 39*(3), 1–15.

## CHAPTER 3

# Individual and Group Psychotherapy with African American Women
## Understanding the Identity and Context of the Therapist and Patient

### JOAN M. ADAMS

Psychodynamic treatment uses the relationship between the therapist and the patient to understand the patient's inner (intrapsychic) life and the patient's relationship with others (interpersonal) via exploration of the patient's history, defenses, conflicts, dreams, and transference to the therapist (Basch, 1980). The therapist uses his or her conscious and unconscious emotional responses to the patient to understand and to contain the patient's experience. The goals of treatment are that the patient develops a more authentic sense of self, has more choices regarding behavior, and develops more adaptive responses to internal and external stress or conflict.

Psychodynamic therapy can be done as individual or group therapy. A psychodynamic understanding of human behavior posits a dynamic interplay between the patient's past and present; unconscious and conscious mind; internal and external world; true, or *authentic*, self and false, or *defended*, self; and symptoms and personality structure.

Two important concepts in psychodynamic therapy are *transference* and *countertransference* (Greenson, 1967). *Transference* refers to a patient's feelings toward the therapist that unconsciously repeat the patient's childhood experiences with significant caretakers. An example of transference is a woman who tells her therapist how angry she is at a colleague who undercut her on a work project and how she confronted the colleague. The patient then becomes anxious in the therapy session and eventually discovers that her anxiety is related to her expectation that the therapist is critical of her expression of anger. Why does she feel this way? Because the patient's mother routinely criticized her whenever she expressed anger, especially anger toward her siblings or parents. This patient had unconsciously *transferred* onto the therapist her experience with her mother. Such transference can then be explored and exposed to the light of the present reality, one in which the therapist encourages the patient to know and explore whatever feelings she has and to be aware of the choices she has about how to handle those feelings. The exploration of transferences in individual therapy and among group members helps free the patient from old repetitive responses to people in her present life.

*Countertransference* is the therapist's unconscious emotional response to the patient's transference or to the patient's general personality style. An important aspect of the therapist's work is to stay attuned to countertransferential responses evoked by the patient and/or related to the therapist's own psychological issues. Suppose the therapist finds herself irritated and impatient with a patient. Upon reflection the therapist realizes that she is resentful and envious of the patient's feelings of entitlement and his tendency to expect others to cater to his wishes. As the therapist recognizes her own wishes to be catered to (a rather universal wish), and her own conflicts about acknowledging such wishes, she is able to understand more about the source of the patient's sense of entitlement and his underlying sense of deprivation.

Countertransference is an inevitable and invaluable source for understanding the patient's inner life. This understanding can be either from the patient's perspective or from the perspective of others to whom the patient relates. In Heinrich Racker's (1968) terms, this is either *concordant* or *complementary* countertransference.

Psychodynamic treatment evolved from psychoanalytic theory and practice, which started with Freud in the early part of this century (Basch, 1980). Current psychodynamic treatment has several major theoretical underpinnings. Many therapists, myself included, incorporate the clinical insights from these major theories: Freudian, ego psychology, object relations, self psychology, interpersonal, and relational. I find that each of these psychodynamic theories has expanded our understanding of the human experience. *Freudian theory* focuses on the key concepts of the unconscious; the structural model of the mind, id, ego, and superego; psychosexual phases of development; instincts and drives; and the conflict model of inner experience (Greenson, 1967). *Ego psychology* focuses on the structure of the ego and the function of psychological defenses (Blanck & Blanck, 1974). *Object relations* deals with the internalization of aspects of significant figures in the patient's life and the way in which people relate to others (Pine, 1985). *Self psychology* looks at the development of the "self" and the centrality of the therapist's empathic attunement to the patient (Pine, 1985). *Interpersonal* and *relational models* focus on the interaction between therapist and patient in the here-and-now of the treatment session to *jointly elucidate* the patient's experience and develop more adaptive modes of behavior (Mitchell & Black, 1995).

More recently I have also been influenced by the systems-centered therapy (SCT) of Yvonne Agazarian (1997). SCT posits an isomorphic relationship in any human system where influence on one aspect of the system impacts all aspects of the system, for example, change in a group member or a subgroup of group members leads to change in the entire therapy group and vice versa. SCT uses nonpathologizing techniques to access patient's feelings, recognizes the close relationship between mind and body, and focuses on the here-and-now of the treatment situation. SCT attempts to systematically undo a person's defenses in a hierarchical sequence in an effort to give that person access to his or her authentic experience. This enables the person to recognize the options he or she has, to be more spontaneous, and to free up energy that he or she can then direct toward his or her goals.

I also insist that the therapist must understand the *context* of each patient. Context includes the race, ethnicity, gender, class, religion, age, sexual orientation, and physical ability of the patient. It also includes the impact of cultural identity and of social, political, and regional environments on the patient and the patient's family of origin. Understanding a patient without attending to his or her *cultural context* is akin to listening to music in mono rather than in stereo: you will miss the rich complex strains that contribute to each person's uniqueness.

The psychodynamic therapy I practice is rooted in an evolved psychoanalytic understanding of people and an appreciation of the sociocultural context of the person. In summary, the work of psychodynamic therapy is for the patient and therapist to explore thoughts, feelings, behavior, fantasies, and dreams in a "safe enough," nonjudgmental relationship with the goal of *understanding meaning and unconscious motivation,* of *experiencing authentic feelings,* and of being able to *choose more adaptive behavior.*

## CRITIQUES OF PSYCHODYNAMIC THERAPY FOR AFRICAN AMERICAN WOMEN

I have heard several criticisms of psychodynamic therapy both from African American clinicians and nonclinicians who consider getting help with psychological problems. I will present the concerns most often expressed and then respond to these critiques.

1. Psychoanalysis and psychodynamic therapy are "elitist" in that they were developed and widely practiced by White clinicians with middle- or upper-class patients of European descent.

2. Analysis and dynamic therapy focus on the *individual* and his or her needs and do not sufficiently consider the patient's attachment to, responsibilities to, and sustenance received from his or her family or cultural group.

3. Analysis and dynamic therapy focus more on a deficit or pathological model of human psychology and not enough on the strengths of the patient or the concept of a human continuum of feelings, impulses, and behavior.

4. The sociocultural and political context of patients, especially people of color, non-Western patients, and until recently women, is not addressed in much of the analytic, dynamic therapy literature or in teaching psychotherapy.

5. Analysis and dynamic therapy, along with other models of mental health treatment (e.g., psychopharmacology, behavior modification, etc.), are experienced as another expression of racism and oppression by the White establishment toward people of African descent. This is related to the power of the medical establishment to label people as "crazy" or "sick" without differentiating behavior that is reactive to oppression (Grier & Cobbs, 1968) from behavior that is culturally normative. Examples of the latter are close extended family ties beyond age 21 or strong spiritual beliefs. There is also a negative expectation related to a historical and continued mislabeling of African American patients who present with symptoms of psychiatric distress, for example, diagnosing African American men as schizophrenic when the accurate diagnosis is bipolar disorder (Thomas & Sillen, 1972). Baker (1988) discusses issues of psychiatric misdiagnosis among African Americans. Another manifestation of racism in the delivery of mental health services is writing off African Americans, especially poor African Americans, as suited only for medication and not psychotherapy (Altman, 1993).

6. The racism that affects everyone in the United States impacts on the therapist–patient relationship. African American patients have difficulty believing that a White therapist will not react to them with negative stereotypes, will understand their experience in the context of being African American, and will not hurt them in overt or subtle ways growing out of conscious or unconscious racist attitudes.

7. A cultural prohibition, though lessened recently, among many African Americans against revealing and discussing personal, often painful "family business" except with family, religious counselors, or close friends, inhibits effective therapy.

8. "Therapy" is perceived as antireligious and as undermining the spiritual institutions and communities that provide very important emotional sustenance, affiliative ties, and ethical/moral structure for many African Americans.

9.  Psychodynamic therapy is historically eurocentric and not relevant to the worldview and emotional needs of African Americans.

## RESPONSES TO THE CRITIQUES OF PSYCHODYNAMIC THERAPY FOR AFRICAN AMERICAN WOMEN

Racism is alive and well at the beginning of the 21st century in the United States. Of course, it is manifested in the practice of psychotherapy with African Americans by White practitioners. It is manifested, subtly or grossly, in *all* areas of American life, including education, the corporate world, housing, religious institutions, and mental health. Racism impacts all of us, White, African American, and other people of color.

Many of the intrinsic values of psychodynamic therapy—for example, an emphasis on freeing people to be authentically themselves, helping people to integrate disparate aspects of themselves so they can be more present, productive, creative and relate more fully with others—are consistent with the values of African Americans. African American people have traditionally valued productivity, creativity, and good relationships within the African American community. Psychodynamic therapy can be used by African Americans to enhance their personal wholeness, their relationship with others, and their ability to contribute their talents and skills to the African American community and the larger United States community.

The critical issue concerning the relevance of psychodynamic therapy to African Americans is the consciousness of the therapist (of whatever color or ethnic group) regarding his or her own cultural context and attitudes, feelings, and behavior toward African Americans.

The critiques cited above include five major attitudes that interfere with the willingness and ability of African American women to use psychodynamic psychotherapy: African Americans often do not trust their personal, emotional "stuff" with White therapists; African Americans think a person has to be "crazy," "sick," or "weak" to seek therapy; African Americans fear that therapists will undermine their spiritual beliefs; African Americans are socialized to keep "personal business" among family, friends, or spiritual advisers; and, finally, psychotherapy is viewed as eurocentric and therefore not applicable to afrocentric people.

It is true that trust is a central initial issue in a White therapist–African American patient dyad, but it is also a key issue for *any* beginning therapeutic encounter. The enduring legacy of American slavery and the continued systemic power differential between "mainstream " Whites and "minority" African Americans intensifies the problem of trust for the African American patient starting to work with a White therapist. It is vitally important, and *possible*, for White therapists to be aware of this and to create an environment for gradually establishing a trusting therapeutic alliance. After all, psychodynamic therapists often have to establish a working alliance in the face of a patient's symptomatic, characterological, and developmental issues, for example, paranoid ideas, narcissistic character, or a history of childhood abuse and neglect, which make the development of trust difficult. The attitudes and skills therapists use to breach these clinical chasms of mistrust can be applied to the mistrust born of the African American patient's experience with racism.

Once a person of African American heritage has reached out to a therapist, it is the responsibility of the therapist to be attuned to any of the patient's fears about revealing family business; fears about being seen as "crazy," "sick," or "weak"; fears that the therapist may challenge his or her religious beliefs; or to a possible assumption that the therapist and the psychodynamic treatment method will be eurocentric and not relevant to a person of African descent. Again, these issues are not unique to African Americans. The adult child of alcoholic parents often comes to therapy with a prohibition against revealing family secrets outside the family; a devout Irish American Roman Catholic or an observant Jew will often have concerns that therapy may compromise or challenge his or her faith; and working-class White Americans may come to therapy with the assumption that dynamic psychotherapy is for elite or middle-class Whites and may not be relevant to their own experience.

Many therapists are attuned to theses issues and develop the ability to establish a good therapeutic alliance and remain *conscious* of their own culture-bound values and stereotypes. Those who have not yet examined these issues in themselves and in their work can certainly learn to do so. One of the tenets of psychoanalytic and psychodynamic therapy is the necessity for the therapist to stay attuned to his or her countertransferences and not *act* on his or her internal responses to patients. Using this tradition of recognizing and working with one's countertransference can help psychodynamic therapists make the transition to recognizing and working with cross-cultural countertransferences. Some excellent examples of cross-cultural countertransference are cited in Comas-Díaz and Jacobsen (1991).

While this chapter focuses on the ways in which psychodynamic therapists can do effective work with African American women, the reader can also use this discussion to identify steps that mental health institutions, professional education institutes, and professional organizations might take in combating manifestations of institutional racism in psychotherapy. Some examples of institutional racism include misdiagnosis of African Americans, treatment of African American women with medication only instead of medication in combination with psychotherapy, and the lack of attention to the sociocultural context of patient and therapist in the training and practice of psychotherapists.

## THERAPIST SELF-AWARENESS AND SOCIOCULTURAL REALITIES: CONDUCTING EFFECTIVE TREATMENT

In my classes and workshops on identity and diversity for mental health professionals and graduate students, I often begin by indicating that these are *not* forums to teach White therapists how to work with patients of color. They provide an opportunity to heighten everyone's awareness about identity—both the therapist and the patient—the sociocultural and political context of each person, and feelings about others from a similar or different background. I examine several dimensions of identity: race, ethnicity, class, gender, age, sexual orientation, religion, and any other dimension relevant to the person. We begin with an experiential exercise in which the workshop participants explore these issues for themselves. I stress the fact that attending to identity, sociocultural and political context, and attitudes about oneself and others should always be a consideration in fully understanding and working therapeutically with *any* patient. I ask each participant to complete a grid indicating the various identity characteristics of each of his or her patients, as a way of focusing the therapist's attention on what he or she does and does not know about his or her patients. We then use these data to examine the way the therapist's and the patient's conscious and unconscious attitudes about their own and different groups affect the therapeutic work.

The class or workshop may also discuss the cultural context of various racial and ethnic groups, often using the experiences of participants. We look at the impact of racism, anti-Semitism, homophobia or heterosexism, and other forms of stereotyping on the group being discussed. I have increasingly devoted some time in the workshop to exploring the way in which staff members from similar and different backgrounds interact in participant's workplaces, with the aim of increasing the level of comfort in those interactions.

My experience in conducting these workshops and classes for many years confirms my belief that working effectively with a person from any background begins with the therapist's conscious awareness of his or her own cultural identity and its impact in his or her life. As I think about what any therapist needs to know to work effectively with African American women, I would focus the therapist's *self-exploration* on particular dimensions in addition to whatever identity characteristics are most salient for him or her. These dimensions, for therapists of all races and genders, include the following:

The therapists' feelings about their own race, class, gender, and sexual orientation.
The therapists' feelings about their own ethnicity and language.
The impact of racism, sexism, and White skin privilege on the therapist.
The therapists' attitudes about complexion and standards of beauty.
The therapists' comfort level with African American language and styles.

How therapists manage assertiveness and competitiveness.
The therapists' attitudes about African American's anger toward Whites and African Americans.
The therapists' ability to be vulnerable and to be powerful.
The therapists' attitudes about spirituality and/or religion.

Although there is no *one* experience for African American women, the themes noted above are particularly relevant to most African American women in this country. There are variations on the themes for Black women from the Caribbean, Central, and South America, but the issues are basically the same. I will elaborate on each theme and its relevance to understanding African American women in therapy.

## The Therapists' Feelings about Their Own Race, Class, Gender, and Sexual Orientation

The self-image of any woman in this society is inextricably related to how she sees herself and how she is regarded by others in terms of race, class, gender, and sexual orientation. To the extent that an African American woman is seen as a racial minority, less privileged in terms of class and gender, and deviant in terms of sexual orientation (if she is lesbian or bisexual), she is an outsider in the mainstream. Audre Lorde, in *Sister Outsider* (1984), describes herself as a "Black lesbian poet" (p. 40) and discusses her experiences as a feminist, activist, mother, and educator in the United States and Grenada.

An African American woman may feel very proud to be African American and female; she may feel shame about or internalize the negative stereotypes attributed to her; she may long to be regarded with the same value publicly accorded to White women; she may be angry at being ignored or devalued; she may feel empowered or powerless about her identity. As the therapist examines his or her feelings about these aspects of identity and considers how they have been regarded by those around them, it will be easier for the therapist to empathize with the complex experience of being an African American woman in this society.

## The Therapists' Feelings about Their Own Ethnicity and Language

Ethnicity (the national group or tribe to which one belongs) and language are critical aspects of how we are regarded and how we regard ourselves. Consider, for example, the tensions that still exist among some Lutherans in this country who identify with either German or Scandinavian forebears. The perception of one's own cultural practices as correct and inherently superior or better than another's cultural practices is age-old and worldwide.

Ethnicity, language, and race are often confused in this society. Hispanic people, for example, are placed in one category, which implies being other, foreign, inferior, and usually darker than White Americans—though not as dark as African Americans. In reality the ethnic identification of a Hispanic person is based on where he or she came from, for example, the Dominican Republic or Ecuador, not just on the language he or she may speak. Also in most Spanish-speaking countries in the Americas people have various racial backgrounds. Hispanics or Latinos tend to come from the same three groups as many African Americans: Africans from different ethnic groups in Africa, Whites from various ethnic groups in Europe, and various indigenous peoples living in the Americas before these lands were "discovered" by Europeans. The relative mixture of these three racial groups has produced a rainbow of colors among peoples of African or indigenous descent throughout North, Central, and South America.

For most African Americans, ethnicity is synonymous with race, because most of us do not know to which African or European ethnic group our ancestors belonged. Consequently, the primary cultural identification for most African Americans is with the African American experience as it has evolved (Adams, 1993). Of course, an individual's regional background, class, age, and degree of involvement with non-African American people will shape his or her particular sense of what it means to be an African American.

It is important for any therapist to pay attention to how his or her African American woman patient views herself in terms of race, ethnicity, and language. If the therapist is unfamiliar with the particular cultural background of his or her patient, he or she should ask the patient to elaborate when she is presenting material for which the therapist has little or no context. The therapist should also learn about the culture and history of the patient's group through reading or talking with colleagues from that background.

## The Impact of Racism, Sexism, and White Skin Privilege on Therapists

Therapists who are either non-White, female, or both will likely recognize that racism and/or sexism have affected them. It is vital for these therapists to consciously reflect on their own experience as the object of stereotyping, denigration, or even violence. The therapist can ask how his or her own voice has been ignored and his or her full access to opportunities denied. Conscious reflection often leads to the surfacing of unconscious memories, feelings, and impulses. As one explores such unconscious material, he or she will reach deeper levels of self-understanding. This understanding allows for greater identification with the African American woman patient. The White American woman therapist who has explored how sexism has limited or demeaned her can more easily make the leap to empathizing with the impact of racism on her African

American woman patient. The same holds true for the African American male therapist who can use his experience with racism to better understand his African American woman patient's experience with sexism and racism.

For those therapists who are fortunate enough to have the privilege automatically bestowed on Whites and males in this society, it is important that they do some work to understand cognitively and affectively how they are privileged in ways that African American women are not. A good place to start is by reading Peggy McIntosh's (1988) work on White privilege and male privilege. She clearly delineates the ways in which our society confers unearned privilege on males and Whites. These privileges are also described by McIntosh (1989) in an essay excerpted from her working paper (McIntosh, 1988). In the essay she describes White privilege as "an invisible package of unearned assets, which I can count on cashing in each day, but about which I was meant to remain oblivious"(p. 10).

It is also helpful for White therapists to consider the economic, social, and psychological cost to themselves individually and collectively of conferring privilege and high expectation on Whites and males and denying the full development and use of the talents of African Americans and women. Bowser and Hunt (1981) discuss the ways in which racism affects White Americans. White therapists can use their personal experiences of being demeaned or negatively stereotyped to begin to understand the impact of racism and sexism on African American women. Finally, therapists who are not familiar with the experience of African American women can get to know African American people in professional and social settings.

## The Therapists' Own Attitudes about Skin Complexion and Standards of Beauty

I grew up with the hyperawareness of skin color gradations common to most African American women, and bombarded by media images that depict female beauty in ways that did not reflect the physical attributes of most African American women. African American attitudes about skin color range from the notion "the blacker the berry, the sweeter the juice" to resentment and envy toward light-skinned African Americans. Many darker skinned African American women assume that their lighter skinned sisters feel superior to them. The wide range of skin color among African Americans, often within the same family, primarily reflects sexual encounters (often rape) between slaves of African descent and White Americans. This has resulted in complex attitudes about skin color among African Americans. Most notably, this country's history of African slavery and the decimation of its indigenous peoples (the Native American nations) has ingrained in the national psyche the notion that darker skinned people are inferior to White-skinned people. African Americans have struggled to define themselves as fully human in their multicolored skins. The

Black power and Black is beautiful movements of the 1960s and 1970s were recent manifestations of this struggle.

Standards of beauty are particularly relevant to self-esteem formation among women in general. Feminist activists and theorists have explored the issues around standards of beauty that do not reflect the reality of most women. Most American women do not have the body size and shape of fashion models, yet most advertising for women's clothes uses tall thin models. African American women still are not represented as often or as accurately in advertising as would help broaden the American standards of beauty.

As a therapist looks at and listens to his or her African American patient, he or she can silently notice his or her internal appraisal of the patient's complexion and physical appearance. Mental health professionals are taught to include a description of physical appearance in their initial assessment of a patient. This is aimed at assessing a patient's level of functioning and affective state. I would encourage the therapist to go beyond this assessment of the patient's *mental* status to a reflection on the therapist's view of the patient's physical characteristics, for example, color and attractiveness. These subjective appraisals happen, consciously or unconsciously, in most human encounters. It is vital that the therapist be aware of these appraisals of patients. Once the therapist is aware of his or her own view of the patient, the therapist can then measure that view against his or her own attitudes about complexion (color) and standards of beauty. Any therapist working with African American women might ask him- or herself how he or she regards the following: African American women who wear dreadlocks, closely cropped hair, braids, straightened hair, naturally curly or kinky hair, or naturally straight hair; African American women with light, brown, or very dark skin; African American women with more African, more European, or more mixed-race facial features; African American women with more round and pronounced behinds, with large or small breasts, with full figures. In fact, it would be useful for therapists to ask themselves how they regard specific types of body structure in any of their male or female patients.

## The Therapists' Level of Comfort with African American Language and Style

In an era of debates about Ebonics and the appropriateness of speaking African American nonstandard English, therapists must also examine their attitudes about these issues in order to work effectively with African American women. I make this observation knowing that African American women who come for therapy will vary greatly in the way they speak English and in the physical style they present to the therapist. Many African American people grew up in homes where standard English was spoken and stressed, so they speak standard English in most settings. They are likely to speak a more idiomatic African American

English when they are in an informal setting where others (African Americans or White Americans) are speaking more colloquially. Many other African American people shift back and forth in everyday usage between standard and more colloquial English. Other African Americans, especially people who did not consistently hear standard English in the home, use varying amounts of nonstandard English in their everyday language. The other aspects of how African Americans use language include the cadence of speech, accents that reflect regional and general African American usage, and the use of specific current slang expressions.

It is common in many African American communities for dress and hairstyles, slang expressions, and body language to develop and become part of African American cultural usage. Often, new styles or language arise from adolescents and young adults, become part of African American usage, and are then adopted by the mainstream and other minority groups. Examples include baggy trousers and shirts among many youth, rap and hip-hop music, giving high-fives and other ritualized handshakes, and braided hairstyles.

There are also some general style practices among African Americans that cut across generational, regional, and class lines. Two major areas of style are attitudes about music and clothes. While African Americans listen to many types of music, music is often an integral part of Black life. Music is often reacted to in a participatory manner. Consider the place of gospel and other choral music in most African American churches, and the importance of music in most African American social gatherings. The centrality of rhythm in African American music, derived from the role of the drum in African music and worship, is another aspect of African American music style (Adams, 1993).

How one dresses is also a long-standing style issue in the African American community. In all regions of this country African Americans tend to "dress up" for church services. Black people regard this as a sign of respect for God, an opportunity to demonstrate their attractiveness and sense of style, and in some cases an opportunity to wear clothes that are not worn at a working-class job. At a recent social gathering of African American and other Black people in New York City one person commented critically about White tourists who annoyed many of the church members by attending services at several large Harlem Baptist churches dressed in sneakers and very casual clothes. Everyone who heard his comment understood that the members of these congregations, middle- and working-class African American people, dressed up for church as had their ancestors in the South and the North for several generations. There is also a tradition for African American women and men to spend time carefully choosing clothes for social events and for jobs where one does not have to get dirty. The goal is to assemble an outfit that looks sharp, often using color and design in a creative way. The style may vary from teenage baggy clothes and the latest sneakers, to a well-designed business suit for the woman or man in a corporate setting, to a beautiful West African dress, but each outfit is arranged with an attention to style.

I want to emphasize that the therapist working with African Americans must be aware of how he or she feels about African American language and style. In fact, he or she must examine what he or she believes and knows about the variety of African American language and styles. Such awareness will help the therapist be more attuned to the cultural nuances of language and style brought in or partially hidden by his or her patient.

## How Therapists Manage Assertiveness and Competitiveness

One might ask why this theme is any more relevant to working with African American women than to working with any patient. While this theme is certainly *an* issue for any patient, African American women have special problems with how they are assertive or competitive. Part of the problem is related to being female in a society that has traditionally expected women to keep a low profile and not compete with men. At the same time African American women have been given more space than African American men by the larger society to assert themselves. African American women have traditionally worked outside as well as inside their homes. In the service jobs that African American women have held since slavery a certain amount of "sassiness" was tolerated as long as the normative power relationship between African and White Americans was maintained. This arrangement consisted of the White male at the top of the hierarchy and included a certain amount of deference to White women.

African American men, who continue to be seen as threatening to White male dominance, are still expected to avoid any open show of assertiveness and competitiveness except in the athletic arena. In a society where males are expected to be competitive and aggressive and to have more social privilege than women, African American men continue to be thwarted in fulfilling these male expectations. This has led to tension between African American women and men, often around the issue of who is in charge. African American women have often sought to compensate for narcissistic attacks on African American men by the White world. This compensation at times takes the form of African American women constricting their own assertiveness and competitive strivings in relating to the African American men in their lives. At the same time African American women, like most women, can be fiercely assertive and aggressive in protecting their families. It is socially expected that women, including African American women, will sacrifice for their families, but women still struggle to place themselves anywhere near the top of their own priority list.

There are two particular ways in which the issues of assertiveness and competitiveness are manifested in the lives of African American women. One is the relationship between African American mothers or primary female care-takers and their sons. African American women continue to struggle to balance their wish to raise strong, self-sufficient sons, their attempts to protect their sons from becoming victims of White racist violence (often in the form of police harassment), and their impulses to coddle and spoil their valued male children. Balancing these competing impulses often stirs up conflict about how assertive to be and resurfaces conflicts about competing with men. These are issues that need to be explored and resolved in psychodynamic therapy if the African American woman patient is to have access to her full range of internal resources.

The other manifestation of issues around competition and assertion that increasingly arise in psychotherapy with Black women is their position in the corporate or professional arenas. A common theme that I hear from my patients and those of colleagues and students is the difficulty they have being accepted as a superior or even as an equal by White colleagues. The authority of African American women is still subtly and grossly challenged in many aca-demic, professional, and corporate settings. One recent reference to this was made by Parker (1997) in a December 1998 lecture about her book *Trespass-ing: My Sojourn in the Halls of Privilege*. She described an incident where she was sent as an in-house consultant from the home office to a branch office of a major corporation. When she convened the initial consultation meeting she was met with consternation by the White males who comprised the entire staff in attendance. They had difficulty accepting her authority. Her White male assistant told her later that when some of the same White male staff saw him in the bathroom, they expressed their disbelief and disapproval about an Afri-can American woman being the consultant. She noted that African American women often indicate at her lectures that a similar challenge to their authority had recently happened to them in a White work setting.

Thinking about some of the ways that African American women struggle with competitiveness and assertion and comparing those with the way the therapist handles these issues will help a therapist be more sensitive to these issues in therapeutic work with African American women.

## The Therapists' Attitudes about African Americans' Anger toward Whites and toward African Americans

African American people's anger has been presented to and perceived by many White Americans in this country as fearsome and threatening since slavery. Stereotypes about African American people as violent toward each other and as violent or potentially so toward White Americans have long been part of the fabric of the White imagination. Terkel opens his book *Race: How Blacks and Whites Think and Feel about the American Obsession* (1992) with a reference to a 1990 survey conducted by the University of Chicago's National Opinion

Research Center. He observes that 56% of non-Blacks believe that African Americans are more violence-prone.

Images about African American anger range from the African American adolescent with his baggy clothes and pulled-up hood with an angry demeanor or voice, to the frustrated young African American mother cursing and yelling at her children in the street, to the African American man or woman in a workplace diversity group expressing anger at the treatment he or she has received from White coworkers. These images, which may have actually been witnessed, tend to merge with the media images of African American men as criminals. I often tell students in my workshops that if I were an alien who dropped onto this planet and learned about Black people only from the print and television news media, I would also be terrified of African American people, especially men.

Another aspect of African American anger, or rejection, which I have heard from White Americans is the experience of being ignored or excluded by African Americans in high school or college. One White therapist, after becoming aware of not asking a young African American woman patient about relevant aspects of her developmental context, recognized that she had feared being angrily excluded by her patient as she had been by African American peers in her high school. A richly layered discussion of the issues around African American adolescents and young adults seeking racially homogenous interactions in integrated settings can be found in Tatum's *Why Are All the Black Kids Sitting Together in the Cafeteria?* (1997).

Just as how a therapist handles his or her own anger requires reflection and for many of us our own therapeutic work, so our attitudes about African American anger toward White Americans, toward African Americans, and toward others requires conscious examination. The mix of attitudes and feelings about race and aggression is powerful for anyone living in the United States and will obviously impact the therapeutic interaction as well. The more the therapist is aware of his or her own feelings in this area, the greater the chance for effective therapeutic work with African American women and men.

## The Therapists' Ability to Experience Vulnerability and Power

Feelings of vulnerability, acknowledgment of one's power, and defenses against one's vulnerability and power are familiar to any psychodynamic therapist who has been practicing for a while. Men and women experience vulnerability to both internal and external phenomena. Vulnerability can be the kind of openness necessary to have an intimate love relationship or it can be a disturbing sense of being at the mercy of harsh internal feelings or dangerous external forces. Unconscious defenses against vulnerability include avoiding intimacy, insisting that one is totally independent, and being rigid.

The ability to experience one's realistic power and to use that power in effective, nonharmful ways is one hallmark of good mental health. Unconscious defenses against one's own power include behaving like a victim, not using one's authority, or maintaining an ineffectual stance.

As a member of a group that is often oppressed or devalued, an African American woman may have particular issues around vulnerability and power. She, like her White sisters, may feel vulnerable and not powerful because of the sexism to which she is subjected. She has the additional burden of being subjected to racism. It is important for the therapist to assess the personal strengths and limitations of an African American woman's ability to be both vulnerable and powerful, and then to examine the impact of external social forces on the patient.

For example, one African American woman patient has internalized harsh negative and vulnerable feelings as a result of childhood sexual abuse. She then finds herself as an adult in a work situation where she is treated abusively by White American or African American men. The therapist will have to attend to the internal issues related to developmental abuse and the impact of the current repetition of abuse. One therapeutic approach would be to explore ways in which this woman has herself or has seen others cope positively with abuse. Group therapy would be an excellent addition to the individual therapy. The right group would offer the patient an opportunity to explore with others the experiences of abuse, of vulnerability, and of being powerful.

Another African American woman in treatment has been raised to trust her instincts and express her voice, and has not been sexually or otherwise abused. This woman then finds herself confronted by subtle but consistent dismissal or devaluing of her ideas and authority by her White female boss. Treatment with this woman will need to explore the ways in which she experiences and handles these challenges to her power and authority. It is likely that such exploration will include the ways in which other African American women and men in her life, and in her ancestral history, have handled threats to their power and authority.

As in the previous issues discussed, the therapist must have a cognitive and affective understanding of how he or she handles vulnerability and powerfulness if he or she is to work effectively with African American women patients.

## The Therapists' Attitudes about Spirituality and/or Religion

Spirituality or religion is so integral to the experience of most African Americans that it is hard to do effective psychodynamic psychotherapy with them without considering the impact of spirituality in their lives. This is not to say that all African American women belong to a religious institution or even believe in God or a Supreme Being. Certainly, there is no one faith tradition among those African American women who do believe in a Supreme Being. What I have found consistently in my work with African American women patients, in my work with therapists who see them, and in my contact with many other African American women is that for most of them some sense of the spiritual is alive in their life.

I have also been aware of the evolving integration of spiritual concerns into the lives and practices of many White colleagues. When I went through psychoanalytic training in the mid- to late 1970s, discussions about religion or spirituality were few and far between in classes and supervision. I had the sense that psychoanalytic theory and practice was regarded as an intellectual and emotional replacement for the function of religion. While I did talk about my own religious beliefs, questions, disbelief, and history in my analysis with an African American man, I remember deliberately not discussing these issues with psychoanalytic peers or teachers. My fear was that I would be regarded as "not psychoanalytic enough" or not intellectually up to par. Now there are many psychoanalytic and psychotherapeutic conference panels and workshops that explore various aspects of the spiritual or religious. This also mirrors the more open discourse about spirituality, particularly of the Eastern and New Age varieties, in the general culture.

Spirituality and religion have played powerful roles in the history of African Americans. Africans who were torn from their traditional cultures, where indigenous religions and/or Islam existed, brought some of their spiritual beliefs with them. Later, as African American slaves were exposed to Christianity of various denominations, they incorporated aspects of their African cultural traditions into the new religions. The use of the drum and other instruments, dancing and singing, and call and response (where the leader says or sings a phrase and the congregation responds out loud) in African American religious services are major carryovers of African cultural traditions. In a number of Caribbean, Central, and South American countries where Roman Catholicism was the religion of the Europeans who colonized the area, African slaves blended African religions (notably the Yoruba religion) and their deities and Catholic saints. The current practice of Santeria in the Spanish-speaking Caribbean, Voudou in Haiti, and Macumbe and Candomble in Brazil are examples of this blending. Again, it is helpful to a therapist working with a Black woman to be aware that part of her family background may be from the Americas outside the United States, and that the spiritual practices just mentioned may be a part of her experience (Adams, 1993).

The "Black" church, of whatever Christian type, has played a crucial role in the social, educational, political, and cultural life of African Americans. It has been one of the most powerful and enduring institutions in the African American community. A full discussion of the African American church is beyond the scope of this chapter; I refer the reader who is interested to Billingsley (1992) and Lincoln and Mamiya (1990). African Americans belong to a number of major historically African American denominations, including several Baptist denominations, several Methodist denominations, Apostolics, Pentecostals, and Church of God in Christ; to African American congregations in major historically White denominations, such as the Roman Catholic, United Methodist, Presbyterian, Episcopalian, and Seventh Day Adventist; and to mixed congregations in historically White denominations, both Roman Catholic and Protestant (Billingsley, 1992). African Americans have also found their way to non-Christian traditions, including Islam, Baha'i, Buddhism, Hinduism, Yoruba, and other traditional African religions, and to spiritual paths not grounded in an institutional religion.

An African American woman in therapy may be closely involved with a religious practice and/or community that gives her spiritual sustenance, social contacts, and support. Another African American woman in therapy may have a personal relationship with God or a spiritual force, but belong to no organized group. Yet another African American woman in therapy may have doubts, negative feelings, anger, and conflicts about God, religion, or spirituality and may want to feel safe about exploring them in therapy. Yet another African American woman may have conflicts about her relationship to spirituality that are imbedded in oppressive, hurtful experiences with family and others in the name of religion. Two common examples of the latter are women who have been shamed and rejected by their families on religious grounds. One was rejected because she was a lesbian and another was rejected for becoming pregnant out of wedlock. The point is that most African American women have grown up in families or communities where religion or spirituality has been a potent force. Their attitudes, feelings, and involvement with spirituality or religion may vary widely, but need to be acknowledged, and explored when they are ready to do so.

## GENERAL CONSIDERATIONS

The role of the therapist is very powerful in any psychotherapeutic encounter. This is one reason why therapists trained in psychoanalytic training institutes are required to participate in their own personal psychoanalytic treatment. Many therapists who do not attend analytic institutes also choose to have personal psychotherapy. The three major professions that train people to become psychotherapists, social work, psychology, and psychiatry, do not require their graduate students to have personal psychotherapy. This is unfortunate. I hope the material I have discussed in this chapter will encourage graduate students who aspire to be therapists to undertake personal therapy. If they would like to get a more in-depth appreciation of psychodynamic therapy I would also encourage them to pursue advanced training in psychotherapy at an institute.

For any therapist working with African American women or men it is vital that he or she examine his or her own attitudes and feelings about his or her own race, ethnicity, class, gender, sexual orientation, and spirituality. The therapist should also explore his or her attitudes and feelings about people who are different and similar, and do some personal work to become more comfortable interacting with patients and colleagues who are from backgrounds different from his or her own. One way to do this is to participate in a group exploration of identity and difference with people from a variety of backgrounds. A group of therapists can also examine the way the therapist's and the patient's conscious and unconscious attitudes about one's own group and about different groups impact on the therapeutic work. If a therapist wants to actively combat racism in his or her home or professional community, Clyde Ford (1994) presents 50 steps to help end racism.

In the therapeutic encounter it is important to acknowledge an obvious difference of race, language, or ethnicity in the first or second session. Since it is often still taboo to talk openly about these differences (especially racial ones) in heterogeneous social settings, the patient should not be expected to know it is safe to acknowledge and explore these differences in the treatment room. When "the elephant in the room" is not acknowledged, the treatment may never get off the ground or it may remain much less than authentic and effective. Near the end of the initial consultation with any new patient I always ask how he or she feels about working with me. If at that time or earlier in our interaction he or she has not mentioned my being an African American woman, I usually ask "How do you feel about working with a Black woman therapist?" The response is rarely extensive, but it opens the door for later exploration of the meaning to the patient of his or her identity and whatever he or she sees or guesses about mine.

It is always vital to listen carefully to what African American women patients say about their experiences being African American, and not to discount any patient's stories about racism, sexism, and other oppression. Any material or experience presented in treatment can be used as unconscious resistance to exploring authentic experience. It is incumbent on the therapist to first listen carefully, and then consider how to use the material therapeutically. The therapist who has had limited personal experience with African Americans should be especially cautious about either deciding material about racism is resistance or focusing on that material only in a literal manner. The material should be worked with as any other material: attend to the manifest information and explore the underlying (latent) feelings and meanings.

If the therapist has not had much experience with African Americans from a variety of class backgrounds, he or she must keep in mind that stereotypes about African American people tend to ignore differences in education, financial status, and class identification and aspiration. A number of African American women come from families where they are second-, third-, or fourth-generation college graduates. Others come from several generations of solidly working-class families. Still other African American women come from materially poor families and have received less-than-adequate public school education, but are richly endowed with love, tenacity, determination, resilience, and creativity. Still other African American women come from families hit hard by poverty, substance abuse, and dysfunction. Some of these women thrive, often due to a family member or church or community figure who was "there" for them. Some do not thrive, but anyone who has made it to therapy has at least some impulse to grow. Many African American and non-African American women from working-class, middle-class, and materially privileged families are also affected by substance abuse, sexual and physical abuse, and other dysfunction. It is important for therapists not to hold on to the stereotypes available in the society about race, class, and gender.

## ILLUSTRATIONS OF EFFECTIVE PSYCHODYNAMIC THERAPY WITH AFRICAN AMERICAN WOMEN

Several descriptions of psychodynamic individual and group treatment with African American women will illustrate the effectiveness of this treatment approach. The stories and vignettes are composites drawn from my clinical, supervisory, and teaching experience.

As with any category of human beings, there is enormous diversity among African American women in the United States. We come from various age cohorts, class and status strata, and regional and family backgrounds. We have various ways of expressing our sexuality and our spirituality. We encompass the entire range of human feelings, psychological mechanisms, and character styles. Yet most of us have a sense of identity that is informed by the fact of being a woman of African descent living in the United States. Many of us experience a sense of sisterhood in relation to other African American women, with all the complexity of feelings between sisters. This sisterhood grows out of our rainbow of skin tones, our shared cultural experiences, and the complex responses we get from Americans outside the African American community. There is an "Mmhmm" experience that resonates among most African American women, often via a look, a murmur, a laugh, or an expression of pain. The following stories and vignettes will illustrate several broad themes encountered in therapeutic work with and in the lives of African American women.

### Mildred Sheds the Blues

Mildred came to therapy complaining of difficulty sleeping, decreased appetite, crying spells, and a general dissatisfaction about her job as a manager in a government bureaucracy. She was in her early 50s, was a widow of several years, and had four young adult children. She had never sought therapy for herself, but had participated in brief family therapy when one of her sons was having behavioral problems in school.

Mildred grew up in the segregated Southwest in a close family with strong Baptist faith and a commitment to education for the children in the family. Her father was a construction contractor, who did work for individuals and businesses in the local African American community. Her mother was a seamstress who worked at home and raised their children. Mildred had several siblings and a large extended family in the vicinity of her parent's home.

Mildred did well in public school and later completed a community college degree. She also took some courses toward a bachelor's degree. She was clearly a bright and creative woman who had the capacity to achieve even more than she had in the workplace. She was a loving and attentive mother, who still struggled with some overprotective impulses toward the son who had problems as a child. Mildred also maintained close ties with her aging parents. Among her siblings she was often the caretaker of their parents.

Mildred began therapy with an African American woman social worker, who had been referred by a work colleague. She began with individual therapy once a week; later, the therapist brought Mildred into her therapy group. Mildred continued in individual and group therapy for several years, then in group alone until a planned termination.

The treatment began with Mildred wondering whether she should be seeing a therapist, because she regarded herself as a strong African American woman who had always taken care of her own responsibilities. She did make a positive connection with the therapist, partly based on her sense that the therapist understood the world she came from and lived in as an African American woman. Mildred was also struck by the therapist's close attention to what she said: she not only listened to the content but always asked about Mildred's feelings about the content she presented. The therapist pointed out that Mildred was taking an active role in handling her current difficulties by choosing therapy. The therapist also pointed out that therapy is a collaborative process between patient and therapist.

As Mildred and her therapist reviewed her personal and family history as the context for her current depressive symptoms, self-image, feelings, and emotional defenses, several themes became clear. Mildred cared for others often to the exclusion of attending to her own wants. She tended to use depression, rationalization (logical explanations denying her feelings), and intellectualization as defenses against her anger and pain. She feared losing control, so she took a back seat or kept silent about her vulnerable or sad feelings. Mildred also underestimated her overall competence.

It emerged in the treatment that Mildred had mixed feelings about her abilities and aspirations while growing up. As a middle "good daughter," she often felt that her charming, assertive older sister and her active demanding younger siblings got much more attention and encouragement from their parents. She was expected to do well and behave in school, and she did. She yearned to be more like her outgoing, popular father, but he did not know how to encourage her active and competitive impulses. He enjoyed her developing domestic skills, valued her even quiet demeanor, and praised her because she looked like her mother. While Mildred's mother took good care of all her children, she paid more attention to their physical needs than to their emotional needs. Mildred learned to soothe herself and to get her parent's approval by caretaking, not by assertively expressing herself or by being playful.

The journey of psychodynamic therapy undertaken by Mildred and her therapist involved continual exploration of the ways Mildred unconsciously moved away from a full range of authentic feelings, most notably her anger, her exuberance, her sexuality, and her intellectual excitement. Mildred's transference to the therapist varied from experiencing her as a somewhat distant and self-involved mother; as the wished-for nurturing and supportive mother or older sister; and as a father who was creative and playful, but gave Mildred the message that this was "all right" for him but not for her. The therapist's countertransference to Mildred centered primarily around her tendency to idealize Mildred's strength and ability to take care of others, and therefore not confront her quietness and intellectualizations. The therapist also experienced anger and impatience at Mildred's tendency to stifle her playfulness and exuberance.

The therapy group afforded Mildred a different opportunity to work on her issues. She explored feelings and impulses in concert with other group members who experienced similar feelings in the group. She was also able to disagree and struggle with group members who had different experiences or who evoked negative transferences.

Mildred moved naturally into the role of caretaker in the group. She had difficulty presenting her own wishes or pain, as had been the case in her family. She learned to express her feelings and views more directly in the group. She was eventually able to cry, be angry, argue, and express sexual feelings in the group. She had the chance in group to challenge others in ways she never felt safe to do in her family. She could express anger toward a member who reminded her of her mother at a moment in the group, and have the group members explore Mildred's anger and explore any narcissistic withdrawal by the other member. Mildred could also "play" with other group members around sexual and intellectual themes and not be ignored or rebuffed as she had been by her father.

In the group that spanned generational, racial, and cultural differences, Mildred contributed her perspective of having grown up an African American female with a strong faith in God in the segregated Southwest. The therapist created a safe-enough environment to explore similarities and differences related to racial, ethnic, gender, and spiritual identity.

Mildred was able to regain her regular sleeping and eating patterns and feel less depressed as she got in touch with her underlying feelings of anger and resentment, and to be aware of her yearning for more self-expression. As Mildred's depression lifted, she and the therapist focused more on her characteristic ways of being in the world, that is, to care for others to the exclusion of herself; and to dampen her expression of wishes, excitement, sexual feelings, playfulness, and intellectual ambition. She gradually began using her intellectual and creative abilities at her church and at her job, eventually deciding to leave the job for a more challenging position. She also began to take college courses that both interested her and advanced her career goals. Mildred was able to begin dating again, after working in the group on sexual and competitive impulses.

## Shameeka Finds Her Voice

Shameeka is a 20-something African American woman who sought therapy to deal with difficulty separating from her parents, self-esteem issues, making her way in the competitive world of jazz singing, and handling negative reactions to her homosexual orientation. She found her way to a nonprofit psychotherapy clinic that had a special unit for treating creative and performing artists. Shameeka requested an African American woman therapist, who would be gay-affirmative, if not lesbian. She was told that no African American woman therapist was available, but that she could see an experienced African American man who was gay-affirmative. Shameeka chose to accept the assignment to the African American male therapist.

Shameeka grew up in the 1970s in an urban northeastern city in a working-class African American/Caribbean family. Her father worked as a toll collector for the city. Her mother, who had emigrated to this country from the English-speaking Caribbean with her family during her early teens, worked as a public school aide. Shameeka's dad grew up in the same city where Shameeka lived. He met his future wife at an event where American and Caribbean Blacks were socializing. Her parents were committed to a college education for both their children. They sacrificed to send them to a Catholic school where they could get a better education than the local public school offered.

A gift for singing was evident even when Shameeka was in grade school. She developed her musical ability with the encouragement of teachers and of her mother, who hoped she would teach music. She won a scholarship to a New York college with strong liberal arts and performing arts programs and finished college with honors. Shameeka moved to New York City to pursue her career and soon found herself struggling to be herself against pulls from her mother to stay closer to home and to settle down and marry.

Shameeka had one younger brother with whom she had a very close relationship, and a number of cousins on both sides of her family. She had an intense relationship with her mother, who alternated between affectionate, nurturing involvement with her daughter and impatient criticism of Shameeka. When things were good with her mother, they were very good, but when things were sour, they were rotten. Her mother's critical and demeaning behavior increased when she was intoxicated with alcohol. She would talk about how pretty the light-skinned family members were and would refer negatively to her husband's dark skin and to Shameeka's dark skin and short natural hairstyle. The mother and many of her family members were light-skinned with naturally straight hair.

Shameeka's curiosity about everything, her athleticism, and her good looks (which reflected her father's looks) left her father feeling somewhat threatened and uncomfortable with his daughter. Consequently, he praised his daughter to his friends, but did not share this praise with Shameeka herself. As her sexual attraction to other females became obvious to him, her father withdrew even more. Since her mother wanted Shameeka to marry an upwardly mobile man and live a traditional middle-class lifestyle, neither parent was available to help Shameeka navigate the difficulties of a lesbian lifestyle in a heterosexist society.

In the first few sessions with her therapist Shameeka was fearful that he would not really hear or understand her and that he would judge her negatively. Her transferential expectation was that the therapist would be critical like her mother and not accept her for herself like her father. She was particularly apprehensive about whether the therapist was really gay-affirmative.

Her therapist was very calm, listened actively and intently, and created a safe environment for the therapeutic work. Two early interventions had a profound positive impact on developing a good therapeutic alliance. As Shameeka talked about the difficulties of being a performer, the therapist quietly revealed that he was jazz musician as well as a psychologist. She was surprised and thought that he might indeed understand a core aspect of her identity. At another point, when Shameeka was expressing her pain at being denigrated by her mother for being dark-skinned and not interested in romance with men, she noticed there were tears on her therapist's face. She told her therapist much later how she felt deeply heard and understood by his silent tears.

Shameeka and her therapist explored her struggles to pursue her career goals and relationship choices, while maintaining a loving connection with her parents. They discovered that her experience of her mother' disapproval contributed to feeling she was not attractive and unentitled to success as a singer. She had picked up her mother's attitude that jazz singing in night clubs and sexual attraction to other women were bad, immoral, and shameful. It also became clear in the therapeutic work that Shameeka had internalized her mother's disparaging comments about dark skin and naturally kinky hair. She had combined these criticisms into a negative self-image.

Unconsciously, Shameeka had come to see herself as a shameful, loose, dark woman who loved the excitement and applause of jazz singing and who loved other women. She identified ambivalently with her equally dark-skinned father who also loved jazz and loved women. His voice, however, had been the more reserved in their household. He had also been humiliated by the mother's hurtful criticism, especially when she was drinking. Since her father was uncomfortable with his daughter's attraction to women, he had not yet developed a way to encourage his daughter to be joyous and enthusiastic about her music and her love life.

In order for Shameeka to separate emotionally from her parents, she had to strengthen and solidify her acceptance of her creativity, passion, musical talent, intelligence, sensitivity, and other positive attributes. As she worked with her therapist to explore these aspects of herself, she came to trust her own instincts and value her hard work and abilities. She was also able to disentangle her mother's internalized racism around skin color and her father's bias against homosexuality from her parents' love for her.

Shameeka became more confident and began to have some success in her singing career. She was then able to offer her parents the opportunity to participate in her life on her own terms. They were gradually able to respond to Shameeka's singing career with pride. She is still finding her voice in establishing a healthy love relationship. She is working with her therapist to build a relationship that does not reenact the masochistic position she saw her father enact with her mother.

The stories of Mildred and Shameeka illustrate in detail the way two African American women used psychodynamic psychotherapy to better understand themselves, increase their self-esteem and the range of emotions available to them, improve their relationships with family and significant others, and become more satisfyingly productive in their work. I will now give brief vignettes about two other African American women who come from opposite ends of the socioeconomic spectrum.

## Daisy Gets Off Welfare

Daisy was in her early 30s when she sought help from a community clinic connected with a psychoanalytic training institute. She had come from a very materially deprived background in the rural South, where she was raised by a great-aunt and great-uncle. They loved her and provided for her as best they could, but they were limited in their ability to guide her schooling and protect her from ridicule about her poverty. She dropped out of high school and flirted with alcohol and substance abuse. She felt abandoned by both parents: her mother died when she was an infant and her father had literally abandoned her to seek his fortune elsewhere. As with many African American families, members of her extended family stepped in to raise her.

Daisy found her way to the big city and began to work in the garment industry. She had some seamstress skills and hoped to start her own business. She became pregnant by a man she imagined would marry her. When she realized he had no intention of caring for her or her child, she applied for welfare benefits to support her family. She came for help with mild symptoms of depression, frustration about repeatedly finding herself with abusive men, and a wish to become financially self-supporting. A report from another clinic where she had been treated briefly with antidepressive medication suggested she was not a good candidate for psychotherapy because of her deprived and difficult upbringing. I wonder if the fact that she was African American and poor contributed to the clinic's limited expectation of her ability to benefit from psychotherapy.

Daisy was assigned to an African American woman therapist who was a social worker in analytic training. Daisy had not requested an African American therapist; in fact, she had expressed the belief that an older White male might be best able to help her. But she was open to trying therapy with the African American woman therapist. Therapist and patient were similar in race and gender, but came from very different class and educational backgrounds. The therapist also recognized that the patient's preference for an older White male therapist indicated something about the patient's self-perception. The therapist's initial task was to engage the patient and try to establish some common ground and safety. Exploring Daisy's request for a White male therapist and her feeling about working with a African American woman therapist immediately acknowledged "the elephant in the room" and addressed the emotional tension. In fact, the exploration led to Daisy's wish for a powerful and loving father who could take care of her and protect her from the dangers of the world. The therapist was able to acknowledge that wish and speak to Daisy's impulses toward self-sufficiency and independence. In time Daisy saw the therapist as a strong and caring figure who was also a role model for her own autonomy.

As the therapist worked with Daisy, she stayed attuned to the similarities and differences between her own and Daisy's internal psychic lives and external life circumstances. On the one hand, the therapist had lived in the South and gone to school where poor African American children were teased by other more fortunate children and had also worked with economically deprived children from different ethnic backgrounds. On the other hand, the therapist grew up with strong family support for getting an education and pursuing a career. She was able to use the similarities and differences in background, coping mechanisms, and general personality style to engage Daisy in building her self-esteem and moving forward in her life.

Daisy was able to complete her high school equivalency certificate and an apprenticeship in the clothes manufacturing industry. She started a full-time job with good union benefits and began plans for doing some freelance dressmaking on the side. She learned to trust her excellent ability to size up a situation and locate resources for herself and her daughter. She also expanded her sense of what was possible for her. The transference toward her therapist become one of a trusted older sister with whom it was also possible to play and laugh. As Daisy worked on a lot of anger and hurt about her unavailable father she was also able to make more appropriate choices regarding the men in her life.

## Cassandra Learns to Compete

Cassandra is an African American woman who was in her late 30s when she sought therapy through her employee assistance program at the corporation where she was a finance manager. She was referred to a White woman psychologist with a private psychodynamic therapy practice. The presenting problem was conflict between Cassandra and her White female supervisor. Cassandra felt the supervisor was being unjustly demanding and critical primarily due to her racism. This was causing Cassandra a great deal of anxiety and stress, which was interfering with her usually solid work performance.

As the therapist listened to Cassandra's family history and her presenting complaints, she recognized that Cassandra's conflict with her boss was reminiscent of her interactions with her mother. Cassandra was fairly passive in both situations and felt undermined and treated like an incompetent child. Cassandra was not fully in touch with her anger at her mother, but did experience a great deal of unspoken anger toward the racist supervisor. The therapist understood that an old parent–daughter scenario was being enacted in the present work situation. She also heard clearly that the supervisor's behavior was unfair and likely racist. She was able to use her own experience with men in the classroom or workplace who behaved in a sexist manner to empathize with Cassandra's experience.

Cassandra had not expressed any preference regarding the race or gender of a therapist. The therapist understood, however, that their racial difference needed to be acknowledged and explored. To the extent that the White therapist–African American patient dyad reflects the societal paradigm of White majority powerful figure and African American minority powerless figure, the issue of trust in this therapeutic dyad is often initially crucial. When the therapist asked how Cassandra felt about having a White female therapist, Cassandra said at first that it did not matter to her. The therapist touched on it lightly again as Cassandra talked more about the "racist, hurtful" supervisor. This time Cassandra was able to acknowledge that she did wonder if the therapist would believe that her boss was racist or instead think that Cassandra was just exaggerating. This exploration helped to create a working therapeutic alliance.

The work in the treatment started with a careful exploration of the facts of the work situation and Cassandra's feelings about those facts. This moved the treatment into Cassandra's feelings about authority (her own and others); how she experienced and handled her aggression; and how she experienced and handled competition. Cassandra was able to resolve her fears about competing with her mother. On one hand, she feared her mother would retaliate and destroy her for the unconscious oedipal strivings she had to take her father away from her mother. On the other hand, Cassandra feared her own rageful impulses toward her mother.

The therapist suggested that Cassandra join a group to further explore and practice using her aggression and competitive strivings with a variety of people. The therapist was not currently running a group, so they talked about what type of group might work best. They decided on a referral to a group that is interracial in composition and led by a African American male therapist. Cassandra added the group therapy to her continuing work with her individual therapist. In the group Cassandra has begun claiming space for herself and joining with others (male and female) to explore competitive, aggressive, and envious feelings. She is also able to explore the racial and gender dimensions of these feelings in the live situation of a safe therapeutic setting. The combination of individual and group therapy maximizes the capacity for Cassandra to feel, understand, and change. The benefits of combined group and individual therapy are elaborated on by Caligor, Fieldsteel, and Brok (1984). While they discuss individual and group with the same therapist, many of the same benefits pertain in addition to the additional transference and real relationship available with an additional therapist.

## SUMMARY

This chapter has provided a current working definition of psychodynamic psychotherapy and has noted other influences, especially systems-centered therapy and a focus on sociocultural context, on the therapy I practice. I have also discussed the critiques of psychodynamic therapy for African American women and responses to those critiques. The next section of the chapter discusses the identity exploration that therapists need to do for themselves, and some of the themes around identity that are particularly salient for African American women. I have suggested some general considerations for the effective practice of dynamic therapy with African American women. Finally, the illustrations of effective psychodynamic therapy with African American women described four hypothetical treatments that represent some of the typical issues and women who come for treatment.

## REFERENCES

Adams, J. (1993). *The Black/African American experience.* Unpublished manuscript, Postgraduate Center for Mental Health, New York.

Agazarian, Y. M. (1997). *Sytems-centered therapy for groups.* New York: Guilford Press.

Altman, N. (1993). Psychoanalysis and the urban poor. *Psychoanalytic Dialogues, 3*(1), 29–49.

Baker, F. M. (1988). Afro-Americans. In L. Comas-Díaz & E. Griffith (Eds.), *Clinical guidelines in cross-cultural mental health* (pp. 151–181). New York: Wiley.

Basch, M. (1980). *Doing psychotherapy.* New York: Basic Books.

Billingsley, A. (1992). *Climbing Jacob's ladder: The enduring legacy of African American families.* New York: Simon & Schuster.

Blanck, G., & Blanck, R. (1974). *Ego psychology: Theory and practice.* New York: Columbia University Press.

Bowser, B., & Hunt, R. (Eds.). (1981). *Impacts of racism on White Americans.* New York: Sage.

Caligor, J., Fieldsteel, N., & Brok, A. (1984). *Individual and group therapy: Combining psychoanalytic treatments.* New York: Basic Books.

Comas-Díaz, L., & Jacobsen, F. (1991). Ethno-cultural transference and counter-transference in the therapeutic dyad. *American Journal of Orthopsychiatry, 61*(3), 392–402.

Ford, C. (1994). *We can all get along: Fifty steps you can take to help end racism.* New York: Dell.

Greenson, R. (1967). *The technique and practice of psychoanalysis.* New York: International Universities Press.

Grier, W. H., & Cobbs, P. (1968). *Black rage.* New York: Basic Books.

Lincoln, C. E., & Mamiya, L. H. (1990). *The Black church in the African American experience.* Durham, NC: Duke University Press.

Lorde, A. (1984). *Sister outsider: Essays and speeches.* Freedom, CA: Crossing Press.

McIntosh, P. (1988). *White privilege and male privilege: A personal account of coming to see correspondences through work in women's studies.* Wellesley, MA: Wellesley College Center for Research on Women.

McIntosh, P. (1989, July–August). White privilege: Unpacking the invisible knapsack. *Peace and Freedom,* 10–12.

Mitchell, S. A., & Black, M. J. (1995). *Freud and beyond: A history of modern psychoanalytic thought.* New York: Basic Books.

Parker, G. M. (1997). *Trespassing: My sojourn in the halls of privilege.* New York: Houghton Mifflin.

Pine, F. (1985). *Drive, ego, object, self.* New York: Basic Books.

Racker, H. (1968). *Transference and countertransference.* New York: International Universities Press.

Tatum, B. D. (1997). *Why are all the Black kids sitting together in the cafeteria? and other conversations about race.* New York: Basic Books.

Terkel, S. (1992). *Race: How Blacks and Whites feel about the American obsession.* New York: Doubleday.

Thomas, A., & Sillen, S. (1972). *Racism and psychiatry.* New York: Brunner/Mazel.

## CHAPTER 4

# The Stone Center Theoretical Approach Revisited
## Applications for African American Women

### YVONNE M. JENKINS

The Stone Center theoretical approach, also known as the "relational theory of women's psychological development," enhances our understanding of relational dynamics associated with most women's relationships in the United States. This theory was renamed *relational/cultural theory* in the mid-1990s, thereby affirming its status as a work in progress that seeks to embrace and respond to the experiences of a diverse population of women. Relational/cultural theory is the basis for relational/cultural therapy, a clinical approach that focuses on defining and understanding connections and disconnections that restrict and block psychic growth. The rationale for this focus is to find ways to move from disconnection to connection within the context of the therapeutic relationship (Miller & Stiver, 1998).

The original conceptualization of relational theory took place in the early 1980s. Despite their intentions, the founders of this particular relational theory have acknowledged limitations of their original theory for intervening with women of color and women from other marginalized groups (Jordan, Kaplan, Miller, Stiver, & Surrey, 1991). The founders attribute these limitations to their White, middle-class, highly educated, heterosexual perspective; the type of clinical work they have done; and particular populations they have worked with over the years. Therefore, for a more inclusive perspective on relational empowerment and a more in-depth understanding of patterns of relationship among those who are oppressed by the dominant culture, the founding theorists have invited "dialogue with those who can teach about other realities and points of view" (Jordan et al., 1991, p. 7). This chapter is a response to that invitation.

## WHY INCLUSION OF THE RELATIONAL/CULTURAL PERSPECTIVE IS ESSENTIAL

Inclusion of the relational/cultural perspective in this text acknowledges a progressive expansion of psychodynamic perspectives on psychotherapy with African American women. Traditional psychodynamic approaches are rooted in vague, dominant cultural assumptions and generalizations that routinely ignore the enormous impact of culture, the environment, and other external factors on therapist–client interactions (Klein, Orleans, & Soule, 1991; Paniagua, 1998). While psychoanalytic models (e.g., Freudian and ego psychology) have failed to incorporate cultural and environmental factors in psychotherapy with people of color, the poor, and gays/lesbians, contemporary analytic models (e.g., object relations and self psychology) espouse an etic perspective of development for both normal personality development and pathology. This perspective and the approaches that have emanated from it actually disguise an Anglo/European emic cultural model. Furthermore, the theories that under-lie traditional psychodynamic approaches focus on accounting for pathological development, while indications of healthy psychological development are merely inferred or overlooked altogether.

The infusion of diversity perspectives with dynamic theories acknowledges the contextual issues relevant for work with African American women. Effective intervention with this population must acknowledge and attend to the roles of race, ethnicity, culture as well as internal *and* external events that shape the identity development, relational development, and current mental status of clients from this diverse population. Psychotherapists must also have the ability to recognize healthy psychological development and other strengths of African American women from a culturally competent perspective.

As increasing awareness of the complexity of human diversity unfolds, the field of psychotherapy progresses toward acknowledging and appropriately responding to sociocultural contexts for problems in daily living, and toward defining and embracing diversity-inclusive frameworks and approaches. Relational/cultural psychotherapy is an intervention in progress that actively avoids replicating the shortcomings of traditional psychodynamic psycho-therapy stated above. Thus, the status of relational/cultural theory as a work in progress acknowledges its openness to continuous examination and development. Psychotherapy based on this approach seeks to give appropriate consideration to sociocultural, environmental/external factors, and internal events that underly presenting problems and shape current functioning. Within these contexts, relational/cultural psychotherapy acknowledges components of healthy psychological development (connections) and disruptions to this process (disconnections) that a woman has experienced. Therefore, when practiced responsibly, relational/cultural psychotherapy does not relegate African American women to the object status allied with traditional psychodynamic theories. Instead, the *real* experiences of *real* women come to life (Miller & Stiver, 1998).

## TURNER'S PERSPECTIVE

In a Stone Center working paper, Clevonne Turner (1987), a former therapist at the Wellesley College Counseling Service, encouraged practitioners to become more aware of ethnic influences on the cultural world views of women of color so that appropriate interventions could be practiced with these populations. In addition, she affirmed the capacity of what has since become known as relational/cultural theory to represent, validate, and legitimize a significant aspect of African American women's psychosocial maturational processes. Turner also acknowledged that racism, sexism, ethnicity, culture, and classism contextualize the relational experiences of this population and provided instructive examples of each. Her attention to race, ethnicity, and culture expanded the original perspective of the founding theorists by naming sociocultural issues that lend complexity to the lives of women of color, particularly African American women. Furthermore, Turner emphasized that the Stone Center approach could be applied within a culturally syntonic context and that such application is an absolute necessity. It is this author's stance that without such application, there is a danger of universalizing White feminist realities at the expense of not responding to the therapeutic needs of African American women appropriately and competently. Hence, there is a danger of perpetuating long-standing theoretical and practice barriers to effective intervention with this population.

Finally, Turner defined clinical guidelines for fine-tuning the application of the Stone Center approach to the therapeutic needs of African American women. Not only was this pivotal to the work of the founding theoreticians but it has also represented a cutting-edge development for therapists who assess and treat African American women. Aspects of Turner's perspective have been echoed by others who have embraced this relational perspective over the years (Coll, Cook-Nobles, & Surrey, 1997; Tatum, 1997).

With the passage of more than a decade since the publication of Turner's paper, and insights gained through the application of her perspective during that period, this chapter further defines the relevance of the Stone Center approach for African American women. It is hoped that more literature on this approach with African American women as well as other women of color shall be forthcoming.

# THE BASIC TENETS OF RELATIONAL/CULTURAL THEORY

The basic tenets of relational/cultural theory are the following:

1. The centrality and continuity of relationships to women's psychological development.
2. Connection and disconnection.
3. Characteristics of growth-enhancing relationships.
4. The "five good things."
5. The belief that a closer examination of women and their development can broaden our understanding of both women and men.

## The Centrality and Continuity of Relationships to Women's Psychological Development

Relational/cultural theory defines a *relationship* as "a set of interactions over a length of time" (Miller & Stiver, 1998, p. 26). Women are thought to add on relationships in age-appropriate ways as they redefine their primary relationships. Therefore, women's relational development is perceived as a dynamic, interactive, and flexible process that may influence higher levels of self-awareness while validating the felt need of women to become more aware of and responsive to others.

## Connection and Disconnection

In contrast to traditional developmental theories, relational/cultural theory also emphasizes the significance of

> connections between people . . . how we create them and how disconnections derail [us] throughout our lives. Just as disconnections restrict us and block psychological growth, connection, which encompasses the experience of mutual engagement and empathy, provides the original and continuing sources of that growth. (Miller & Stiver, 1998, p. 3)

Relational/cultural theory posits that "an inner sense of connection to others is the central organizing feature of women's [psychological] development" (Miller & Stiver, 1998, p. 16). Healing and growth are outcomes of *connection*, while pain, suffering, and psychological problems are outcomes of *disconnection*. Prominent sources of disconnection, according to Miller and Stiver (1998), are early parentification, emotional inaccessibility, and family secrets.

As Turner and the Stone Center theoreticians have emphasized, women's experiences of the self seem to contradict most developmental theories. For example, traditional theories emphasize the prominence of disconnection from early relationships toward achieving a separate and bounded sense of self. In contrast, relational/cultural theory highlights the relational self as the outcome of an evolutionary process that begins early in life and that develops *within*, *rather than outside of,* mutually empathic relationships (Surrey, 1984).

Connection and differentiation are also foci of this theory, rather than separation and individuation, which are emphasized by traditional theories. Relational/cultural theory associates positive relational development and the ability to participate in growth-enhancing relationships with *connection to others and the self.* Furthermore, a differentiated, rather than a separate, sense of self is thought to enhance connection to others and the self. Thus, differentiation permits connection to self and the other simultaneously. This is a distinct departure from the "either–or" stance of traditional theories that emphasize separation within a self or other context. It is also a departure from the separation and disconnection that has resulted from the definition of African American women's identity by the dominant culture rather than by those who belong to this population.

## Characteristics of Growth-Enhancing Relationships

The characteristics of growth-enhancing relationships as defined by relational theory include engagement, authenticity, mutual empathy, and mutual empowerment.

*Engagement* involves attention to and expressed interest in the relationship (Surrey, 1991, p. 30). The impact of engagement on connection is evident in "the gradual evolution of a differentiated self, a self with its own clear properties, wishes, impulses . . . that achieves articulation through participation in and attention to the relational process." Furthermore, engagement "leads to the possibility of speaking one's true thoughts and feelings" (p. 54). Engagement, as defined in this context, is particularly necessary for African American women since some (1) are routinely silenced, rendered invisible, and not taken seriously by institutions, or their relational development has been squelched by parents' and others' efforts to disprove stereotypes; (2) endure the pressure of the fishbowl effect; and (3) are subjected to countless other oppressive processes that take place throughout the life cycle.

*Authenticity* involves the genuine capacity to state one's feelings and thoughts directly or to represent one's experience as it arises. This process enables the woman to develop courage, defined in this context by Miller and Stiver (1998) as "the ability to put forward her feelings and thoughts . . . and to stand by them" (p. 30). However, the authors caution that authenticity "is not a static state that is achieved at a discrete moment in time; it is a person's ongoing ability to represent her/himself with increasing truth and fullness" (p. 54). For many African American women, the perception of authenticity in the therapist is very significant in the early stages of therapy, for it is an indication of the therapist's capacity "to be real," to understand/to connect with the client, and to be trusted.

*Mutual empathy* allows knowledge of the inner cognitive and affective state of the other (Jordan, 1991, p. 82). "It is a joining together based on the authentic thoughts and feelings of all participants in a relationship" (Miller & Stiver, 1998, p. 29). Because mutual empathy facilitates "adding something more" to the dialogue, "each person can receive and then respond to the feelings and thoughts of the other . . . to enlarge one's own feelings and thoughts and the feelings and thoughts of the other person" (p. 29). Mutual empathy requires real knowledge of the client's experiences as influenced by social realities (e.g., prejudice, sexism), cultural differences, and standard clinical factors (e.g., family relational dynamics).

*Mutual empowerment*, that is, empowerment of the self and other, is the outcome of mutual empathy (Miller & Stiver, 1998). The five components of mutual empowerment, also known as the "five good things" (discussed below), may be expressed similarly or differentially from one ethnocultural group to another.

For African American women, engagement, authenticity, mutual empathy, and mutual empowerment promote positive relational development and increase the capacity for connection via (1) the purging of debilitating relational images such as stereotypes and other misconceptions about African Americans; (2) acknowledging individual and group strengths within a culturally competent purview; and (3) growth-fostering approaches to vulnerabilities.

## The Five Good Things

The five good things include the following:

1. *Zest or high energy*: the feeling of vitality, aliveness, and energy that results when a real sense of connection, togetherness with, and joining by the other person(s) is experienced. The relational/cultural approach has the capacity to move the client from a diminished energy level for relationships to zest or high energy.

2. *Action*: the ability to choose, to move, or to do "in the moment of the immediate exchange" (Miller & Stiver, 1998, p. 31). Each participant in the dialogue has an important impact on the other that leads to change. Mutual empowerment also leads to action beyond the immediate interaction. The inability to act progressively changes the capacity to act progressively in the interest of the self and others.

3. *Knowledge*: the enlarged and more accurate picture of self and the other that develops in relationship. Each participant learns more about her relationship with another/others and how it influences her own relational experience.

Such understanding promotes clearer differentiation of feelings and promotes positive self-image development.

4. *Self-worth*: this develops out of recognition, acknowledgment, and understanding of one's experience by those who are important to her. The sense of connection felt while feeling emotions nurtures self-worth as well as social esteem, one's value for one's own reference group (e.g., ethnocultural, racial, gender) (Jenkins, 1993b).

5. *A greater sense of connection and a desire for more connection*: this involves the strong bond that develops between participants in the relationship and their desire for more connection based on interactions that have taken place until the present. The relational/cultural approach also enhances motivation for action in the larger community.

In contrast to the "five good things," disconnection ultimately leads to (1) a diminished energy level, (2) disempowerment or an inability to act, (3) confusion, (4) a diminished sense of worth, and 5) avoidance of relationships/isolation.

## Closer Examination

A closer examination of women and their development can broaden our understanding of both women and men. While relational/cultural theory is inspired by a theoretical framework based on the relational development of women, it also acknowledges commonalities in the relational needs of men and women based on the fundamental human condition. Yet attention is also paid to key differences in the socialization of girls and boys and the ways in which these influence relational norms for women and men differentially. Race, ethnicity, and social class lend other complexities to differential socialization and relational processes.

Influenced by its collective orientation, traditional African American culture values (1) egalitarianism between men and women in many aspects of work and family life, (2) the extended family, and (3) spirituality. Because of this, relational/cultural theory has tremendous potential to enhance our understanding of relational development among African American women, adaptive behaviors within this group, and how social factors function as connectors and disconnectors.

### CONNECTION, DISCONNECTION, AND
### AFRICAN AMERICAN WOMEN

## Connection

My work as a psychotherapist has repeatedly revealed that connection to or disconnection from African American heritage are central to how African

American women perceive themselves and the world, how they cope, and their ability to move or take progressive action in the world. The extent of their connection to or disconnection from African American heritage also seems to be associated with their mental and social health status. For some women, this connection is strong, deliberate, and passionate, while for others it is more naturally a way of life or a way of being influenced by upbringing and lifelong exposure to afrocentric values, traditions, and customs. Some women in the latter group develop this connection without much awareness of how it influences their daily living until exposed to African American women who have had a different experience or women from other racial and ethnocultural groups. Yet, the benefits of this connection to identity development and relational development are obvious.

Those women who are raised with positive images of who they are racially and ethnoculturally appear to have more positive self-concepts, particularly higher levels of self-esteem and social esteem, than those who do not. The same group appears to be less conflicted about body-image issues related to differences between African and eurocentric standards of beauty. In addition, these women cope more progressively with racism, prejudice, and discrimination than those with vulnerable racial or ethnocultural identities. Furthermore, they more often rely on afrocentric coping mechanisms, such as spirituality, the extended family, reverence for hard work and education, dual socialization of offspring, and creative approaches to survival despite limited economic resources at times.

It is also important to call attention to significant relational dynamics between African American women and other groups. A dramatic demographic shift in the population of people of color and other diverse populations in the United States is presently occurring where those ethnocultural groups that have been considered nontraditional are becoming the numerical majority. Intrinsic to this is the reality that the White middle-class heterosexual male population is being redefined to a less dominant status. Increasingly evident during this transitional period is the openness of many African American women to embrace diversity in the workplace, the community, and the family. Yet this is not a new phenomenon since African Americans have historically embraced other groups, including many of those from the dominant culture who have shared this objective. This tendency to embrace racial and ethnocultural diversity has often been passed on to African American youth.

As carriers of African American culture, African American women nurture a vital connection for their young. Turner (1987) observed that African American women often pass afrocentric values on to their children. Also, some socialize their children to survive or even prosper in a world where they are not always valued as highly as their White peers or children from some other racial and ethnocultural groups. Sadly, the basis for such rejection tends to be racism, colorism, and a history of prejudice and discrimination against African Ameri-

cans in the United States. Yet some women insure that their children's socialization includes exposure to other African Americans and people from other
ethnocultural groups. This connection is particularly vital for children of color
who live in predominantly White communities where such exposure may not
easily occur.

Some parents drive their children considerable distances to schools, music
or dance lessons, or athletic practices to insure that they are "not the only ones"
and that they are exposed to school personnel and other role models from a
variety of racial and ethnocultural backgrounds. Some parents also join Black
inner-city churches and/or Black civic, service, or social organizations, and seek
out Black-owned businesses in an effort to provide their children with such
connection. Without this, there is a high risk of estrangement from African
American culture, and thus a high risk of psychosocial disconnection.

## Disconnection

Disconnection, a break in connection, restricts and blocks psychological growth
as well as social identity development. Disconnection for some African American
women involves internalized dominance/oppression that damages the connection to the self and others. This surfaces in various forms of self-hatred such as
rejecting African physical characteristics, or "passing for White" (Turner, 1987);
a belief in intellectual and moral inferiority of African Americans and other
people of African descent; and low social esteem, that is, little value, respect
for, and pride in one's own racial and/or ethnocultural group. Such self-hatred
may also surface in the perception that another racial group is generally superior to peoples of African descent. Lack of social esteem is often the basis for
low self-esteem, low self-confidence, and a poor body image. Other sources of
disconnection for African American women mentioned elsewhere are the dual
trauma of racism and sexism (Walker, 1999), and overly strict upbringing
intended to protect from to downplay stereotypes about hyper sexuality (Wyatt,
1997). Self-defeating beliefs about one's possibilities of experiencing satisfying and fulfilling relationships, repeated romantic failures, and social isolation
are common outcomes of the latter (Jenkins, 1993a).

In view of racism and all the other societal problems that African Americans routinely contend with, Miller and Stiver's (1998) stance that "a relational approach can lead to changes in the larger world" (p. 5) is indeed
optimistic. Yet some African Americans might embrace this view with caution in light of their struggles associated with intractable societal problems
that systematically challenge their well-being. These struggles have often impacted negatively on possibilities to engage in growth-enhancing relationships. While it may be uncomfortable and painful for the therapist to recognize, name, and accept responsibility for his or her personal participation in
the perpetuation of such problems along with transforming such barriers,

taking these steps is imperative toward building growth-enhancing connections that influence the demise of societal problems and the psychological disorders they engender.

## OTHER KEY RELATIONAL PROCESSES

The tone and quality of women's relationships is also influenced by other relational processes. These include (1) "power over" versus "power with" the other, (2) relational images, and (3) the central relational paradox.

### "Power over" versus "Power with": The Position of Relational/Cultural Theory on Power

Central to the oppression of African American women is the "power over" stance associated with White privilege, the double bind of racism and sexism, and other forms of oppression. The "power over" stance is embedded in the standard practice of psychotherapy and perpetuates the oppression of this population by promoting disconnection from self, others, and society. This prevents some African American women from developing or sustaining a positive and empowered view of self and other African Americans. Not only is such disconnection associated with many of the problems in daily living and the social and psychological disorders experienced by this group, but these disconnections also deny some women the sense of agency that is so vital to their relational development and well-being.

Miller (1991) suggests that *agency* is an active and assertive state that uses all of one's resources. Agency involves increased powers to do for others while developing a greater sense of one's own capacities. Agency also permits more clarity about one's choices within a relationship. The empowered sense of self gained is experienced *in connection with* others rather than *during separation/ disconnection from* others. Therefore, agency allows the African American woman to experience a broader range of feelings and actions, and a more competent and dynamic sense of self. The affirmative stance that underlies this perspective is infectious. It promotes connection through development of self-esteem and social esteem, meaningful relationships with other African Americans as well as members of other ethnocultural groups, use of effective coping strategies, and therefore healing and recovery.

As an alternative to the "power over" stance of traditional theories, relational/cultural theory applies a "power with" approach to therapy intended to increase the connection that is so conducive to growth-enhancing relationships. This involves "a power that grows, as it is used to empower others" (Miller & Stiver, 1998, p. 16). The actualization of mutuality is central to this approach.

Jordan (1991) contends that "in a mutual exchange one is both affecting the other and being affected by the other; one extends oneself . . . to the other and is also receptive to the impact of the other. There is openness to influence, emotional availability, and a constantly changing pattern of responding to and affecting the other's state. There is both receptivity and active initiative toward the other" (p. 82). In this context, the process of mutuality does not mean that the client and the therapist have equal power in their relationship. However, it does acknowledge that both persons contribute, have value, may learn from, and may be moved by the other while in their relationship. The practice of mutuality represents a distinct departure from the societal and personal disconnection that African American women routinely experience in this society. One outcome of such disconnection is internalization of pejorative relational images that block possibilities for mutual empowerment.

## Relational Images

Relational images portray patterns of relational experience and their meanings. Such images also include expectations of what will happen in future relationships as they unfold and explanations of why relationships are the way they are. In *The Healing Connection*, Miller and Stiver (1998) describe the powerful influence of relational images on what may become lifelong relational patterns:

> If we have built images that allow us . . . to take in new relational experiences, our images and meanings can keep growing, and this can . . . encourage us to change further and to explore new experiences in our relationships. . . . If we have experienced many disconnections, our relational images will lead us away from engagement with other people. If this is the case, our relational images will not grow and change; they can become quite fixed. (p. 41)

Positive relational images of African American women are more often promoted within the African American culture. Extended families are highly valued and women are central to this family structure (Collins, 1990). Ironically, racism and sexism are among the factors that also promote these images. This is evident in Turner's (1987) observations concerning how societal problems have shaped mother–daughter relationships, and how African American mothers nurture positive survival- and prosperity-oriented relational self-concepts that enable daughters to succeed despite the perils of racism and sexism:

> [African American mothers] are constantly working in a "relational" context to instill in their daughters deeper feelings of self-esteem, awareness of . . . how to nurture and how to achieve more self-confidence, resourcefulness, and racial pride. . . . These mothers work to build . . . a sound base of

inner strengths and coping mechanisms which they hope will fit well with the minority and majority cultures. Values are taught and reinforced continually even though ... daughters are ... raised in a society that often devalues both them and their mothers in every stage of each other's development. [Daughters] are usually taught very early in life to rely on themselves as well as to care for others. (pp. 2–3)

## Stereotypes and Mythical Images

In contrast to growth-fostering relational images that facilitate survival and prosperity, stereotypes and mythical images of African American women are destructive to the relational image development of this population and that of society at large. Stereotypes portray African American women as sub- and superhuman beings who have "their place"; that is, they are not to hold any authentic power or to be taken seriously, they are to be used and discarded, and they are fundamentally unacceptable. Majority culture distortions of African American women's identities as influenced by racism, the societal projection process (Bowen, 1978), and anxiety about difference still underlie the relational images of some African American women. Stereotypes, such as the following, and their meanings, still play a prominent role in shaping such images (Boyd, 1993; White, 1994; Wyatt, 1997):

1. "Mammy": a selfless caretaker, the epitome of trustworthiness, but also not very smart and often a buffoon.
2. "Matriarch": strong, but domineering/controlling.
3. "Sapphire": evil, bitchy, hard and tough, domineering, castrating.
4. "She-Devil"/"Jezebel": impulsive, promiscuous, seductive, and a loose woman/ immoral.
5. "Welfare Mother": controlling, lazy, and irresponsible.
6. "Superwoman": a strong workhorse who values performance and achievement, does all things perfectly simultaneously, and has no needs of her own for interpersonal and sexual intimacy.

African American women have also been portrayed as long suffering, as saintly, as confused about their identities, and as passive victims.

Stereotypes and mythical images disempower and oppress via (1) images that grossly distort the experiences, strengths, vulnerabilities, and potentials of African American women; (2) perpetuating internalizations that negatively impact development of self–other perceptions; and (3) fostering relational styles that perpetuate disconnection. Yet stereotypes and mythical images may be catalysts for developing growth-fostering relationships via (1) promoting accurate relational images of African American women, (2) social activism, (3) effective parenting and socialization of children, (4) articulating one's experiences, and (5) determination to not succumb to distortions and the disconnection these engender through bitterness, hopelessness, and social isolation (Collins, 1990; Fleming, cited in Gillem, 1983).

Many African American women have learned to find "a way out of no way."[1] This resilient mind-set is often nurtured by exposure to positive and effective role models, resistance to internalization of negative relational images, spirituality, and other ethnocultural values.

## Negative Relational Images and Relationships with African American Men

Many African American women and men enjoy positive and long-standing relationships together. Hopson and Hopson (1994) emphasize that mutual love in relationships is preceded by learning to love the self. However, the imagery of stereotypes and associated social problems challenge the development of self-love and growth-fostering relationships between African American men and women. Hopson and Hopson (1994) suggest that some women succumb to destructive relational images that result in (1) repetitive involvement in violent or abusive relationships, (2) efforts to change or "fix" the man one becomes involved with, (3) constant criticism and bullying of the man, (4) overindulging a male partner, (5) repetitive participation in relationships with married or otherwise committed men, and (6) increased disrespect for the self and others. In addition, the nodal role, as described by Pinderhughes (1982), seems to be another outcome of destructive relational images. This role involves a selfless form of caretaking that confuses self-care with selfishness. Women in the nodal role feel obliged to compensate for the wounds and burdens of African American men associated with racism via caretaking that includes understanding, sympathizing with, and sharing their partners' burdens at the expense of neglecting their own needs and encouraging responsibility.

At the core of many destructive relational patterns for African American women are the following relational images:

1. That of an absent parent or a parental figure who expected his or her needs to come before those of his or her children or others.

---

[1]This concept is borrowed from the African American spiritual and historical traditions. In the African American church, it is often used to describe the power of faith toward creating options and opportunities for those without obvious or visible resources. This concept has also been used to describe the social, political, and economic survival of the African American population since slavery days despite the odds of displaced families, lost languages and cultures, and the loss of other key organizing structures.

2. Exposure to a preference for male siblings or other male relatives.
3. Repetitive exposure to the manipulation by, disrespect from, or abuse of a parent or one's self.
4. That of a passive–dependent parent.
5. Confusion of love with domination/abuse, sex, or money.
6. Exposure to an overly strict or overly permissive stance toward expression of sexuality and toward dating.
7. The perception that all Black men are lazy and not to be trusted.
8. The perception that to be loved is to be spoiled.
9. The perception that the primary role of men is to satisfy all of women's psychological and financial needs.


Relational meanings of such images include (1) self-perceptions of inadequacy and low self-esteem; (2) the belief that it is better to avoid commitment and intimacy/illusions of intimacy; (3) the belief that most Black men are unworthy of trust, but worthy of exploitation; (4) doubt concerning one's capacity to love or worthiness to be loved. Obviously, the aforementioned images have negative meanings and expectations for the women and men who internalize them. Disconnection seems to be a natural outcome for those who become immobilized by these mind-sets.

## Relational Images of Psychotherapy

Until the late 1960s, the mental health professions assumed a destructive stance toward African Americans. Rooted in racism, sexism, ethnocentrism, and other deeply embedded societal problems, this stance involved gross preconceptions of what constitutes difference, substandard mental health care, and miseducation. Therefore, some African American women fear mental health practitioners and assume that psychotherapy is only appropriate for "crazy" or "sick" people, White people, or those who are too weak or inadequate to manage their lives effectively on their own. These images infer a lack of mutuality in that they are based on the standard practice assumption that therapists are "all-knowing" while consumers of color are defective, inferior, and enter psychotherapy with little or nothing of value to contribute to healing or recovery processes. Yet, it is important to acknowledge that fewer women embrace such images than before as more culturally competent and politically astute therapists become available, and as more African American women are exposed to positive word-of-mouth appraisals of psychotherapy and how it benefits others like themselves. Another factor that has prevented African American women from seeking therapy is the central relational paradox.

## The Central Relational Paradox

The central relational paradox involves a process of increasingly building restrictive relational images and meanings. This takes place while seeking connections to others via keeping more and more of one's experiences and one's responses to those experiences out of connection (Miller & Stiver, 1998) with others and even the self. Some African American women avoid therapists of other races because they assume that it will be necessary to educate them about sociocultural factors that contextualize their experiences at the risk of still not being understood or perceived accurately. Where there has been no alternative but to see a therapist from another race, some clients have never revealed such assumptions over the course of treatment. This process of seeking connection while keeping such assumptions out of the relationship constitutes a central relational paradox. This paradox includes the "requirement" to live in two worlds.

*Dual socialization,* the process of learning to survive and to succeed in both Black and White worlds, is a common and necessary bicultural process for many African American children that begins as early as the toddler years. One of the earliest messages taught during this period is that African Americans must be more competent/effective than their White counterparts to receive equally positive credit or attention. The requirement to excel becomes a tremendous source of pressure for some women in that it is costly to both relational development and efforts to sustain supportive connections to others. Survival and success in two worlds often demands the isolation of more and more of the African American woman's total experience from a variety of settings (e.g., school, the workplace, social service agencies) where it is assumed that diversity is not fully embraced. The woman may transfer to the therapist the belief that she cannot reveal painful experiences associated with societal problems nor her true thoughts and feelings concerning these if she is to survive, be approved of, or accepted. Some women decide that it would be a waste of time to reveal these aspects of the self since previous experiences have taught them not to be hopeful about change. Hence, an illusion of intimacy passes for true intimacy.

The central relational paradox has impacted much of the African American woman's experience since slavery. For instance, the basic survival of slaves was dependent on their abilities to endure their own and their loved ones' psychological and physical neglect, abuse, and trauma without protest or retaliation. Those who did protest or retaliate often suffered permanent physical and/or psychological injuries or paid with their lives.

Some contemporary women find it difficult to be assertive in relationships with men due to their belief that to do so would be disloyal or lead to the immediate loss of the relationship. Another common but underacknowledged example of the central relational paradox is associated with negative changes that some women's relationships with family members undergo secondary to social class transitions attributed to education, occupational advancement, or marriage. The woman's world changes from one that is more familiar to her family to one that is not. Such changes are often unexpected and complicated and may involve decreased intimacy and empathy, fewer shared interests or experiences, different value orientations, or resentment and jealousy of the woman's experiences. These changes may surface without any awareness of those involved until they become serious threats to the woman's relationships. In response to this, some women begin to keep more and more of their experience out of their family relationships in an effort to sustain at least some semblance of connection. Engagement may become strained while authenticity may be compromised. This illusion of intimacy promotes considerable anxiety, sadness, and conflict.

Turner (1987) noted that Black women represent cultural variations within the relational model due to the impact of racism and sexism. Therefore, accurate understanding of the past and present relationship between African American women and the central relational paradox, as well as culturally competent judgment concerning the complex interplay between social and intrapsychic factors, are central to effective clinical work with this population.

Despite its limitations, the central relational paradox is a complex dynamic in that it is adaptive in its capacity to increase the survival and success of this population. Understandably, some women are reluctant to completely relinquish this coping mechanism.

*Naming* cultural representations of the central relational paradox as well as other cultural variations of relational experience is essential to effective intervention with African American women and other nontraditional populations.

## Naming the "Unnamable"

Much of the African American woman's experience was historically denied, omitted, or ignored before the 1960s. *Naming the "unnamable,"* a powerful form of acknowledgment, has been proposed by M. Maureen Walker (1995) as an alternative to and remedy for the impact of the central relational paradox. Naming the "unnamable" is essential to overcoming social obstacles to growth-fostering relationships. The potential value of such acknowledgment is highlighted in Walker's (1999) comments on the racial and sexual traumatization of African American women. It is also suggested by other authors' attention to how stereotypes, definition and rejection by the dominant culture, and internalized dominance and oppression impact on stress levels, sexuality, and self-perceptions of loveability (Boyd, 1993; Greene & Hucles-Sanchez, 1994; Jenkins, 1993a; Richardson & Wade, 1999; Wyatt, 1997).

As an alternative, *naming* facilitates growth-enhancing relationships for African American women via acknowledging and validating all of their experience, thereby influencing authentic, positive, and differentiated connections to the self, others, and society-at-large. Naming also challenges the destructive superwoman image by increasing African American women's tolerance for "being held," comforted, and emotionally supported without confusing such needs with inadequacy/failure, weakness, or justification for exploitation.

Behaviors associated with the superwoman image symbolize internalizations of dominance or oppression. Those who have internalized this stereotype often seek to undo perceptions of African American women as incompetent, unworthy of serious attention, and incapable of success. Furthermore, sometimes these internalizations are an attempt to suppress uncomfortable affect. Thus, some women are overextended in the workplace and/or at a personal level in an effort to respond to the needs or to gain the approval of authority figures, friends, and family. As a consequence, many neglect their own interpersonal needs.

African American women's internalizations of the stereotypes that have been discussed are also associated with chronic and debilitating mental, social, and physical health problems. Among these are workaholism, loneliness, depression, anxiety, eating disorders, substance abuse, hypertension, obesity, and interpersonal problems. Stereotypes are constructed to make chronic societal problems appear to be natural, normal, and an inevitable part of everyday life (Collins, 1990). Naming these images and the conditions that influence and perpetuate them in a woman's life are major steps toward her empowerment to move beyond them.

## ETHNOCULTURAL ORIENTATION OF AFRICAN AMERICAN WOMEN AND THE RELATIONAL APPROACH: THE INTERFACE

There seems to be a natural interface between the ethnocultural orientation of African American women, as shaped by historical and ethnocultural factors, and the relational/cultural approach. Despite the vast degree of heterogeneity within this population, its worldview continues to be influenced by perceptions of the relational self as expressed by the African proverb "I am because we are, and since we are, therefore, I am." Therefore, perceptions of connection for many African American women are deeply embedded in the interdependent, collective, affiliative, and spiritual orientation of traditional African American culture. Indeed, positive ethnocultural group identification and positive relationships with other African Americans are central to positive self-image and social esteem development of this client population (Jenkins, 1993b).

From a relational/cultural therapy perspective, this interface is evident in its theoretical stance on the centrality and continuity of relationships to women's identity development, their relationships, and life experiences in general. Yet critical sociocultural factors that influence these aspects of African American women's lives must not be ignored.

## TOWARD GREATER INCLUSIVENESS

There is much potential for the relational/cultural clinical approach to effectively address the therapeutic needs of African American women if guided by an authentic and empathic understanding of critical societal problems (e.g., racism, sexism, classism) that shape the identity and relational development of this population. Appropriate self-understanding and cultural competence are the foundation of such understanding.

Cultural competence (Greene & Hucles-Sanchez, 1994) is a measurable professional standard that evaluates the incorporation of the differential historical, political, socioeconomic, psychophysical, spiritual, and ecological realities, their interaction, and its impact on individuals or groups. Here culture is used in its broadest sense to include race, ethnicity, gender, and sexual orientation and considers other dimensions of an individual's or group's experiences that are salient to their understanding of the world and of themselves. This definition also suggests that factors that are prominent in contextualizing the identity and relational development of one racial/ethnocultural group may differ significantly from that of another. For example, Jenkins, De La Cancela, and Chin (1993) contends that culture, inclusive of customs, traditions, and language of origin, is the most prominent determinant of Asian Americans' experience while race, gender, and social class are the most prominent for African American women.

As relational/cultural theory progresses toward more inclusivity, authenticity, and optimal effectiveness, ethnospecific acknowledgment of variability is imperative to guard against applying universal assumptions about women that have misguided the standard practice of psychotherapy.

## CONCLUSION

The interface between the ethnocultural orientation of most African American women and basic tenets of relational/cultural theory suggest that interventions based on this approach are of use to this population. However, it is imperative for critical nuances in the identity development, relational development, and therapeutic needs of this population to be understood within appropriate sociocultural contexts. The absence of this perspective is certain to distort clinical impressions and prompt intervention that is harmful rather than helpful. Last but not least, in order for the therapist to achieve the authenticity, empathy, and mutual empowerment that are so integral to relational/cultural intervention, ongoing active attention to his or her own personal internalized dominance and oppression is primary to effective intervention with this population. Thus, Cook-Nobles (Coll, Cook-Nobles, & Surrey, 1997) emphasizes that "knowledge without action is merely an intellectual task which sustains diversity issues in a marginal rather than centralized position" (p. 6). With a similar voice, Tatum (1997) contends that therapists must be "prepared to hear, see, and understand [Black women's] authentically told experience" (p. 6). Concrete suggestions on how to prepare for this are made by several authors (Chin, De La Cancela, & Jenkins, 1993; Coll et al., 1997; Pinderhughes, 1989).

## REFERENCES

Bowen, M. (1978). *Family therapy in clinical practice.* New York: Jason Aronson.

Boyd, J. (1993). *In the company of my sisters.* New York: Dutton.

Chin, J. L., De La Cancela, V., & Jenkins, Y. M. (1993). *Diversity in psychotherapy: The politics of race, ethnicity, and gender.* Westport, CT: Praeger.

Coll, C., Cook-Nobles, R., & Surrey, J. (1997). *Diversity at the core: Implications for relational therapy* (Work in progress, No. 75). Wellesley, MA: Stone Center Working Papers Series.

Collins, P. H. (1990). *Black feminist thought.* New York: Routledge.

Gillem, A. R. (Ed.). (1983). *Beyond double jeopardy: Female, biracial, and perceived to be black. Is this double jeopardy?* Unpublished manuscript.

Greene, B., & Hucles-Sanchez, J. (1994). Diversity: Advancing an inclusive feminist psychology. In J. Worell & N. Johnson (Eds.), *Feminist visions: New directions in education and training for feminist psychology practice* (pp. 173–202). Washington, DC: American Psychological Association Press.

Hopson, D. S., & Hopson, D. P. (1994). *Friends, lovers, and soulmates.* New York: Simon & Schuster.

Jenkins, Y. M. (1993a). African American women: Ethnocultural variables and dissonant expectations. In J. L. Chin, V. De La Cancela, & Y. M. Jenkins, *Diversity in psychotherapy: The politics of race, ethnicity, and gender* (pp. 117–136). Westport, CT: Praeger.

Jenkins, Y. M. (1993b). Diversity and social esteem. In J. L. Chin, V. De La Cancela, & Y. M. Jenkins, *Diversity in psychotherapy: The politics of race, ethnicity, and gender* (pp. 45–64). Westport, CT: Praeger.

Jenkins, Y. M., De La Cancela, V., & Chin, J. L. (1993). Historical overviews: Three sociopolitical perspectives. In J. L. Chin, V. De La Cancela, & Y. M. Jenkins, *Diversity in psychotherapy: The politics of race, ethnicity, and gender* (p. 34). Westport, CT: Praeger.

Jordan, J. (1991). The meaning of mutuality. In J. Jordan, A. Kaplan, J. B. Miller, L. Stiver, & J. Surrey, *Women's growth in connection: Writings from the Stone Center* (pp. 81–86). New York: Guilford Press.

Jordan, J., Kaplan, A., Miller, J. B., Stiver, L., & Surrey, J. (1991). *Women's growth in connection: Writings from the Stone Center.* New York: Guilford Press.

Klein, R. H., Orleans, J. F., & Soule, C. R. (1991). The Axis II group: Treating severely characterologically disturbed patients. *International Journal of Group Psychotherapy, 41*, 97–115.

Miller, J. B. (1991). The development of women's sense of self. In J. Jordan, A. Kaplan, J. B. Miller, L. Stiver, & J. Surrey, *Women's growth in connection: Writings from the Stone Center* (pp. 11–28). New York: Guilford Press.

Miller, J. B., & Stiver, L. (1998). *The healing connection.* Boston: Beacon Press.

Paniagua, F. A. (1998). *Assessing and treating culturally diverse clients.* Thousand Oaks, CA: Sage.

Pinderhughes, E. B. (1982). Minority women: A nodal position in the functioning of the social system. In M. Ault-Riche (Ed.), *Women and family therapy* (pp. 51–63). Rockville, MD: Aspen.

Pinderhughes, E. B. (1989). *Understanding race, ethnicity, and power.* New York: Free Press.

Richardson, B., & Wade, B. (1999). *What Mama couldn't tell us about love.* New York: HarperCollins.

Surrey, J. (1984). *The "Self-in-Relation": A theory of women's development* (Work in progress, No. 13). Wellesley, MA: Stone Center Working Papers Series.

Surrey, J. (1991). The self-in-relation: A theory of women's development. In J. Jordan, J. B. Miller, L. Stiver, & J. Surrey, *Women's growth in connection: Writings from the Stone Center* (pp. 51–66). New York: Guilford Press.

Tatum, B. (1997). *Racial identity development and relational theory: The case of Black women in White communities* (Work in progress, No. 63). Wellesley, MA: Stone Center Working Papers Series.

Turner, C. (1987). *Clinical application of the Stone Center theoretical approach to minority women* (Work in progress, No. 28). Wellesley, MA: Stone Center Working Papers Series.

Walker, M. M. (1995, May 3). Comments made at Stone Center colloquium offered by Jean Baker Miller and Irene Stiver on *Relational images and their meanings in psychotherapy*, Wellesley, MA.

Walker, M. M. (1999). Dual traumatization: A sociocultural perspective. In Y. M. Jenkins (Ed.), *Diversity in college settings: Directives for helping professionals* (pp. 51–66). New York: Routledge.

White, E. C. (1994). Love don't always make it right: Black women and domestic abuse. In E. C. White (Ed.), *The black woman's health book* (pp. 92–97). Seattle, WA: Seal Press.

Wyatt, G. E. (1997). *Stolen women.* New York: Wiley.

## CHAPTER 5

# African American Lesbian and Bisexual Women in Feminist–Psychodynamic Psychotherapies
## Surviving and Thriving between a Rock and a Hard Place

### BEVERLY GREENE

> Passing is an obscene form of salvation. . . . Just as a Black woman passing for white is "required to deny everything about her past," a Black lesbian who passes for heterosexual is required to deny everything about her present. . . .
> —JEWELLE GOMEZ (1999 p. 164)

This chapter focuses on the issues of race, gender, and sexual orientation in psychodynamic psychotherapy with African American lesbian and bisexual women. Neither the burgeoning literatures on psychotherapy with lesbian, gay, and bisexual (LGB) people, nor the developing field of multicultural psychotherapy has much to say specifically about many issues intrinsic to psychotherapy with African American lesbians. While the psychotherapy with women literature gives African American women marginally more attention than the LGB or multicultural psychotherapy literature, little is said about African American lesbians at all (Hall & Greene, 1996). In Greene and Boyd-Franklin (1996) we observed that African American women are barely a footnote in American psychology; here I might add that African American lesbians are less than a footnote to the footnote.

Paradoxically, however, there have been many long-standing discussions questioning whether psychodynamic psychotherapy approaches, and more recently even feminist therapy approaches, are appropriate for any African American female client. While psychodynamic theories and feminist therapy theory have at times presented themselves as if they were universal and free of cultural bias, we know that they are not. We also know that there is no theory of psychotherapy that is not embedded in the sociopolitical matrix that spawned it, and as such none can be culture-free.

Therapists using psychodynamic modalities have overlooked and often disputed the importance of integrating the contextual and environmental factors that interact with and shape intrapsychic structures and dynamics and their development as well as their role in shaping behavior, particularly in members of societally disadvantaged groups. Contributors to this volume would argue that this is not an inevitable outcome of psychodynamic technique. Rather, it is a function of what Thompson (1987, 1989) argues is a manifestation of the therapist's countertransference resistance, his or her own personal discomfort addressing issues that require an acknowledgment and examination of societal racism, sexism, and heterosexism and their effects. Examining any of these phenomena requires acknowledging the power differentials that are associated with ethnicity, gender, class, and sexual orientation, as well as the social structures that keep these differentials in place.

I operate from the perspective that relational (see Jenkins, Chapter 4, this volume) and feminist–psychodynamic psychotherapy theory and techniques (Glassgold, 1995; Gould, 1995; Kassof, Boden, deMonteflores, Hunt, & Wahba, 1995) can be useful in assisting African American lesbians and bisexual women in exploring their conscious and unconscious contributions to their dilemmas as well as the effects of societal disadvantages or challenges that compromise their optimal functioning. Sociopolitical, intrapsychic, and interpersonal issues are always interrelated in the lives of African American lesbian and bisexual women. When therapists do not understand the complexity of these issues or are either uninformed or unskilled at disentangling them, the result is often an exclusive focus on intrapsychic dynamics *or* societal barriers, as if they are mutually exclusive or as if either exists or develops in isolation.

## AFRICAN AMERICAN LESBIANS AND BISEXUAL WOMEN

African American lesbians and bisexual women are a large and diverse group. Members cut across the lines of age, class, education, physical ability, geographical region, and other characteristics. Therefore, these aspects of diversity must be considered in the therapy process. Members of this group have multiple identities and the therapist may not presume which identity is most important or that any *one* is more important than others. Information presented in this chapter therefore should be considered as general guidelines and not absolutes about every African American lesbian or bisexual woman.

African American lesbians and bisexual women share cultural origins that are rooted in the tribes of Western Africa and in ancestors forcibly brought to the United States as slaves (Boyd-Franklin, 1989; Greene, 1986, 1990c, 1994a, 1994b, 1997). Historically, all Black women in the diaspora share the horrific legacies of the slave trade. However, Wekker (1993) points out that even before leaving Africa and becoming slaves African women were far from homogeneous as a group. The mixed preslavery lineages of African women include membership in different tribes, speaking hundreds of different languages, and growing up with different systems of family values, relations, and tribal customs. Another feature of these diverse lineages included subtle to stark differences in the kinds of slavery policies practiced in different countries, as well as the presence of cross-ethnic relationships/marriages. All these preslavery diversities and postslavery realities gave rise to a wide range of expressions of female homosexuality among Black women in the diaspora (Blackwood & Wieringa, 1999; Kendall, 1998; Wekker, 1993).

The heterogeneity of African women notwithstanding, Wekker (1993) observes that Black lesbians in the diaspora have been integral members of Black communities, experiencing varying levels of tolerance for their sexual orientation, and sharing the same devalued position borne of racism and sexism as heterosexual Black women. While the presence of Black women who have sex with other women throughout the diaspora and their experiences is worthy of attention, a comprehensive discussion of them is beyond the scope of this chapter, which focuses primarily on African American women.

Like their heterosexual counterparts, African American lesbians and bisexual women share African cultural derivatives that include the presence of strong family ties encompassing nuclear and extended family members in complex networks of mutual obligation and support (Boyd-Franklin, 1989; Greene, 1986, 1994a, 1997; Icard, 1986). They also reflect more flexible gender roles than White and other ethnic minority groups. This flexibility may be attributed, in part, to cultural values that stress interdependence and a greater gender egalitarianism in some precolonial African tribes.

U.S. Census reports in 1990 suggested that by the millennium there would be 18 million African American women living in the United States. Gonsiorek and Weinrich (1991) estimate that a range of 4–17% of the general population is lesbian and gay, depending on how one defines *sexual orientation*. Overall the figure of 10% is regarded as an acceptable estimate. Based on this conservative estimate of 10%, we may assume that there are some 1.8 million African American women who could be defined as lesbian and bisexual in the United States. This is not an inconsiderable population.

Bass-Hass (1968), Bell and Weinberg (1978), Croom (1993), Mays and Cochran (1988), Mays, Cochran, and Rhue (1993), and Jackson and Brown

(1996) are among the few published empirical studies in psychology that include all or significant numbers of African American lesbian and bisexual respondents. Croom (2000) discusses the negative implications of the absence of such material on understanding the psychologies of all LGB people. The findings in the studies mentioned suggest that African American lesbians are more likely to have children; to maintain close relationships with their biological and extended families; to depend more on family members or other Black lesbians for support than their White counterparts; and to have greater contact with men and heterosexual peers than their White counterparts. The latter finding has also been observed among African women who have sex with women (Kendall, 1998; Wekker, 1993). African American lesbians and bisexual women have also been noted to have a greater likelihood of experiencing tension and loneliness but were seen as less likely to seek professional help. This particular combination of observations is troubling, as it may leave them more vulnerable to the effects of chronic stressors with perhaps a higher rate of negative psychological outcomes when professional help is finally sought (Greene, 1994a, 1998a).

All characteristics of African American lesbians and their families cannot be attributed to their African legacies alone. For example, certain aspects of their family structures and a lack of rigid gender-role stratification within families and couples were also responses to racism and the patriarchal culture in the United States (Boyd-Franklin, 1989; Greene, 1997). Slavery, institutional racism, and a lack of employment opportunities made it difficult for African American men to conform to the Western ideal of male as provider. This ideal devalued women who worked and men who required their female partners to work outside the home to support the family and survive economically. Slavery, however, required that African American women work outside the home from the very moment they arrived on these shores to a greater degree than their White counterparts. This may have facilitated a level of cultural gender role flexibility (Boyd-Franklin, 1989). That flexibility notwithstanding, sexism continues to exist in African American communities (Greene, 1994a, 1994b, 1997).

An understanding of the meaning and reality of being an African American woman who is lesbian or bisexual requires a careful exploration of the impact of factors such as ethnic identity, gender, and lesbian sexual orientation, and their dynamic interactions in the individual. The nature of the traditional gender-role stereotypes within African Americans, the role and importance of family and community, and the role of religion and spirituality in the lives of African Americans are also salient factors. Other powerful factors include the role of racial stereotypes about African Americans; the degree of sexism, internalized racism, and homophobia within African Americans as a group; racist and sexist barriers and challenges from the dominant culture; and how all these contribute to the ethnosexual myths imposed on African American lesbian and bisexual women.

The sexual objectification of African Americans during slavery has been reinforced by images propagated concerning this population, fueling negative stereotypes and myths of excessive sexual desire, promiscuity, and moral looseness (Clarke, 1983; Collins, 1990; Dyson, 1996; Greene, 1986, 1990a; Icard, 1986; Loiacano, 1989; Wekker, 1993; West, 1993). Such conceptions are relevant to the development of the images that African American lesbian and bisexual women have of themselves, how the larger family and African American community views its lesbian and bisexual members, as well as their own sexuality. The strength of family ties often mitigates against the outright rejection of lesbian and bisexual family members. However, the African American community is viewed by its lesbian members as extremely homophobic, generating pressures for many women to remain closeted (Clarke, 1983; Croom, 1993; Dyson, 1996; Gomez, 1999; Gomez & Smith, 1990; Greene, 1990b, 1994a, 1994b, 1995b, 1998a; Icard, 1996; Jackson & Brown, 1996; Loiacano, 1989; Mays & Cochran, 1988; Poussaint, 1990; Smith, 1982).

In therapy with African American lesbian and bisexual clients, family history and community context must be explored. The therapist should consider a range of questions. For example, how much do parents or family of origin continue to control or influence children in the family, even when they are adults? How important is the family as a source of economic and emotional support? Other factors to be explored include the degree to which procreation and continuation of the family line is valued, as well as the closeness and importance of ties to the African American community.

African American communities across the United States are often very different from one another. Urban and rural locales differ in many ways, and both the harshness and the restrictions that are a product of racism vary from place to place too. The components of racism and other institutional discrimination will not be identical and the mechanisms needed to address it will also vary from locale to locale. Hence, African American lesbians and bisexual women will have different experiences of what it means to be an African American that are often a function of a locale. Where, in the United States, if at all, the client was raised and socialized must be considered an important contextual element of the client's history.

Another important area to inquire about is the client's degree of acculturation or assimilation into the dominant cultural community, as well as how the client's family regards this issue. For example, is the client's class or educational standing similar or significantly different from that of other family members? If these things are different, how do family members feel about the difference and how do they explain it? Another question to raise is the extent to which, if at all, the client's work, class, or education places her in primarily dominant culture working and/or social environments. To what extent do differences in the class, education, or race of colleagues or social peers of the lesbian family member differ from the peers of other family members? How do family members feel about that issue? It is not uncommon for African American family members to respond to disclosures that a family member is a lesbian with the charge that she "acquired" this "decadent White sickness" from being in too great a proximity to Whites or from trying to be like them. African American lesbian and bisexual women who work, live, or play in predominantly White environments may be more vulnerable to taking this challenge to their "blackness" seriously. The concept of lesbian sexual orientation as "the White man's disease" may seem deceptively harmless. However, in my clinical and personal experience, it is often connected to more pernicious beliefs the client may harbor about herself and about other African Americans. This issue and its connection to those beliefs will be explored more comprehensively later in this chapter.

The history of racial discrimination and oppression that African Americans have endured from the dominant culture and direct experiences with racism and their meaning to the client are also important areas of inquiry. When analyzing the history of discrimination against any ethnic group, it is essential to consider the group member's understanding of that oppression and her sense not only of how she copes, but of where and how she learned to cope. In therapy, you can use elements of the client's strategies for coping with one form of stigma and discrimination to teach her how to cope with other forms. African American lesbian and bisexual women who correctly understand the adverse ways in which they are affected by institutional racism and sexism and who develop affirming and adaptive coping strategies in response to them can use these strategies to negotiate and better understand their devalued position as lesbians. They may then use those understandings to assist in the resolution of their internalized homophobia when it is present. The client's effective strategies for coping with one form of discrimination, or resisting the internalization of one set of negative stereotypes, for example, can be a most potent psychological resource in a person who has multiple stigmatized identities. The skills learned and used to understand and deflect one form of stigma may be used to develop adaptive coping strategies for negotiating other forms of stigma.

It is not helpful to limit one's understanding of African Americans to dominant cultural analyses of them and their behavior. This may only reinforce preexisting ethnocentric, sexist, and homophobic biases found in the mental health literature (Greene, 1994a, 1994b, 1998a). When analyzing the history of discrimination against any ethnic group, group members' own understandings of their history, oppression, and coping strategies must be incorporated into that analysis. Reviewing the dominant culture's perspectives on such groups may only reinforce preexisting racist, sexist, and heterosexist biases (Greene, 1994a, 1994b, 1996a).

Another important dimension that must be considered is how sexuality and gender interrelate with culture. Espin (1984) suggests that in most cultures a range of sexual behaviors is tolerated. It is important for the clinician to determine where the client's behavior fits along the spectrum of sexual behavior for African Americans in general (Espin, 1984; Greene, 1996a). In exploring the range of sexuality tolerated by African Americans, one needs to know whether or to what extent formally forbidden practices are tolerated as long as they are not discussed and labeled, or if they are not tolerated under any circumstances.

It is also important to determine the relationship of the ethnosexual mythologies applied to African Americans to an African American lesbian and bisexual client's understanding of her sexuality in general, and a lesbian sexual orientation in particular (Greene, 1996a). Ethnosexual myths were created and perpetuated by the dominant culture and often represent a complex combination of racial and sexual stereotypes. These negative stereotypes have been used to objectify African American men and women, isolate and degrade African American women in comparison to their idealized White counterparts, and promote their sexual exploitation and control (Cohen, 1999; Collins, 1990; Dyson, 1996; Greene, 1994a, 1994b, 1996a; hooks, 1981; West, 1999). The symbolism of these stereotypes and its interaction with stereotypes held about lesbians play an important role in the stereotypes and myths perpetrated against and often internalized by African American lesbians and bisexual women. Therefore, they are important areas of inquiry in psychotherapy. I will return to the discussion of ethnosexual stereotypes after briefly reviewing characteristics of African American families that are relevant to African American lesbian and bisexual women's lives.

## FAMILY OF ORIGIN

The African American family has functioned as an important refuge to protect group members from the racism of the dominant culture. It has also served as an important socializing tool for African Americans as an oppressed group in a hostile environment. The family teaches its young how to recognize and negotiate racial barriers, and offers positive cultural mirroring to mitigate against internalizing negative images. Greene and Boyd-Franklin (1996), Jackson and Brown (1996), Smith (1997), Villarosa (cited in Brownworth, 1993), and Walters (1996) observe that the importance of African American family and community as a survival tool makes the "coming out" process for African American lesbians fraught with greater difficulty and perhaps with greater risk than that of their White counterparts (Smith, 1997). Because of the strength of family ties, there may be a reluctance to formally "expel" a lesbian from the family despite an undisputed rejection of a lesbian sexual orientation. This may be a result of varying levels of tolerance for nonconformity, denial of the person's sexual orientation, or even culturally distinct ways of conveying negative attitudes about a family member's sexual orientation (Greene, 1994a, 1994b, 1998a). In African American families, lesbians are not typically "disowned," to the extent that their White counterparts may be. We believe this is a reflection of the importance of family members to one another. Villarosa (cited in Brownworth, 1993) observes that instead of throwing someone out of the family, they "keep you around to talk you out of it" (p. 18).

## COMING OUT: A DEVELOPMENTAL CHALLENGE

Mental health clinicians should not view the apparent "tolerance" of some families as if it constitutes approval or as if there are no African American families who do "throw out" or disown a lesbian family member. What we observe as a kind of quiet tolerance is usually contingent on a lesbian's silence about her sexual orientation. Serious conflicts *may* occur within the family or between family members if a lesbian family member openly discloses, labels herself, or discusses being a lesbian. For example, a lesbian family member's lover may have been "accepted" in the family in ways that lead the lesbian member to assume that the family "knows" she is a lesbian. This may go along smoothly until the relationship is openly labeled as lesbian. If the lesbian family member moves out of the family's household (depending on her age) and establishes a household with a female partner, or makes any other overt acknowledgment of her lesbian sexual orientation, the response may be problematic. Even when family members are accepting and supportive, the broader African American community or the woman's heterosexual friends may not be (Greene, 1996a, 1998a; Walters, 1996). West (1999) observes that the "closeted sexuality" that exists in African American communities "should be seriously interrogated" because it contributes significantly to internalized homophobia within lesbian and gay persons (p. 293).

Because of the extended nature of African American families, close and emotionally intense ties between adult women are common. There is a culturally defined role within the African American community for the nonrelated adult girlfriend who has an often very intense but nonsexual, spiritual, and emotionally connected relationship with an African American woman friend and her family (Greene & Boyd-Franklin, 1996). This is reflected in the greeting "girlfriend" that acknowledges and confers kinshiplike status on a close adult female friend who is not blood-related but is experienced as intensely as if she were "blood family." These women are often informally "adopted" by the family and are referred to by children and younger family members as "Aunt." Sometimes this relationship is formalized when this girlfriend asked to serve as a godparent to a child in the family.

The role of the close female friend among adult women in African American culture can make it even easier for African American families to avoid acknowledging the lesbian nature of a relationship between two adult women, even when it is right within their midst (Greene & Boyd-Franklin, 1996). African

American lesbian clients can sometimes collude in this denial by never actually *saying* anything to pierce the family's denial. Others may not keep the information a secret per se but still never fully "come out" to their family members. Other clients may come out to their families, and then find that the family continues to pretend that the lesbian relationship does not exist, accepting the lover in the culturally accepted role of "girlfriend." Of course, in some African American families a lesbian family member and her relationship may be openly accepted by both the nuclear and the extended family.

It is important for clinicians to keep in mind that there is a tremendously wide range of responses, and not all family members respond in the same way. When clients discuss the possibility of coming out to loved ones, it is important that the therapist explores the potential responses of specific persons in the family, rather than the "family" as a whole group. The client cannot presume a general rejection or general acceptance from everyone in the client's family at once. The prospect of coming out to the entire family at once can be overwhelming but is unnecessary (Greene & Boyd-Franklin, 1996). The therapist can help the client to anticipate potentially painful reactions to the disclosure, especially if the client's partner is White. In interracial relationships, the White partner's race may become a more comfortable target for the family's anger about the disclosure and may be scapegoated (Greene & Boyd-Franklin, 1996).

The client should be warned not to overreact to the initial negative response of a family member. The client who is at the stage of coming out is at a very different developmental stage than the person to which they come out. An individual's acceptance of her own lesbian orientation has rarely taken place without hesitation or private doubts, nor typically will it for loved ones. Its absence at the stage of coming out does not mean that it can never take place; rather, it may require time to develop (Greene, 1994a; Greene & Boyd-Franklin, 1996). The therapist must assist the client in anticipating and preparing for the worst as well as the best scenarios. At the end of each scenario problem solving about different outcomes is advisable. In spite of the most thoughtful preparation, outcomes will be as diverse as African American families themselves.

## DOMESTIC RELATIONSHIPS AMONG AFRICAN AMERICAN LESBIAN AND BISEXUAL WOMEN: ISSUES AND THERAPEUTIC CHALLENGES

There is great diversity among African American lesbian and bisexual women where their domestic relationships are concerned. The race/ethnicity of the partner of an African American lesbian can greatly effect the dynamics of the relationship as well as its level of visibility, and therefore how it is perceived and received. Many African American lesbians' relationships are largely unsupported outside of the broader, predominantly White lesbian community and the much-smaller African American lesbian community. The latter may be nonexistent outside of large urban centers. These women may encounter unique challenges in relationships with partners who have the same gender socialization, in a hostile environment, that conspicuously devalues their person, that devalues their relationships on multiple levels, and where there are few open, healthy models of such relationships. Those in lesbian relationships may find some support for their relationship within the African American community. However, this "support" is often marked by an often conspicuous collusion of silence, ambivalence, and denial. African American lesbian and bisexual women have usually received family support for their struggles with racism, and perhaps for their struggles with sexism, but they may not presume that this support will extend to their romantic relationships. Nor can they assume that their families will empathize with their appropriate distress if the relationship is troubled or ends. For some family members, the end of a lesbian relationship will be cause for rejoicing. This is compounded upon seeking professional assistance, where many African American lesbians and bisexual women find few, if any, therapists who have been trained in addressing issues in lesbian relationships with women who are not White (Greene, 1994a, 1994b, 1994c; Greene & Boyd-Franklin, 1996).

African American lesbians and lesbians of color in general have relationships with women who are not members of their same ethnic group to a significantly greater degree than their White counterparts (Croom, 1993; Greene & Boyd-Franklin, 1996; Mays & Cochran, 1988; Tafoya & Rowell, 1988). This has been attributed in part to the larger numbers of White lesbians (Tafoya & Rowell, 1988). While heterosexual interracial relationships often lack the support of each member's family and community, lesbian interracial relationships face even greater challenges in a situation already fraught with difficulty (Greene, 1994a, 1994b, 1995a; Greene & Boyd-Franklin, 1996).

An interracial lesbian couple may be more publicly visible and hence more recognizable as a "couple" than two women of the same ethnic group. Such a couple has a greater potential to elicit homophobic reactions. Both may be perceived by others as lacking loyalty to their own ethnic/racial group, and either member or both may even feel ashamed of their involvement with a person of a different group (Clunis & Green, 1988; Falco, 1991; Greene, 1994a, 1998a; Greene & Boyd-Franklin, 1996; Walters, 1996). This both complicates the resolution of issues within the relationship and intensifies the complex web of loyalties and estrangements for African American lesbians.

While racial issues and cultural differences between partners offer realistic challenges to lesbian relationships, they are not responsible for every problem within them. Visible differences like race may be scapegoated as the cause of problems simply because they are so visible. This can allow the client to avoid looking at more complex and often painful issues in the relationship (Greene, 1994b, 1995a).

Choices of partners and feelings about those choices may but do not automatically reflect an individual's personal conflicts about racial and ethnic identity. When such conflicts are present, they may be expressed by African American lesbian women who choose or are attracted to White women exclusively or who devalue African American or lesbians of color as unsuitable partners. Or African American lesbians who experience themselves as racially or culturally deficient or ambiguous may seek a partner from their own ethnic group to compensate for their perceived deficiency or to demonstrate their cultural loyalty. There may also be a tendency for an African American lesbian in a relationship with another African American lesbian, or with a lesbian of color who is not African American, to presume that they are more like one another than is realistically warranted. While their common oppression as women of color and as lesbians may be similar, and may facilitate an intense emotional bond in the early development of the relationship, their views on their respective roles in the relationship, on maintaining a household, on the role of other family members in their lives, and so on, may be very different (Greene, 1994b, 1995a; Greene & Boyd-Franklin, 1996). Beyond this general assessment, the kinds of assumptions the client holds about other women of color or White women within an intimate relationship and their meanings should be explored (Greene, 1994a, 1994b).

Exclusive choices in this realm may also reflect a client's tendency to idealize people who are like her and to devalue those who are not or its corollary. When this is the case, the reality often does not live up to the fantasy, resulting in the client's intense disappointment and even feeling of failure. It is important to remember that such decisions and preferences have many different determinants that are often made outside of her conscious awareness (Greene, 1994b).

A therapist should never presume that participation in an interracial lesbian relationship is an expression of cultural or racial self-hate in the African American lesbian. Similarly, the therapist cannot accurately presume that her presence in a relationship with another African American woman is anchored in either loyalty or respect for that culture. Nor are any of the aforementioned problematic premises necessarily present at all. What is of significance is that therapists should be aware of a wide range of clinical possibilities and explore them accordingly (Greene, 1994b).

## THE ROLE OF ETHNOSEXUAL STEREOTYPES IN HETEROSEXISM

Since their origins in America as objects of the U.S. slave trade (Greene, 1990c, 1992, 1994a, 1994b), African-American women were considered to be property wherein forced sexual relationships with African males and White slave masters were the norm.

Ethnosexual stereotypes about African American women have their roots in images created by a White society that struggled to reconcile the contradictions between its ideals and espoused values and its inhuman treatment of African Americans (Greene, 1996a). African American women clearly did not fit the traditional stereotypes of women as fragile, weak, and dependent, as they were never allowed to be "dependent" on anyone. The "Mammy" figure is the historical antecedent to the stereotype of African American women as assertive, domineering, and strong. Assertiveness was considered the equivalent of antimale and even castrating attitudes and behaviors.

Popular images of African American women, and any other strong assertive women, as "castrating" were created in the interest of maintaining the status quo arrangement of social power. In this arrangement African American men and women are subordinate to Whites, and women are subordinate to men. Psychological theories that depicted assertive women as castrating were used to stigmatize any woman who wanted to work outside the home or to cross the gender-role stereotypes of a patriarchal culture (hooks, 1981). Today's stereotypes are a product of those myths and depict African American women as not sufficiently subordinate to African American men, inherently sexually promiscuous, morally loose, assertive, matriarchal, defective, and "other" when compared to their White counterparts (Christian, 1985; Clarke, 1983; Cohen, 1999; Collins, 1990; Greene, 1986, 1990a, 1994a, 1994e, 1996a, 1998a; hooks, 1981; Icard, 1989; Monroe, 1998; Silvera, 1991).

Stereotypes of lesbians as masculinized females converge with stereotypes of African American women as "too strong" and "domineering." Both are depicted as defective females who want to be men or who act like men and are sexually promiscuous. It is important to understand the history of institutional racism and its role in the development of the myths and distortions regarding the sexuality of African American lesbians (Greene, 1994d, 1994e).

African American males are encouraged to believe that strong women, rather than the practices of racist institutions, are responsible for their oppression. Racism, sexism, and heterosexism converge to cast the onus on African American women for the failure of their men to live up to the Western ideal of the male role, and consequently for the "failure" of African American families. In this analysis, the prescribed remedy for liberating people of African descent is male dominance and female subordination (Collins, 1990; Greene, 1994a, 1994e, 1996a, 1998a; hooks, 1981; Monroe, 1998; Riggs, 1995). Many African American women, including lesbians, have internalized these myths. Their internalization intensifies the negative psychological effects on African American lesbians and further compromises their ability to be affirming of themselves, to protect themselves, and to obtain support from the larger African American community (Cohen, 1999; Collins, 1990; Greene, 1994a, 1994b, 1994d, 1996a; Monroe, 1998).

African American men and women who have internalized the racism, sexism, and heterosexism inherent in the patriarchal values of Western culture may scapegoat any strong women, that is, any women who defy traditional gender role norms. As women whose primary romantic and emotional attractions are to other women, lesbians and bisexual women are easy targets.

## BETWEEN THE ROCK AND THE HARD PLACE: MULTIPLE JEOPARDIES

### Understanding Challenges to Optimal Psychological Development

African American lesbian and bisexual women develop, work, play, and love in a climate of ubiquitous hostility toward them. The need to negotiate pervasive environmental antagonism and discrimination creates a range of psychological challenges to the optimal development and functioning of this group's members. Despite the odds against them, African American lesbian and bisexual women are not inevitable psychological cripples. Clearly, many African American lesbian and bisexual women survive and even thrive despite the wide range of social disadvantages and obstacles they face. However, therapists must appreciate the tenacity of their resilience under what are most challenging circumstances. Survival in a ubiquitously hostile environment always requires the use of psychological resources, and thus always carries a price. That price is paid even among those who thrive. The antagonism that confronts African American lesbians and bisexual women comes from personal, family, and institutional sources. These sources, unfortunately, include the theory and practice of organized mental health.

The underpinnings of traditional approaches to psychology and psychotherapy are replete with racist, sexist, classist, and heterosexist biases (Garnets & Kimmel, 1991; Glassgold, 1992, 1995; Greene, 1994a, 1994b, 1995c, 1996a, 1998a, 1998b). These approaches often reinforce rather than mitigate the beliefs and rationales that support the multiple levels of discrimination that African American lesbians and bisexual women routinely encounter.

### The Rock: Feminist and Psychodynamic Therapy Theories As Challenges to Culturally Competent and Lesbian Affirmative Practice

Feminist therapy theory, a derivative of feminist political ideology, has traditionally questioned the validity of rationales that maintain institutional patterns of male dominance and female subordination. The analysis of race, class, sexual orientation, and other inequities, and their interactive effects on women, have not been routinely accorded this attention and its omission has been problematic in the practice of feminist therapy (Greene, 1994b, 1994e, 1996c). Feminist formulations, which traditionally have focused on gender inequality as the primary locus of social oppression of women, have been criticized for their failure to reflect the full spectrum of diversity among women (Brown, 1990, 1995; Espin, 1995; Greene, 1994b, 1994e, 1995a; Mays & Comas-Díaz, 1988). This failure to reflect greater diversity among women has been problematic in understanding the unique lives of women, such as African American lesbians and bisexual women, who have multiple identities and who share more than one socially disadvantaged identity.

Revisions of traditional feminist theory reflected in contemporary feminist theory add a concern with the relationship of sexism to other forms of societal disadvantage to their therapeutic focus (Brown, 1994; Daugherty & Lees, 1988; Lerman, 1996; Lerman & Porter, 1990). When feminist political theory explored the relationship between women's oppression and the patriarchal systems of the dominant culture, those explorations logically extended to institutional mental health.

Feminist psychotherapy approaches explicitly acknowledge the reality that societal disadvantages resulting from social hierarchies play a prominent role in creating and maintaining many of the problems presented by female clients in psychotherapy (Brown, 1994; Lerman, 1996; Lerman & Porter, 1990). Conspicuously absent from traditional psychotherapies has been this explicit acknowledgment of the role of institutional oppression in contributing to such problems. Instead, there has been an almost exclusive focus on the degree to which an individual should "adjust " to the particular context that the existing power structure defined as "healthy" or "normative." In this context, the diagnostic and treatment process of institutional mental health is used as a social tool whose purpose is to legitimize both the stigma and the subsequent punishment of women who do not conform (Brown, 1994; Daugherty & Lees, 1988; Lerman, 1996; Marecek & Hare-Mustin, 1991). Two key aspects of the socially constructed sex-role expectation is to be heterosexual and to conform to the Western White female ideal of beauty (West, 1995). In the United States, mental health institutions also served to stigmatize the appropriate responses of women to oppressive circumstances, rather than to explore and appropriately stigmatize the pathology of societal oppression.

Glassgold (1995), and other lesbian and feminist–psychodynamic clinicians (Daugherty & Lees, 1988; Gould, 1995; Kassoff et al., 1995) critique classical psychodynamic theories because such theories claim to be separate from society and politically neutral. This is particularly problematic when the behavior of the dominant group is pathological and the appropriate response to the dominant group's oppressive behavior is viewed as the problem. If norms are organized around dominant group characteristics and values, any pathological behavior of the dominant group is obscured. Theories that privilege the dominant culture's values and position, and presume objectivity, are less likely to be helpful to clients who are abused by societal pathology. Such perspectives give African American lesbian and bisexual women no tools with which to analyze either themselves, their sociopolitical context, or the relative contributions of each to their sense of self as well as their current dilemma.

Psychodynamic theories of psychotherapy have their origins in the psychoanalytic theory of neurosis, of which Sigmund Freud was the chief architect (Blatt & Lerner, 1983). It should be noted that in many of Freud's original writings he expressed his contentions in a manner that suggests that they were regarded by him as hypotheses, speculations, and tentative explorations. It is noteworthy that later interpretations of his work have not always been expressed with the same level of tentativeness. Many psychodynamic principles are still reported and interpreted by many contemporary theoreticians who seek to elaborate on them. They are often communicated with a level of certainty that is not only inconsistent with earlier writings but is not in keeping with the very nature of what a theory is: an attempt to explain a phenomenon or phenomena that constantly evolves with the acquisition of new knowledge, rather than being the final word on an issue.

Psychodynamic and psychoanalytic theories have also been criticized for their assertion that reproductive sexuality is the only normal outcome of psychosexual development. Despite Freud's early assertions that men and women were innately bisexual, psychoanalytic theories tend to privilege reproductive sexuality as the only healthy outcome of psychosexual development (Glassgold, 1995; Gould, 1995; Kassoff et al., 1995). Glassgold (1992) observes that just as psychoanalytic theories of gender evolved out of traditional, stereotyped views of gender roles, its theory of the etiology of sexual orientation has its origins in the same traditional views of gender. In this framework, heterosexuality is so much a part of the definition of psychological normalcy that it is also assumed to be a part of the definition of normal gender identity (Glassgold, 1992). In this framework, sexual attraction to men is embedded in the definition of what it means to be a normal woman. Therefore, lesbian sexual orientation is presumed to evolve out of problems or abnormalities in the early mother–daughter relationship. By claiming that reproductive sexuality equals normalcy, one assumes that trauma or pathology offers the only explanation for any other outcomes. Moreover, most of these observations have been used to support contentions based on isolated, selective clinical cases that are not representative samples of the lesbian and bisexual population.

The view that reproductive sexuality is normative mirrors the long-standing bias against lesbian and gay sexual orientations in the broader culture, in Western psychology, and in much of organized mental health. It was not until 1973 that the American Psychiatric Association removed the diagnosis of homosexuality from its *Diagnostic and Statistical Manual of Mental Disorders*. Similarly, it was not until 1975 that the American Psychological Association adopted its new official policy that homosexuality per se implied no psychological impairment. While psychodynamic theories and practice have not been alone in views that pathologize lesbian and gay sexual orientations, psychoanalysts have been the slowest of organized mental health professionals, training programs, and theoretical perspectives to alter the view that a lesbian sexual orientation is the result of a developmental arrest or trauma and that its expression is pathological. In fact, it was not until 1991, after 5 years of discussion and debate, that the American Psychoanalytic Association, the dominant psychoanalytic organization in the U.S., finally modified its official policy on the subject. While the association passed a resolution that formally opposed public and private discrimination against lesbians and gay men in 1991, words that included training and supervising analysts were not added to the resolution until 1992 (Lamberg, 1998). Prior to 1991, in psychoanalytic circles, lesbian and gay sexual orientations were considered perversions that required a cure. Open lesbian and gay applicants to psychoanalytic training institutes were regarded as undesirable candidates and turned away. Despite its slow pace in altering its view of lesbian and gay sexual orientation as pathological, the association endorsed same-sex marriage in 1997 (Lamberg, 1998). Haldeman (2000) observes that while organized mental health professions once uniformly assumed that lesbian and gay sexual orientations were mental disorders, they now dismiss pathology theories as "scientifically indefensible." In 1997, the American Psychiatric Association's Board of Trustees, and in 1998 the American Psychological Association's Council of Representatives, passed resolutions condemning reparative, conversion, or any psychiatric or psychological therapies that are based on the assumption that lesbian or gay sexual orientation is a mental disorder. Both organizations cite a lack of credible scientific evidence to support the efficacy of such therapies. They also warn that these therapies are not benign and carry potential risks that include depression, anxiety, and self-destructive behavior, as well as reinforcing societal prejudice against lesbians and gay men. Despite these official changes in organizational policy and in the diagnostic nomenclature, negative bias and misinformation continue to infuse the practice of psychotherapy with lesbians (Brown, 1996; Garnets, Hancock, Cochran, Goodchilds, & Peplau, 1991; Garnets & Kimmel, 1991).

The legacy of pervasive bias and discrimination against lesbians and gay men, women, and people of color—among other socially disadvantaged group members in society—creates a wealth of challenges to their optimal development as well as to their optimal treatment in psychotherapy. This is particularly true for African American women who are lesbian or bisexual. Prior to changes in the diagnostic nomenclature, most practitioners would engage in unquestioned attempts to "convert" lesbian or bisexual clients to heterosexual sexual orientation via what are known as the "conversion therapies." These attempts represent one of many manifestations of institutional bias against lesbian clients. Haldeman (2000) reviews the history and discusses the ethical implications of conversion therapies. Most clients expect psychotherapy to provide a safe, nonjudgmental haven for them. Lesbian clients, however, could expect to find themselves pathologized and ill-treated by the very professionals we would expect to be helpful to them. In addition to the discrimination they face in day-to-day life, bias against lesbians in the basic theoretical and practical structures of organized mental health institutions leaves members of this population at risk for more psychological abuse.

It is fair to say that the needs of African Americans, women, and lesbians have been ill considered in American mental health. It is also fair to say that these institutions have often contributed to the stigma associated with these identities. They also facilitate the development of biased attitudes in therapists in the form of negative countertransference. A comprehensive discussion of the various manifestations of countertransference and their resolution in psychotherapy with African American lesbian/bisexual women is beyond the scope of this chapter. The reader interested in this topic is referred to Greene (1994a, 1994b, 1994d, 1995a, 1995c) and Greene and Boyd-Franklin (1996).

Overall, an exclusive focus on intrapsychic dynamics runs the risk of ignoring important social and cultural realities that shape the lives and functioning of women, as well as the interactions between those realities. The therapist who has a personal need to avoid the anxiety this material may often evoke may focus exclusively on inquiries about intrapsychic material as if they have a universal context. It is safe to assume that the relationship between childhood trauma and adult pathology has many determinants, not simply one, and that the very notion of pathology itself is socially and culturally determined as well (Altman, 1995; Chodorow, 1989; Glassgold, 1992, 1995; Gould, 1995; Kassoff et al., 1995; Maracek & Hare-Mustin, 1991; Thompson, 1987).

Institutional mental health has played a distinct role in supporting heterosexist beliefs and values. These beliefs often result in misconceptions about lesbians and appear to be as common among people of color as they are in the dominant culture. Some of these questionable beliefs are that lesbians either want to be or naturally look like men (Taylor, 1983); are unattractive or less attractive than heterosexual women (Dew, 1985); are less extroverted (Kite, 1994); are unable to attract or have had traumatic experiences with men that presumably "turned" them against men, or are simply defective females (Christian, 1985; Collins, 1990; Glassgold, 1995; Gould, 1995; Greene, 1994a, 1994b, 1994d; Kite, 1994). In African American communities the assumption that sexual attraction to men is intrinsic to being a "normal" woman is as acceptable as it is in the dominant culture. Acceptance of this assumption often leads to a range of equally inaccurate conclusions. Two of the most significant assumptions are that reproductive sexuality is the only form of sexual expression that is both psychologically normal and morally correct (Garnets & Kimmel, 1991; Glassgold, 1992, 1995; Greene, 1994a, 1994c, 1994d, 1996a, 1998a), and that there is a direct relationship between sexual orientation and conformity to traditional gender roles and physical appearance within the culture (Kite & Deaux, 1987; Newman, 1989; Whitley, 1987). In the latter example, women who have not voiced the desire or attempted to conform to traditional gender-role stereotypes run the risk of being seen as lesbians; conversely, those who do conform do not arouse as much suspicion. These assumptions are also used to threaten women with the stigma of being labeled "lesbian" if they do not adhere to the traditional gender-role stereotypes of the African American community in which males are supposed to be dominant and females are supposed to be submissive (Collins, 1990; Gomez & Smith, 1990; Monroe, 1998; Smith, 1982). This often occurs in African American communities despite the history and tradition of gender role flexibility within African American families.

Being labeled a lesbian can prevent women, whether they are lesbian or not, from seeking nontraditional gender roles or engaging in nontraditional gender behaviors. Some scholars who are also women of color feel that simply acknowledging, writing about, or analyzing lesbian themes in African American women's literature; correctly identifying significant historical and literary figures as lesbians; or acknowledging lesbian themes in literature will raise questions about their own sexual orientation. The concern is that they will be viewed negatively as a result (Clarke, 1993). Such an atmosphere can perpetuate the invisibility of African American lesbians and bisexual women. In a society where, for women, attraction to men only, male dominance, and female subordination have been viewed as normative, the fears of being labeled as a lesbian and the negative consequences of the label maintain the patriarchal status quo.

This leads to a discussion of heterosexism/homophobia in African Americans. Heterosexism/homophobia among African Americans has multiple determinants. I will explore them in detail because I contend that there is often a connection between homophobia and the internalized racism that resides in the psyches of many African Americans. Both are psychologically destructive to individuals as well as to the African American community.

## The Hard Place: Homophobia/Heterosexism among African Americans

Cornel West (1999) observes that "it seems to me to talk about the history of heterosexism and the history of homophobia is to talk about ways in which various institutions and persons have promoted unjustified suffering and unmerited pain" (p. 290). This discussion does not presume that homophobia is any greater in African Americans than it is in other people of color or in their White counterparts. Boykin (1998) observes that an April 1993 Gallup Poll reports that greater numbers of African American respondents favored equal rights for lesbians and gay men in job opportunities and the lifting of military bans against them than their White counterparts. Congressman Barney Frank (cited in Boykin, 1999) also observes that the Congressional Black Caucus has been most supportive of lesbian and gay rights. It is possible that the homophobic voices are the loudest in many African American families and communities but are not necessarily representative. What must be clear to clinicians is that African American gays, lesbians, and bisexuals are harmed by homophobic rhetoric and action in their communities, no matter how large or small the source.

Many authors (Boykin, 1998; Clarke, 1983; Jeffries, 1992; Wekker, 1993; West, 1999) observe that there was once a greater tolerance for lesbians and gay men in some poor African American communities, such as Harlem, New York, in the 1940s through the1950s. Clarke (1983) offers as one explanation for this tolerance "seizing the opportunity to spite the White man" (p. 206). Jeffries (1992) attributes it to the empathy African Americans may have experienced, as oppressed people, toward members of another oppressed group. The dissolution of that tolerance may have multiple origins. A strong component to this tolerance was the relative invisibility of lesbians and gay men within the African American community and the dominant culture. The heightened visibility of lesbians in contemporary environments may place greater tension on the invisibility and denial that has been a large component of that tolerance in the past (Greene, 1994a, 1994b, 1994d, 1996a). West (1999) suggests that during the earlier periods referred to, homophobia was "thick" in the Black community. However, the survival of that community, when it was more cohesive and under siege, was a higher priority than its homophobia. In that context, a greater sense of tolerance was created and warranted. In West's (1999) analysis, as Black communities' undergo crisis and disintegration, paranoid dispositions develop and the communities' most vulnerable members—Black women, lesbians and gay men, and children (Lipsky, 1987)—become scapegoats. When scapegoating occurs, vicious forms of violence against these members increase and in some quarters are even viewed as acceptable or even necessary.

Historically oppressed groups, specifically African American and Native Americans, have accorded reproductive sexuality great importance (Clarke, 1983; Greene, 1994a, 1994d, 1996a). Many group members view it as the way to guarantee their continued presence in a society that wants to be rid of them and uses racist and genocidal practices to accomplish that goal. Nonreproductive sexual practices are seen by many African Americans as another way that the group's survival is threatened (Kanuha, 1990; Monroe, 1998). Lesbian and gay sexual orientation is sometimes viewed as part of a larger scheme on the part of White America to accomplish this goal (Monroe, 1998). In this context, women's primary role is to reproduce. Women who reject this role are viewed as traitors to the race (Cohen, 1999; Monroe, 1998). Kanuha (1990) describes these beliefs as "fears of extinction" (p. 176). Although fears of genocidal practices against African Americans as a group are warranted, this view scapegoats lesbian and gay members of the community rather than holding the proponents of racist and other discriminatory practices more accountable.

Furthermore, having a lesbian or bisexual sexual orientation does not preclude having children, particularly among African American lesbians and other lesbians of color. Despite this reality, the internalization of this myth may make it harder for an African American lesbian who wishes to have children to reconcile this desire with that of her sexual orientation. It may also be used as a barrier between members of the African American community that affects the kind and degree of support a lesbian or bisexual member may obtain (Cohen, 1999; Greene, 1994a, 1996a, 1998a; Monroe, 1998). When this occurs, it must be addressed by the clinician as a therapeutic issue (Greene, 1994a, 1994b, 1998a).

Homophobia may assume many diverse forms. Many are based on distortions of lesbian sexuality. One form of homophobia is represented in the belief that lesbian sexual orientation is a "chosen lifestyle." Many African Americans, like members of the dominant culture, believe strongly that lesbian or gay sexual orientation is a poorly chosen "lifestyle" rather than a human inclination that is as "natural" as heterosexuality. As a "chosen lifestyle," the resulting discrimination is viewed as if it were an "inconvenience" rather than the protracted, involuntary hardship of being Black (Gates, 1993). This stands in stark contradiction to the assumption that heterosexuality is not chosen. Heterosexuality is presumed to be the only "natural" expression of sexuality, because it is the only form that leads to procreation. The belief that lesbian sexual orientation is chosen and that race is not is a factor in the resentment expressed by many African Americans at the comparison between racial oppression and homophobia.

I contend that the relative visibility of race/ethnicity among African Americans and the invisibility of lesbian sexual orientation plays a significant role in the belief that lesbian sexual orientation is chosen. It is as if lesbians are not lesbians, or are at least invisible until they make their sexual orientation known to others. People who have these beliefs also believe that if lesbians would simply be quiet and hide, they would not be discriminated against and there would be no need for legal protection of their civil rights. This line of reasoning can suggest that lesbians who are "out" are inviting negative treatment and that perhaps they even deserve it. Gomez (1999) describes the demand within the Black community to be invisible as "a demand for a lie I was able to tell by not telling . . ." (p. 163).

In African American communities and families, the simple act of "telling" someone that you are a lesbian, expecting a lesbian relationship to be recognized, or engaging in any other behavior that is routine among heterosexuals is often regarded as "flaunting" something distasteful (Gomez, 1999). The message put forth is that lesbian sexual orientation, unlike racial identity, is something that can and should be concealed. Any hardship that would result from identification presumably could be avoided, making homophobia appear to be more controllable than racism. It is assumed that the problem rests in being known and that there is no cost in remaining silent. This position is a stark representation of heterosexual privilege and homophobia and is a contradiction to what we know about passing for White among African Americans. Both of these assumptions require what West (1993) describes as a serious interrogation.

The first and perhaps most important consideration is the psychological cost of passing, invisibility, hiding, and remaining closeted. Both the lesbian and gay literature and both the cultural and psychological literature on people of color document the negative psychological effects of passing as a long-term mechanism for managing discrimination (Gomez, 1999; West, 1999). Kitzinger (1996) observes:

> [W]hen you are *not* dismissed from work because you stayed in the closet; when there is *no* anti-lesbian explosion from your parents because you have de-dyked your apartment before their visit. . . heterosexism is functioning in its most effective and deadly way. . . . It is not necessary to murder or torture us to ensure our silence and invisibility . . . because a climate of terror has been created in which most gay people will *choose* to remain silent. (p. 11)

Aside from the stress that accompanies a constant threat and fear of being discovered, there is a price to be paid in the form of physical and psychic energy that a person is forced to expend if they live a fraudulent life, and is forced to conceal and compartmentalize important aspects of that life. There is also an ongoing level of vigilance and a concomitant lack of spontaneity required for authenticity in interpersonal relationships. Furthermore, when a climate of terror gives rise to the kind of silence that is required for people to become invisible, the act of silencing itself represents another form of social oppression and fuels the development of internalized homophobia.

Finally, sexual orientation is not routinely visible in the way that race/ethnicity is among most African Americans. However, the assumption that race is always equally visible among African Americans or that they are always identifiable is not valid. This assumption ignores the presence of African Americans, now and throughout history, who can and do pass for White. Individuals who can claim African ancestry, but who pass for White, are often the objects of scathing contempt from other African Americans. In fact, many people who are biracial or multiracial, who can claim some but perhaps not a majority of African ancestry, are often disparaged by some members of the African American community if they do not claim their African ancestry as their primary ethnic identification. This suggests that many Black people feel it is important to claim one's African ancestry with pride and feel that those who do not are at the very least lacking in integrity. However, the same principle is not applied to sexual orientation and in this manner constitutes an exercise in heterosexual privilege. In this case, heterosexual African Americans exercise a kind of heterosexual dominance or privilege by defining being "out" racially and ethnically as healthy and imperative, while being "out" as a lesbian is equated with inviting abuse and thus deserving of it. When a person is discriminated against because they are a descendent of Africans, racism is clearly defined as the problem, not the person who is harmed. In fact, when an African American feels that they deserve mistreatment because of their race, we consider it an expression of internalized racism. However, when a lesbian is harmed by discrimination, it is as if the heterosexism that spawns the discrimination is not even seen; it is the victim who is defined as the problem. This kind of behavior exemplifies heterosexual privilege in that the very behavior that is defined as laudable in a dominant or privileged group—heterosexuals— is deemed a defect in lesbians, the disadvantaged group. Heterosexism is not defined as the problem, the person who identifies herself as a lesbian is considered the problem. While African Americans may be righteously seen as a socially disadvantaged group, these examples inform us that all African Americans are not equally disadvantaged, nor are they immune to behaving in oppressive ways just because they are members of an oppressed group.

The maintenance of heterosexual privilege also represents a source of homophobia for some African Americans. This form of homophobia can be a function of maintaining both the privileges and the status that are derived from being heterosexual in this society, while denying the existence of an identity that is privileged. Clarke (1983), Silvera (1991), and Smith (1982) write that sexism in both the dominant and African American cultures, and racism in the dominant culture, leave heterosexual privilege (aside from class privilege for middle- and upper-middle-class African American women) the only privilege that African American women may have (Greene, 1994a, 1994b, 1996a). As such, they may be reluctant to jeopardize the privileges associated with this status.

Another more pernicious form of homophobia among African Americans is based on religious and theological grounds. One of the most frequent sources of internalized homophobia among African American lesbians, and a frequent source of conflict between them and other family members, is an objection to their lesbianism on "religious grounds." Family members may report that their acceptance of the lesbian family member's sexual orientation is a betrayal or repudiation of their faith; that a lesbian relationship violates the teachings in Scripture, God's law, or intent. Many clients themselves report feeling great conflict about whether or not they can be of good moral character if they are lesbian. The degree and intensity of these feelings of conflict or ambivalence about being a lesbian vary with the client's degree of involvement (present or past) with formal religious practice. These conflicts are not limited to African American lesbian or bisexual women who regularly attend church; they are a reflection of the extent to which religious beliefs, their own or those of significant others, have been internalized. For strict adherents to Western Christian theology, selective interpretations of biblical scripture have been historically used to reinforce homophobic attitudes (Claybourne, 1978; Gomes, 1996;

Greene, 1994a, 1994b; Icard, 1986; Monroe, 1998; Moses & Hawkins, 1982; Weatherford & Weatherford, 1999). African Americans have a strong Christian spiritual and religious orientation (Boyd-Franklin, 1989; Dyson, 1996; West, 1993). It is no surprise that religious derivatives are often a part of the conflict for clients who are ambivalent about or who do not accept their sexual orientation, particularly those who seek solace from their church. Weatherford and Weatherford (1999) observe: "The African American church sweeps eroticism under the rug, but most congregations don't even give homosexuality a foot in the door" (p. 21).

While the Black church has served as a haven for many African Americans in their struggles with racism, and has often been a potent force in liberation theology, it has been less than hospitable toward its lesbian, gay, and bisexual members. Silvera (1991) writes that when her grandmother discovered that she was a lesbian, she took out her Bible and explained: "This was a 'ting only people of mixed blood was involved in" (p. 16). Shaka Zulu (1996) reflects on her life and struggles as an African American lesbian growing up in a Black fundamentalist church. She notes that a "Don't ask, don't tell" policy of denial was a part of an atmosphere in which compulsory heterosexuality was strictly enforced. Her description of different kinds of fundamentalist believers may prove useful to therapists in conceptualizing and developing responses to the challenges presented by fundamentalist family members of lesbian clients or clients who have internalized such beliefs themselves.

There is a great variance among African American mainstream denominations in their official policies on homosexuality (Weatherford & Weatherford, 1999). The Weatherfords write that the Roman Catholic, Southern Baptist, and Pentecostal denominations maintain the most conservative positions on the subject, while the United Church of Christ is most welcoming to lesbian and gay members. Other denominations fit in between these extremes. The reader is referred to Weatherford and Weatherford for more detailed information about the official policies of other specific denominations.

Many congregations that belong to national religious organizations have a measure of local autonomy in their execution of the organization's policies (Weatherford & Weatherford, 1999). Hence there may actually be some latitude in the degree to which official denominational policies are followed. Certain non-Christian religious sects view homosexuality as a decadent Western practice as well.

For adherents to Western Christian religiosity, homophobic interpretations of biblical scripture may be used to express indirectly a family member's discomfort with other aspects of the lesbian family member's person or life choices. Objections to lesbian sexual orientation can mask difficulty that parenting or other figures may experience over the loss of control over or healthy separation/individuation of an adult child. There is great potential for this when a lesbian member is establishing a "family" of her own with another woman and leaves the household of her family of origin. If parenting figures are not "ready" for healthy separation, objections to their daughter's relationship on the grounds that it is a lesbian relationship are apt to gain more support from peers than it would if a daughter "leaves" her parents to live with or marry a man. Clearly, marrying a man would be regarded as a normal developmental expectation. Objections might be more easily recognized as the parent's, not the adult child's, problem. In close-knit families or those where most of their time is spent together, introducing a lesbian significant other may be problematic for other reasons. Some family members may feel threatened by the presence of someone who is so important to their loved one and fear that they will have less time, access, and perhaps influence over their child or sibling. There may be a concrete fear that the significant other will have greater access to the resources of their loved one as well. Expressions of religious indignation about the person's lesbian sexual orientation can serve to mask their feelings about these other issues. In these cases, the outraged family member would probably not welcome anyone who they perceived as threatening to displace them in importance to their loved one. A parent or sibling may focus on sexual orientation as a point of outrage, as it may garner more support, than acknowledging their jealousy of the significant other. It is important to scrutinize the behavior of the family members who object so vehemently to lesbian sexual orientation on religious grounds. Rarely is their own behavior completely consistent with their espoused beliefs. Assisting the lesbian client in understanding this discrepancy can be important. Family objections may also mask a family member's characterological discomfort with her own sexuality or sexual matters altogether. These and other forms of discomfort may be expressed via the rationale of religious conviction. The therapist must be aware of a wide range of possibilities.

It is important that therapists be aware of the role of selective interpretation of biblical scripture in homophobia. Perhaps of even greater importance is the awareness that there is a lack of absoluteness and certainly no sense of uniformity with which Christian theologians or biblical scholars interpret these issues. When a client expresses absolute certainty about them, their defensive use should be explored. The therapist must attempt to discern how the Scripture or belief is being used defensively rather than argue the specifics of the interpretation with either the client or a family member. For example, is the belief being used in the interest of bringing family members together in a peaceful and mutual reconciliation? Or is the belief used to promote further splitting between family members into "good" and "bad," exacerbating preexisting conflicts between members or between other factions of the family, or in any of the ways previously mentioned? The therapist must also have access to members of the clergy in the community both to personally consult with and to refer clients. For some clients, hearing alternative theological positions from a member of the clergy may be more validating and supportive than support from a therapist alone. It can be helpful if the therapist has some working background knowledge of what Christian biblical scriptures used to support homophobia *actually* say about the subject, rather than only what is reported to them. There may be conspicuous leaps between the client's reading of Scripture, the actual content of such material, and the wide range of interpretations of it. The client's choice of meaning, even when it is self-depreciating, and how it is defensively used is of dynamic significance. It can be symbolic of a wider range of ways that the client views herself and other family figures. Gomes (1996) observes:

> The legitimization of violence against homosexuals, Jews, women and Blacks, as we have seen, comes from the view that the Bible stigmatizes these people and therefore they are fair game. . . . If the Bible expresses such a prejudice, then it can't be wrong to act on that prejudice. . . . every anti-Semite and racist has used this argument with demonstrably devastating consequences, as our social history all too vividly shows. (p. 146)

Gomes (1996) and Weatherford (1999) and Weatherford write that no credible case against homosexuality or homosexuals can be made from the Bible unless one chooses to interpret Scripture in ways that presume the preexisting prejudices against homosexuality are true. Gomes argues that the subject of homosexuality is not even mentioned in the early texts of the Bible and that the word "homosexual" itself, an invention of the late 19th century, is never mentioned until the 1946 Revised Standard version. Gomes and Weatherford and Weatherford challenge the notion that the Bible's failure to mention homosexual relationships warrants condemning them. They point out that the Bible does not discuss celibacy, the single state, friendships, or other kinds of relationships that we do not hold in contempt. That heterosexuality is dominant does not warrant the assumption that it is the only form of sexuality that is morally correct.

Cone (1990), Dyson (1996), Fielding-Stewart (1994), and West (1993, 1999) observe that the African American church espouses a "profoundly" conservative theological position on sexuality and that this "rigid" perspective creates a repressive climate. It is within that repressive climate that African Americans are taught *not* to question or apply a critical analysis to biblical scriptures or religious doctrines. Rather than question interpretations of Scripture, they are expected by church authorities to accept what is given at face value, particularly about sexual matters. Dyson (1996), Monroe (1998), and West (1993, 1999) suggest that this conservative theology regarding sexual matters is a derivative of a legacy of slavery, misogyny, and racism. I contend that "theological homophobia," often expressed in the rejection of lesbians (and gay men) in both the Black church and the African American community, has some of its roots in internalized racism and sexism among African Americans.

Dyson (1996), Monroe (1998), and Simmons (cited in Weatherford & Weatherford, 1999, p. 32) observe that gay-friendly roles (the choir master, etc.) in the Black church, and by extension in the Black community, are tolerated as long as they are nonthreatening and as long as there are no open "displays" of homosexual behavior. As long as lesbians are not a part of the governing, administrative, or power hierarchy, and as long as they are silent about who they are, lesbian members are tolerated. Monroe describes the ministry of misogyny and homophobia in the Black church as one in which social action is predicated on the devaluation of women and lesbian, gay, bisexual, and transgendered people. In Monroe's thesis, this practice rests on the belief that Black men are the most endangered members of the Black community, and that they must be protected by and at the expense of African American women, as well as other members of the community. Male superiority and dominance is an active ingredient in homophobia, for it supports the preservation of traditional gender roles and the hierarchies that accompany them (Cohen, 1999; Dyson, 1996; Greene, 1996a; Monroe, 1998). Roles and hierarchies that maintain female subordination are not viewed appropriately as a construction of society but rather are seen as "God's will." In this analysis, African American lesbians are blamed for not upholding what are perceived to be roles given by God rather than the dictates of a patriarchal society. Lesbians act in defiance of the rule that establishes sexual pleasure as a male domain, a domain that maintains the status quo of dominance and submission between Black men and women, and eroticizes female submission to men (Cohen, 1999; Monroe, 1998).

Lesbian and gay sexual orientations among African Americans have long been attributed to the assimilation of decadent Western practices or the White man's disease. These are positions that find support in the African American community, in the hierarchy of some organized Black churches, and among select Black nationalists. Smith (cited in Riggs, 1995) suggests that homophobic beliefs among African Americans are also a function of Black nationalist efforts to claim an African heritage. These beliefs, however, are based on the assertion that there was (and is) no homosexuality in Africa. Myths are created about an Africa and an African past that most contemporary African Americans have no direct connection to, whose accurate historical depiction has been obscured, and—depending on the period of African and American history one examines—was alternately devalued and then idealized by African Americans.

I now briefly address the contention that lesbian (and gay) sexual orientations are inauthentic in African-descended people based on the assertion that there is no evidence of them in Africa. Overall, this view is not supported by careful study of African peoples. It is important to note, however, that the way a culture defines sexuality will determine whether or not the African and Western constructs of sexual orientation are conceptually equivalent. What we in the West mean when we label someone "lesbian," "gay," or "bisexual" is often conceptualized and constructed differently in other cultures and may be less visible to the Western observer. Blackwood and Wieringa (1999) review a range of methodological obstacles and blinders that interfere with the identification of "lesbians" in Africa and their appropriate study. Chief among these obstacles are the influence of Western taboos and erroneous beliefs about homosexual behavior that have led many anthropologists to presume that sex between women only takes place when there are no men around. Armed with these biases, researchers fail to ask appropriate questions during interviews in studies that might illuminate the existence of lesbian women and their relationships. The reader is referred to the aforementioned authors for a more comprehensive review of these factors.

Despite methodological obstacles, anthropological evidence reveals that there have always been forms of female homosexuality in Africa and in all other human cultures (Blackwood & Wieringa, 1999; Gevisser, 1998; Kendall, 1998; Murray & Roscoe, 1998; Potgieter, 1997; Wekker, 1993). For example, anthropologists have examined marriage between Nandi women of Kenya and mummy–baby relationships in Lesotho, where older women whose husbands are migrant mine workers take younger women as their "spouses" (Potgieter, 1997). They have also examined Modjadji, the "Rain Queen" of the Lovedu in the Northern Province of South Africa, a female hereditary leader who keeps as many as 40 wives (Gevisser, 1998). Wekker (1993) observes two different ways that Black women in the diaspora expressed what we would consider lesbian relationships. Wekker's research reveals that in a number of West African regions where slaves were taken from Dahomey and Ashanti, women who had sex with other women were not the target of negative sanctions and prohibitions. For example, in Dahomey, a woman could formally marry another woman and the children of one were considered to be the children of the other. In Suriname, lesbian relationships were tolerated as long as they were not named. Wekker compares "lesbian relationships" among Black women in the United States with those among Black women in Suriname. Her findings suggest that *mati* (the Suriname Tongo name for women who have sex with women) retained more African cultural derivatives and working-class elements than Black lesbians in the United States, who were observed to have more Eurocentric and middle-class features. Wekker concludes that *matisma* (the Sranan Tongo word for women who have sex with women) display lesbian *behavior* while Black lesbians in the United States view themselves as having a lesbian *identity*.

In some parts of Southern Africa lesbians are often considered traditional healers (as they were in many Native American tribes). Their "difference" in some cultures is seen as something that gives them a special connection to the supernatural (Gevisser, 1998). Their healer status also means that they are not required to marry. Not having to marry allows them to live independent lives as unattached women (Gevisser, 1998; Kendall, 1998). It is important to understand the economic structure of a society and its role in defining marriage. Women who must marry men in order to attain economic viability may construct their relationships with other women differently than the "lesbian" couples structure we observe in the West (Kendall, 1998). It is also important to consider the effect of colonization on indigenous cultural practices. In Africa, the advent of Christianity and the influx of Christian missionaries that facilitated Africa's colonization stigmatized the kinds of people and relationships whom Westerners would currently regard as lesbian. If and when they were stigmatized, punishment by death was often the price paid for this identity. For this reason, many became hidden members of society. Gevisser (1998) and Potgieter (1997) observe that as more African nations turn to democracy lesbian and gay Africans have become more visible and assertive, putting them in conflict with conservative African leaders (Aarmo, 1999). Indeed, South Africa under the leadership of Nelson Mandela is the only nation that includes protection from sexual orientation discrimination in its constitution (Potgieter, 1997).

In any cross-cultural examination of sexual behavior it is crucial to understand that the biological underpinnings of any sexual behavior is always experienced, mediated, and interpreted through the lens of culture and cultural values (Aarmo, 1999; Blackwood & Wieringa, 1999; Wekker, 1993). Many contentions about the absence of lesbian or other forms of nontraditional sexuality in contemporary and precolonial Africa are more representative of social fiction than of reality. Despite this, many African Americans believe these contentions, forgetting that they are social creations. I contend that many of the social creations represented in myths about the presence or absence of lesbian sexuality in Africa also serve a defensive purpose. Because of the important role these ideas play in the psyche of African Americans, and the degree to which they are accepted as fact among many African Americans, I think it is important to briefly address them. Many of these beliefs are significant ingredients in the internalized racism and homophobia of the African American community, as well as in the internalized homophobia of African American lesbians. As such, this warrants the serious attention of clinicians.

We must begin by asking: What are the psychological consequences of developing in a society that objects to and negatively stigmatizes significant elements of African Americans' sexual and other identities? The sexuality of African American women has been defined and depicted by the dominant culture as excessive, dangerous, and bestial and conjures up the image of a lascivious, promiscuous woman who not only lacks virtue, but is undeserving of the protections of "feminine virtue" offered White women. African American women's images are often dichotomized between the poles of two extremes. One is the former image of the lascivious woman and the other is the devout, asexual Mammy/virtuous woman of the church (Cohen, 1999; Collins, 1990; Davis, 1998; Dyson, 1996; Monroe, 1998; West, 1995). Cohen (1999) argues that these depictions have been used to justify the implementation of marginalizing social systems. Images of "reckless, irresponsible, dangerous, black sexuality" are used to maintain stigmatized images of African American women and simultaneously support and sustain their exploited position in the social hierarchy (Cohen, 1999; Monroe, 1998; West, 1993). While race plays a role in defining Black sexuality, sexuality has also always played an important role in defining blackness. This is evident in the ethnosexual mythologies used to stigmatize African American sexuality (Greene, 1996a; Wyatt, Strayer, & Lobitz, 1976).

Cohen (1999), Gomez (1999), Higginbotham (1993), and West (1993) observe that for many African Americans, respectability and acceptance by the dominant group came to be equated with distancing themselves from any image or behavior found in racist stereotypes of African Americans. This, of course, meant distancing themselves from any members of the African American community who cannot or who refuses to attempt to live up to the dominant culture's proscription for respectability. West writes:

> Black survival required accommodation with and acceptance from White America. . . . Struggling black institutions made a Faustian pact with White America: avoid any substantive engagement with black sexuality and your survival on the margins of American Society is, at least, possible. (p. 86)

West's conceptualization describes behavior that in psychological terms can be seen as an attempt to act *against*, or to disprove, a stereotype. The problem, of course, is that one cannot disprove a contention that is a lie to begin with. Some individuals who behave as West describes do not necessarily believe the essence of the stereotypes that degrade Black sexuality. They may, however, feel required to give the appearance of imitating the dominant culture's values, whether or not they believe in them. However, there are many other individuals who engage in this behavior because they do believe that degrading stereotypes about Black sexuality are true. In clients who believe the degrading stereotypes of Black sexuality, and who behave as West describes, this can be understood as a form of psychological defense against the belief that one is actually inferior. The belief in racial stereotypes of one's own inferiority represents a form of internalized oppression referred to as "internalized racism."

Lipsky (1987) defines *internalized oppression* (racism) as a reenactment of an old hurt or trauma that will create a distress pattern if it is not healed or discharged (p. 3). The distress pattern consists of varied kinds of rigid, destructive, or ineffective feelings or behaviors in the victim, which may be directed at the victim him- or herself or at someone else. Lipsky suggests that African Americans as victims of racism have been denied the safe conditions needed to discharge racial distress in healthy ways. As a result, they may direct their distress at themselves or at targets who are even more vulnerable than they are—often other African Americans. Self-invalidation, fear, despair, embarrassment, or shame; feeling "not as Black as thou" or "Blacker than thou"; or the need to live up to unrealistic (or arbitrary) standards often form the substance of the behavior described as internalized racism. The shame and distress that many African Americans experience around the mythical but negative depictions of Black sexuality and the need to negate those depictions can lead to the disparaging of African American lesbians and gay men. Hence, internalized racism and homophobia share important underpinnings among African Americans.

For African Americans who have internalized the negative stereotypes of their sexuality, sexual behavior outside of dominant societal norms can be experienced as a negative reflection on all African Americans. There may be an exaggerated desire or pressure to model "normalcy" to the dominant culture (Clarke, 1983; deMonteflores, 1986; Gomez, 1983; Greene, 1986a, 1994a, 1994b, 1996a, 1996b, 1998a; Higginbotham, 1983; Wyatt et al., 1976). Gomez (1999) writes that convincing White people that African Americans were just like them was a strategy used by African Americans in an evolving political arena, but was not useful as a long-term survival strategy. Furthermore, Gomez suggests that this strategy facilitated the development of a personal mythology among African Americans about who they were. This self-created mythology is observed to be as narrow and misleading as many of the mythologies that Whites created about African Americans. Lipsky (1987) suggests that narrow, limited views of Black culture, of what "authentic" Black behavior is, and anger about anything that differs too much from the mythical ideal of the middle class of the majority culture exemplifies internalized racism.

Defensive responses to attacks on African American sexuality are reflected in part and supported by the African American church's demonizing of sexuality and idealizing the need for sexual purity (Dyson, 1996; Higginbotham, 1993; Lipsky, 1987; Monroe, 1998; Weatherford & Weatherford, 1999). Since acceptance of lesbian sexual orientations is inconsistent with the dominant culture's ideal, African American lesbians may be experienced as an embarrassment to African Americans who strongly identify with the dominant culture (Cohen, 1999; Greene, 1994a; Poussaint, 1990; West, 1993). Indeed, the only names for lesbians in the African American community, "funny women," or "bulldagger women," are derogatory (Jeffries, 1993, p. 44; Omosupe, 1991).

Homophobia allows African Americans who have internalized sexual/racial stereotypes to distance themselves personally, and as a Black community to distance themselves as a society, from the sexual stigma that the dominant culture has associated with Black identity, particularly Black sexuality (Cohen, 1999; Dyson, 1996; West, 1993, 1999). This allows some segments of the African American community to maintain their hope for legitimacy and full incorporation into the dominant culture's power structure (Cohen, 1999; Dyson, 1996; Monroe, 1998; West, 1993, 1999). For other African Americans, their homophobia and subsequent distancing from lesbian and gay members when rooted in African nationalist arguments represent a distortion of African cultures and African descendency. This distortion, intended to "normalize" Africans and their descendants, appears to be based on the assumption that the presence of lesbian and gay members in one's ethnic group is a bad thing or a negative reflection on the group. Hence, claims of African conformity to exclusive heterosexuality represent a denial of the realistic presence of lesbian, gay, bisexual, and transgendered people among Africans—just as they are present among every other human group. Despite the fact that same-gender sexual attractions and relationships occur in all cultures, they may be constructed and understood in ways that differ from the Western concept of lesbian and gay identities (Blackwood & Wieringa, 1999; Kendall, 1999; Wekker, 1993).

The notion of a monolithic racial identity that excludes lesbian sexual orientation represents an attempt to exercise a form of social control designed to establish unilateral conformity among oppressed group members (Cohen, 1999; Gates, 1996; Monroe, 1998; Walters, 1996; West, 1993). However, this mythical uniformity is maintained by keeping elements of the community and group silenced, invisible, and denied. If a model of the African American community requires that members of the community be silenced, or their presence denied, we are left with a model of the group that is neither authentic nor representative. Lesbian members of the African American community who attempt to deny healthy parts of themselves, such as their sexuality, commit a form of psychological suicide. This behavior at its core illustrates a derivative of internalized racism. Rejection of African American lesbians by other African Americans, for the reasons previously discussed, represents a kind of pathology in the group that will neither tolerate nor accept the realistic diversity of its members. African American lesbian and bisexual women are not pathological for failing to live up to a mythological cultural, and some would argue false, moral standard.

One method for silencing nonconforming group members is the accusation of racial disloyalty, lack of authenticity, or the incompatibility of lesbian sexual orientation and true blackness. Such accusations often lead clients to experience conflicts of allegiance and the need to compartmentalize and conceal different parts of themselves (Greene, 1994a, 1996a; Walters, 1996). The concept of racial loyalty presumes that a lesbian sexual orientation is incompatible with a Black identity, or at least an authentic Black identity. This charge is extremely painful for many African Americans. Those who organize other aspects of their identity around being African American are particularly vulnerable. In therapy these issues should not be regarded as frivolous or tangential. It is important for the therapist to understand what it is like for an African American lesbian or bisexual client to face the stated or implied charge of racial disloyalty or of failing to be "Black enough." The client who is African American and lesbian is a member of a visible oppressed ethnic group, as well as a member of a less visible oppressed minority, in a racially hostile society. Most members of these groups have other identities as well, and those multiple identities further complicate their dilemma. Because of the racism in the predominantly White lesbian and gay community, this community is no substitute for the protective function of the African American family and community (Walters, 1996). However, African American lesbians may be forced to be silent about their sexual orientation to obtain the protection and support offered by the African American community and their families. Gomez (1999) writes: "I could be a lesbian in what they imagine is my dark secret world but when I'm in the [Black] community, the message to me is: don't bring that mess" (p. 163).

It is important to understand what happens when the client is relegated to the margins or pushed outside of the group that has been necessary to her survival, or, worse yet, when she is accused of belonging to the enemy camp or of being "confused" or a traitor to her race. African American lesbians who internalize these beliefs are indeed between a rock and a hard place. The loss of tangible and emotional support, the special buffering function and protection from racism that is withdrawn from some African American lesbian and gay members on disclosure, is real, and its impact should not be underestimated. However, we must ask why these assertions of racial disloyalty carry such emotional weight and are so painful to many clients when on the surface their manipulative function may appear obvious. Gates (1996) observes:

> Blacks across the economic and ideological spectrum are often astonishingly vulnerable to charges of in-authenticity or disloyalty to the race. . . . This vulnerability and the pain associated with it attests to the enduring strength of our feelings of guilt, and our anxiety about having been or having the potential to be false to our people, having sinned against our innermost identity. (p. 118)

I believe that some of this sensitivity resides in our own psyche as descendants of Africans, a group that was and remains far from monolithic. A part of our heritage is that of being descendants of stolen people, an identity that most African Americans readily claim. We are also, however, descendants of the Africans who sold other Africans, an ancestry for which there is no rush to claim. The participation of some Africans and African tribes in the selling of Africans into slavery does not relieve the dominant culture in America for its establishment and operation of institutional chattel slavery nor of the responsibility for the destructive effects of hundreds of years of American apartheid and institutional racism.

African Americans share a complex legacy. Descendants of Africans do not inherit an ideal legacy. Indeed, none exists for any ethnic group, nor is one required to demonstrate human worth. One way of "idealizing" African legacies is to deny the existence of group members or behaviors that the majority culture disapproves of, disparages, or uses to rationalize the validity of our exploitation. The need of some African Americans to construct an "idealized" but incomplete version of African ancestry, one that is devoid of the sexuality that is condemned by the West, is understandable. It is a logical defense against the overwhelming barrage of negative images and distortions of Africa and African descendants and the harsh treatment based on those depictions. Similarly, the attempt to distance from community members that appear to fulfill negative stereotypes of the dominant culture about Black sexuality begin, at least, as understandable attempts at accommodation and survival. The danger is that they lead communities to deny many of their members and leads those members to deny or experience shame about legitimate and important parts of themselves. Furthermore, these attempts do not leave us with a realistic legacy of the African past, or understanding of contemporary African America. The denial and subsequent rejection of lesbian and gay members of the African American community does not represent an affirmation of African cultural derivatives or of Africans themselves. It simply reflects the blind acceptance of the White majority cultural norm of heterosexism that is a function of the gender-based hierarchies of a patriarchal culture. In the long run, it does not serve the interests of the African American community as the diverse community that it really is.

Baldwin (cited in Goldstein, 1984) observed that "there is nothing in me that is not in everybody else, and nothing in everybody else that is not in me" (p. 182). Baldwin's eloquence draws our attention to the reality that African Americans have all of the potential in terms of behavior and emotions that all other human beings have; that these are a part of being totally human; and that they need not apologize for any of those elements. Distortions of what it means to be authentically "Black," particularly when internalized by lesbian clients, that rest on silencing elements of our contemporary communities and eradicating pieces of our history must be deconstructed. Just as there is no ideal family, there is no ideal nation family, and none is warranted. However, idealization represents a defense mechanism. It is a manifestation of a need to be defensive about self and nation and to subsequently deny certain aspects of the self/nation whether they are really toxic or not (i.e., being African American lesbian and gay persons).

Psychological health is predicated on the acceptance and integration of the disparate elements of the self and "family," in both the biological and nation or ethnic sense. Thus, assisting clients, when appropriate, in identifying and acknowledging both healthy nurturing and unhealthy toxic elements in the "family," among or within loved and trusted members, as well as within hated figures, is an active component of most psychotherapies. It includes both the repudiation or appropriate management of toxic or unhealthy elements of the self, family, and community. The failure to identify, acknowledge, and accept the real toxic elements of African heritage (i.e., the selling of its own people), the realities of external oppression and internalized racism, and the defense against them leads many African Americans to simply deny whatever behavior or identities that are *perceived* to be toxic, whether they really are or not. The spiritual and emotional reconciliation of those disparate elements as well as the client's own ambivalence about them must take place in order for a healthy therapeutic transformation to occur. In psychotherapy, this is an appropriate goal of treatment.

Techniques that integrate psychodynamic and feminist therapies are most useful in this area. Just as reconciliation takes place in therapy around mixed and multiple legacies among a client's biological family, it may for some clients need to take place when it applies to the nation family that they have internalized as well. This is particularly important when it is connected to such beliefs about core aspects of the client's identity. This means accepting in the nation context, just as one must in the family context and in the self, a mixed heritage. The identities of African American's ancestors and descendants need not be distorted to redeem them or demonstrate their worth. When reconciliation is successful, there is no need to distort and silence those members of the community or elements of the self that do not maintain images borne of shame or defensiveness. The internalized racism that is a significant ingredient in the need for the distortions discussed above can be transformed into a healthy acceptance of a wider range of ways of being in the world that do not mitigate the authenticity of one's identity as an African-descended person.

## INTEGRATING FEMINIST AND PSYCHODYNAMIC THERAPIES IN PRACTICE WITH AFRICAN AMERICAN LESBIANS AND BISEXUAL WOMEN

Despite problematic aspects of both of these therapeutic approaches, particularly when used in isolation, they may be used in an integrated fashion to explore the vicissitudes of racism, sexism, and heterosexism and their interactions with development and the inner life of African American lesbians and bisexual women in therapy. Glassgold (1995), Glassgold and Iasenza (1995), and Kassoff and colleagues (1995) provide a detailed and comprehensive review of feminist and lesbian feminist revisions of psychodynamic theories that may be useful as background information for clinicians who are unfamiliar with their use. The idea that is most salient in the integration of these approaches is that every individual is capable of developing a subjective understanding of both her inner and her outer worlds, and how each shapes or affects the other. Individuals are shaped by the societal and familial conditions and circumstances that surround them during their development. Yet they also have the capacity to alter the results of their particular experiences and, at the very least, their understanding of their circumstances; they are not inextricable prisoners of them. Furthermore, no one set of circumstances may be seen as inevitably giving rise to pathological outcomes. Nor can a pathological outcome be consistently attributed to one determinant. It is important that clients in therapy be able to distinguish between societal realities and circumstances that are within their control, those that are not, and those whose control is relative to the context they occur in. The very real existence of societal oppression does not mean that the client has no control over the strategies she uses to cope with that oppression or how she understands it. However, solutions based on the client's conscious and deliberate strategies are more desirable than those based on responses made outside of the client's awareness. To make conscious decisions the client must be able to appreciate the strategies that she uses and why she uses them. She must also be able to analyze whether or not they are effective. Feminist approaches have demonstrated an effectiveness at assisting clients in recognizing and understanding the nature of the social oppression that they confront. Psychodynamic approaches can be useful in helping the client determine how she responds to societal oppression and to what extent, if any, it intensifies or is connected to other personal or familial issues and if their manifestations are a problem for her.

Therapists who treat African American lesbians using an integrated approach must themselves be able to make distinctions between internal psychological conflicts that interfere with the client's ability to problem solve and how problem-solving ability is affected by the social context. In addition, the complex interplay between these two overlapping phenomena must be appreciated.

In addition to maintaining an awareness of social barriers, the therapist must be simultaneously aware of significant figures, relationships and their patterns, and events in the client's life. It is important to understand the extent to which those previous relationships and events bear on the development of the client's personality, current actions, and perception of solutions and alternatives in addressing current realistic problems. While there are realistic institutional barriers in the world that African American lesbian and bisexual women must face as a group, each individual has her own unique experience and understanding of that reality. That reality is central to what the therapist must attempt to discern. The therapist should not romanticize the struggles against the often painful effects of institutional barriers simply because they are often a factor in the development of resilience, nor should they be used to explain away all of a client's problems.

Rarely is racism, sexism, or heterosexism the exclusive source of a client's difficulty. For some clients, societal oppressions may be less painful to focus on than other problems, such as personal histories of abuse or maltreatment at the hands of loved ones. Exploring a client's personal or characterological contributions to her problems does not mean that the client is to blame for everything that happens to her. Traditionally trained therapists often have difficulty with this concept when it involves institutional oppression. Therapists who are members of dominant groups may have particular difficulty unraveling these complex and interconnected issues. The therapist cannot explore the role of oppression in a client's life without having explored the role of oppression and privilege in his or her own life, particularly where he or she is positioned on the spectrum of privilege and oppression relative to the client (Green, 1996c, 2000). This can be particularly difficult when the therapist is on the more privileged end of the social hierarchy. Understanding the role of societal oppression in a client's life, for members of dominant groups, may elicit feelings of guilt, shame, or anger and trigger avoidance of this material (Greene, 1996c, 2000; Holzman, 1995; Wildman, 1996). When discrimination is finally accepted as the real reason for the problem, this realization is often accompanied by the therapist's sense of helplessness, being overwhelmed, or feeling of guilt. Therapists must understand and work through these painful reactions to their client's life circumstances because the failure to do so often leads them to overlook, avoid, or deny that such circumstances exist.

African American lesbians and bisexual women have the opportunity in therapy of having their accurate perceptions of discrimination and unfair treatment validated; identifying and understanding the conscious and unconscious methods they employ in confronting and negotiating systemic and personal barriers; analyzing the effectiveness of their methods; and developing a wider range of personally compatible options.

## SUMMARY

For African American lesbian and bisexual women, the effects of racism, sexism, and heterosexism (among other forms of discrimination) cannot be neatly separated from one another. Sexism and heterosexism affect African American and White women differently. Racism affects African American heterosexual and lesbian and bisexual women differently. Being an African American shapes the construction and understanding of the client's sexuality in a reciprocal fashion. It also shapes the construction and manifestations of heterosexism and internalized homophobia as well. Gender, race, and sexual orientation oppression interact with one another in particular ways, and all shape and interact with the personality dynamics of each individual. Any analysis that fails to take this complex interaction of experiences and their effects into account can neither sensitively nor appropriately address the treatment of African American lesbian and bisexual women.

The appropriate use of feminist and psychodynamic therapies with African American lesbians and bisexual women explicitly requires a special blend of cultural literacy and competence of its practitioners. This cultural literacy includes understanding the plight of African American lesbians and bisexual women in the context of:

1. The prevailing reality of the convergence of race, gender, and sexual orientation bias and the interpersonal and institutional barriers that result in a client's life. This includes a familiarity with the dominant culture's view of African American women's roles and histories as distinct

from its view of White women's roles and histories and their respective roles in the ethnosexual mythologies about African American women.

2. A willingness on the part of the therapist to validate the client's accurate perceptions of discrimination and bias and their impact on the client's life.

3. The wide range of similarities and diversities that exist within African American lesbians and bisexual women as a group.

4. The individual client's intrapsychic and familial endowments and personal history as they are embedded in the aforementioned context.

5. An acknowledgment of the therapist's value system and its potential impact on the therapist's ability to maintain an empathic, therapeutic relationship with the client. This includes the therapist's personal scrutiny about his or her feelings and motivations for working with clients who are African American and lesbian, the biases inherent in the theoretical orientation(s) employed, the therapist's analysis of his or her position on the spectrum of social privilege and disadvantage, and both his or her understanding of and feelings about that position relative to each client's position on that spectrum. What should follow is a careful analysis of the developmental interactions of these variables, how they shape the African American lesbian/bisexual woman's view of the world, her strategies for negotiating both her external and inner world, and her relationships with other persons (Greene, 1996b, 1998a).

## ACKNOWLEDGMENT

I thank Dr. Kathy Gainor and Lawrence Greene for their generous assistance, helpful comments, and discussions during the preparation of this chapter.

## REFERENCES

Aarmo, M. (1999). How homosexuality became "un-African": The case of Zimbabwe. In E. Blackwood & S. E. Wieringa (Eds.), *Same sex relationships and female desires: Transgender practices across cultures* (pp. 255–280). New York: Columbia University Press.

Altman, N. (1995). *The analyst in the inner city: Race, class, and culture through a psychoanalytic lens.* New York: Analytic Press.

Bass-Hass, R. (1968). The lesbian dyad: Basic issues and value systems. *Journal of Sex Research, 4,* 126.

Bell, A., & Weinberg, M. (1978). *Homosexualities: A study of diversity among men and women.* New York: Simon & Schuster.

Blackwood, E., & Wieringa, S. E. (1999). Sapphic shadows: Challenging the silence in the study of sexuality. In E. Blackwood & S. E. Wieringa (Eds.), *Same sex rela-*

*tions and female desires: Transgender practices across cultures* (pp. 39–63). New York: Columbia University Press.

Blatt, S. J., & Lerner, H. (1983). Psychodynamic perspectives on personality theories. In M. Hersen, A. E. Kazdin, & A. S. Bellack (Eds.), *The clinical psychology handbook* (pp. 87–106). New York: Pergamon Press.

Boyd-Franklin, N. (1989). *Black families in therapy: A multisystems approach.* New York: Guilford Press.

Boykin, K. (1998). Gay and lesbian movements in the United States. In K. A. Appiah & H. L. Gates, Jr. (Eds.), *Microsoft encarta africana: Comprehensive encyclopedia of Black history and Black culture* [CD-ROM]. Redmond, WA: Microsoft.

Brown, L. S. (1990). The meaning of a multicultural perspective for theory building in feminist therapy. In L. Brown & M. Root (Eds.), *Diversity and complexity in feminist therapy* (pp. 1–21). New York: Haworth Press.

Brown, L. S. (1994). *Subversive dialogues.* New York: Basic Books.

Brown, L. S. (1995). Antiracism as an ethical norm in feminist therapy practice. In J. Adleman & G. Enguidanos (Eds.), *Racism in the lives of women: Testimony, theory, and guides to antiracist practice* (pp. 137–148). New York: Haworth Press.

Brown, L. S. (1996). Preventing heterosexual bias in psychotherapy and counseling. In E. Rothblum & L. Bond (Eds.), *Preventing heterosexism and homophobia* (pp 36–58). Thousand Oaks, CA: Sage.

Brownworth, V. A. (1993, June). Linda Villarosa speaks out. *Deneuve*, pp. 16–19, 56.

Chodorow, N. J. (1989). *Feminism and psychoanalytic theory.* New Haven, CT: Yale University Press.

Christian, B. (1985). *Black feminist criticism: Perspectives on Black women writers.* New York: Pergamon Press.

Clarke, C. (1983). The failure to transform: Homophobia in the Black community. In B. Smith (Ed.), *"Home girls": A Black feminist anthology* (pp. 197–208). New York: Kitchen Table Women of Color Press.

Claybourne, J. (1978). Blacks and gay liberation. In K. Jay & A. Young (Eds.), *Lavender culture* (pp. 458–465). New York: Jove.

Clunis, M., & Green, G. D. (1988). *Lesbian couples.* Seattle, WA: Seal Press.

Cohen, C. (1999). *The boundaries of blackness: AIDS and the breakdown of Black politics.* Chicago: University of Chicago Press.

Collins, P. H. (1990). Homophobia and Black lesbians. In P. H. Collins, *Black feminist thought: Knowledge, consciousness, and the politics of empowerment* (pp. 192–196). Boston: Unwin/Hyman.

Cone, J. (1990). *A Black theology of liberation: Twentieth century edition.* Maryknoll, NY: Orbis Books.

Croom, G. (1993). *The effects of a consolidated versus non-consolidated identity on expectations of African American lesbians selecting mates: A pilot study.* Unpublished doctoral dissertation, Illinois School of Professional Psychology, Chicago.

Croom, G. L. (2000). Lesbian, gay, and bisexual people of color: A challenge to representative sampling in empirical research. In B. Greene & G. L. Croom (Eds.), *Education, research, and practice in lesbian, gay, bisexual, and transgendered psychology: A resource manual* (pp. 263–281). Thousand Oaks, CA: Sage.

Daugherty, C., & Lees, M. (1988). Feminist psychodynamic therapies. In M. A. Dutton-Douglas & L. Walker (Eds.), *Feminist psychotherapies: Integration of therapeutic and feminist systems* (pp. 3–11). Norwood, NJ: Ablex.

Davis, A. (1998). *Blues legacies and Black feminisms.* New York: Pantheon Books.

deMonteflores, C. (1986). Notes on the management of difference. In T. Stein & C. Cohen (Eds.), *Contemporary perspectives on psychotherapy with lesbians and gay men* (pp. 73–101). New York: Plenum Press.

Dew, M. A. (1985). The effects of attitudes on inferences of homosexuality and perceived physical attractiveness in women. *Sex Roles, 12,* 143–155.

Dyson, M. E. (1996). When you divide body and soul, problems multiply: The Black church and sex. In M. E. Dyson, *Race rules* (pp. 77–108). New York: Addison Wesley.

Espin, O. (1984). Cultural and historical influences on sexuality in Hispanic/Latina women: Implications for psychotherapy. In C. Vance (Ed.), *Pleasure and danger: Exploring female sexuality* (pp. 149–163). London: Routledge & Kegan Paul.

Espin, O. (1995). On knowing you are the unknown: Women of color constructing psychology. In J. Adleman & G. Enguidanos (Eds.), *Racism in the lives of women* (pp. 127–135). New York: Haworth Press.

Falco, K. L. (1991). *Psychotherapy with lesbian clients.* New York: Brunner/Mazel.

Fielding-Stewart, C. (1994). *African American church growth: Twelve principles for prophetic ministry.* Nashville, TN: Abington Press.

Garnets, L., Hancock, K. A., Cochran, S. D., Goodchilds, J., & Peplau, L. A. (1991). Issues in psychotherapy with lesbians and gay men: A survey of psychologists. *American Psychologist, 46,* 964–972.

Garnets, L., & Kimmel, D. (1991). Lesbian and gay male dimensions in the psychological study of human diversity. In J. Goodchilds (Ed.), *Psychological perspectives on human diversity in America* (pp. 137–192). Washington, DC: American Psychological Association.

Gates, H. L. (1993, May 17). Blacklash. *New Yorker, 69*(13), 42–44.

Gates, H. L. (1996, April 29–May 6). The charmer. *New Yorker, 72*(10), 116–131.

Gevisser, M. (1998). Homosexuality in Africa: An interpretation. In K. A Appiah & H. L. Gates, Jr. (Eds.), *Microsoft encarta africana: Comprehensive encyclopedia of Black history and culture* [CD-ROM]. Redmond, WA: Microsoft.

Glassgold, J. (1992). New directions in dynamic theories of lesbianism: From psychoanalysis to social constructionism. In J. Chrisler & D. Howard (Eds.), *New directions in feminist psychology: Practice, theory, and research* (pp. 154–163). New York: Springer.

Glassgold, J. (1995). Psychoanalysis with lesbians: Self-reflection and agency. In J. Glassgold & S. Iasenza (Eds.), *Lesbians and psychoanalysis: Revolutions in theory and practice* (pp. 203–228). New York: Free Press.

Glassgold, J., & Iasenza, S. (Eds.). (1995). *Lesbians and psychoanalysis: Revolutions in theory and practice.* New York: Free Press.

Goldstein, R. (1994). Go the way your blood beats: An interview with James Baldwin. In Q. Troupe (Ed.), *James Baldwin: The legacy* (pp. 173–186). New York: Simon & Schuster.

Gomes, P. J. (1996). The Bible and homosexuality: The last prejudice. In P. J. Gomes, *The good book: Reading the Bible with mind and heart* (pp. 144–172). New York: Morrow.

Gomez, J. (1983). A cultural legacy denied and discovered: Black lesbians in fiction by women. In B. Smith (Ed.), *"Home girls": A Black feminist anthology* (pp. 120–121). New York: Kitchen Table Women of Color Press.

Gomez, J. (1999). Black lesbians: Passing, stereotypes, and transformation. In E. Brandt (Ed.), *Dangerous liaisons: Blacks, gays, and the struggle for equality* (pp. 161–177). New York: New Press.

Gomez, J., & Smith, B. (1990). Taking the "home" out of homophobia: Black lesbian health. In E. C. White (Ed.), *The Black women's health book: Speaking for ourselves* (pp. 198–213). Seattle, WA: Seal Press.

Gonsiorek, J., & Weinrich, J. (1991). The definition and scope of sexual orientation. In J. Gonsiorek & J. Weinrich (Eds.), *Homosexuality: Research implications for public policy* (pp. 1–12). Thousand Oaks, CA: Sage.

Gould, D. (1995). A critical examination of the notion of pathology in psychoanalysis. In J. Glassgold & S. Iasenza (Eds.), *Lesbians and psychoanalysis: Revolutions in theory and practice* (pp. 3–17). New York: Free Press.

Greene, B. (1986). When the therapist is White and the patient Black: Considerations for psychotherapy in the feminist heterosexual and lesbian communities. *Women and Therapy, 5,* 41–66.

Greene, B. (1990a). Sturdy bridges: The role of African American mothers in the socialization of African American children. *Women and Therapy, 10*(1–2), 205–225.

Greene, B. (1990b, December). African American lesbians: The role of family, culture, and racism. *BG Magazine,* pp. 6, 26.

Greene, B. (1990c). Stereotypes of African American sexuality: A commentary. In S. Rathus, J. Nevid, & L. Fichner-Rathus (Eds.), *Human sexuality in a world of diversity* (p. 257). Boston: Allyn & Bacon.

Greene, B. (1992). Still here: A perspective on psychotherapy with African American women. In J. Chrisler & D. Howard (Eds.), *New directions in feminist psychology: Practice, theory, and research* (pp. 13–25). New York: Springer.

Greene, B. (1994a). Ethnic-minority lesbians and gay men: Mental health and treatment issues. *American Psychological Association, 62*(2), 243–251.

Greene, B. (1994b). Lesbian women of color: Triple jeopardy. In L. Comas-Díaz & B. Greene (Eds.), *Women of color: Integrating ethnic and gender identities in psychotherapy* (pp. 389–427). New York: Guilford Press.

Greene, B. (1994c). Lesbian and gay sexual orientations: Implications for clinical training, practice, and research. In B. Greene & G. Herek (Eds.), *Psychological perspectives on lesbian and gay issues: Vol. 1. Lesbian and gay psychology: Theory, research, and clinical applications* (pp. 1–24). Thousand Oaks, CA: Sage.

Greene, B. (1994d). African-American women. In L. Comas-Díaz & B. Greene (Eds.), *Women of color : Integrating ethnic and gender identities in psychotherapy* (pp. 10–29). New York: Guilford Press.

Greene, B. (1994e). Diversity and difference: The issue of race in feminist therapy. In M. P. Mirkin (Ed.), *Women in context: Toward a feminist reconstruction of psychotherapy* (pp. 333–351). New York: Guilford Press.

Greene, B. (1995a). Lesbian couples. In K. Jay (Ed.), *Dyke life: From growing up to growing old. A celebration of the lesbian experience* (pp. 97–98; 100–101; 103–104; 106). New York: Basic Books.

Greene, B. (1995b). An African American perspective on racism and anti-Semitism within feminist organizations. In J. Adleman & G. Enguidanos (Eds.), *Racism in the lives of women* (pp. 303–313). New York: Haworth Press.

Greene, B. (1995c). Addressing racism, sexism, and heterosexism in psychodynamic psychotherapy. In J. Glassgold & S. Iasenza (Eds.), *Lesbians and psychoanalysis: Revolutions in theory and practice* (pp. 145–159). New York: Free Press.

Greene, B. (1996a). Lesbians and gay men of color: Ethnosexual mythologies in heterosexism. In E. Rothblum & L. Bond (Eds.), *Preventing heterosexism and homophobia* (pp. 59–70). Thousand Oaks, CA: Sage.

Greene, B. (1996b). African American women: Considering diverse identities and societal barriers in psychotherapy. In J. A. Sechzer, S. M. Pfafflin, F. L.Denmark, A. Griffin, & S. Blumenthal (Eds.), *Annals of the New York Academy of Sciences: Women and Mental Health, 789*, 191–209.

Greene, B. (1996c, November). *Psychotherapy across the cultural divide: Barriers to addressing power and privilege in the psychotherapeutic relationship.* Invited keynote address, Center for Women's Development Conference, Cultural Competence, Boston.

Greene, B. (1997). Psychotherapy with African American women: Integrating feminist and psychodynamic models. *Smith College Studies in Social Work, 67*(3), 299–322.

Greene, B. (1998a). Family, ethnic identity, and sexual orientation among African American lesbians and gay men. In C. Patterson & A. D'Augelli (Eds.), *Lesbian, gay, and bisexual identity: Psychological research and social policy* (pp. 40–52). New York: Oxford University Press.

Greene, B. (1998b). Sexual orientation. In M. Hersen & A. Bellack (Eds.), *Comprehensive clinical psychology: Vol. 10. Sociocultural and individual differences* (pp. 207–232). Oxford, UK: Elsevier Science/Pergamon Press.

Greene, B. (2000). Developing an inclusive lesbian, gay, and bisexual psychology: A look to the future. In B. Greene & G. L. Croom (Eds.), *Education, research, and practice in lesbian, gay, bisexual, and transgendered psychology: A resource manual* (pp. 1–45). Thousand Oaks, CA: Sage.

Greene, B., & Boyd-Franklin, N. (1996). African American lesbians: Issues in couples therapy. In J. Laird & R. J. Green (Eds.), *Lesbians and gay men in couples and families: A handbook for therapists* (pp. 251–271). San Francisco: Jossey-Bass.

Haldeman, D. (2000). Therapeutic responses to sexual orientation: Psychology's evolution. In B. Greene & G. L. Croom (Eds.), *Education, research, and practice in lesbian, gay, bisexual, and transgendered psychology: A resource manual* (pp. 244–262). Thousand Oaks, CA: Sage.

Hall, R. L., & Greene, B. (1996). Sins of omission and comission: Women, psychotherapy, and the psychological literature. *Women and Therapy, 18*(1), 5–31.

Higginbotham, E. (1993). *Righteous discontent: The women's movement in the Black Baptist Church, 1880–1920.* Cambridge, MA: Harvard University Press.

hooks, b. (1981). *Ain't I a woman? Black women and feminism.* Boston: South End Press.

Holzman, C. (1995). Rethinking the role of guilt and shame in White women's antiracism work. In J. Adleman & G. Enguidanos (Ed.), *Racism in the lives of women: Theory, testimony, and guides to practice* (pp. 325–332). New York: Haworth Press.

Icard, L. (1986). Black gay men and conflicting social identities: Sexual orientation versus racial identity. *Journal of Social Work and Human Sexuality, 4*(1–2), 83–93.

Jackson, K., & Brown, L. B. (1996). Lesbians of African heritage: Coming out in the straight community. *Journal of Gay and Lesbian Social Services, 5*(4), 53–67.

Jeffries, I. (1993, February 23). Strange fruits at the purple manor: Looking back on "the life" in Harlem. *NYQ, 17,* 40–45.

Kanuha, V. (1990). Compounding the triple jeopardy: Battering in lesbian of color relationships. *Women and Therapy, 9*(1–2), 169–183.

Kassoff, B., Boden, R., deMonteflores, C., Hunt, P., & Wahba, R. (1995). Coming out of the frame: Lesbian feminism and psychoanalytic theory. In J. Glassgold & S. Iasenza (Eds.), *Lesbians and psychoanalysis: Revolutions in theory and practice* (pp. 229–263). New York: Free Press.

Kendall, K. (1998). Women in Lesotho and the Western construction of homophobia. In E. Blackwood & S. E. Wieringa (Eds.), *Same sex relations and female desires: Transgender practices across cultures* (pp. 157–178). New York: Columbia University Press.

Kite, M. (1994). When perceptions meet reality: Individual differences in reactions to lesbians and gay men. In B. Greene & G. Herek (Eds.), *Lesbian and gay psychology: Theory, research, and clinical applications.* (pp. 25–53). Thousand Oaks, CA: Sage.

Kite, M., & Deaux, K. (1987). Gender belief systems: Homosexuality and the implicit inversion theory. *Psychology of Women Quarterly, 11,* 83–96.

Kitzinger, C. (1996). Speaking of oppression: Psychology, politics, and the language of power. In E. Rothblum & L. Bond (Eds.), *Preventing heterosexism and homophobia* (pp. 3–19). Thousand Oaks, CA: Sage.

Lamberg, L. (1998, August 12). Gay is okay with APA—Forum honors landmark 1973 events. *Journal of American Medical Association, 280*(6), 497–499.

Lerman, H. (1996). *Pigeonholing women's misery.* New York: Basic Books.

Lerman, H., & Porter, N. (1990). The contribution of feminism to ethics in psychotherapy. In H. Lerman & N. Porter (Eds.), *Feminist ethics in psychotherapy* (pp. 5–13). New York: Springer.

Lipsky, S. (1987). *Internalized racism.* Seattle, WA: Rational Island.

Loiacano, D. (1989). Gay identity issues among Black Americans: Racism, homophobia, and the need for validation. *Journal of Counseling Development, 68,* 21–25.

Maracek, J., & Hare-Mustin, R. (1991). A short history of the future: Feminism and clinical psychology. *Psychology of Women Quarterly, 15,* 521–536.

Mays, V., & Cochran, S. (1988). The Black Women's Relationship Project: A national survey of Black lesbians. In M. Shernoff & W. Scott (Eds.), *The sourcebook on lesbian/gay health care* (2nd ed., pp. 54–62). Washington, DC: National Lesbian and Gay Health Foundation.

Mays, V., Cochran, S., & Rhue, S. (1993). The impact of perceived discrimination on the intimate relationships of Black lesbians. *Journal of Homosexuality, 25*(4), 1–14.

Mays, V., & Comas-Díaz, L. (1988). Feminist therapy with ethnic minority populations: A closer look at Blacks and Hispanics. In M. Dutton-Douglas & L. Walker (Eds.), *Feminist psychotherapies: Integration of therapeutic and feminist systems* (pp. 228–251). Norwood, NJ: Ablex.

Monroe, I. (1998). Louis Farrakhan's ministry of misogyny and homophobia. In A. Alexander (Ed.), *The Farrakhan factor: African-American writers on leadership, nationhood, and Minister Louis Farrakhan* (pp. 275–298). New York: Grove Press.

Moses, A. E., & Hawkins, R. (1982). *Counseling lesbian women and gay men: A life issues approach.* St. Louis, MO: Mosby.

Murray, S. O., & Roscoe, W. (Eds.). (1998). *Boy wives and female husbands: Studies of African homosexualities.* New York: St. Martin's Press.

Newman, B. S. (1989). The relative importance of gender role attitudes toward lesbians. *Sex Roles, 21,* 451–465.

Omosupe, K. (1991). Black/lesbian/bulldagger. *differences: A Journal of Feminist and Cultural Studies, 2*(2), 101–111.

Potgieter, C. (1997). From apartheid to Mandela's constitution: Black South African lesbians in the nineties. In B. Greene (Ed.), *Psychological perspectives on lesbian and gay issues: Vol. 3. Ethnic and cultural diversity among lesbians and gay men* (pp. 88–116). Thousand Oaks, CA: Sage.

Poussaint, A. (1990, September). An honest look at Black gays and lesbians. *Ebony,* pp. 124, 126, 130–131.

Riggs, M. (Producer/Director). (1995). Interview with bell hooks and Barbara Smith. In *Black Is . . . Black Ain't* [Videotape]. (Available from California Newsreel, 149 Ninth St./420, San Francisco, CA 94103)

Shaka-Zulu, N. (1996). Sex, race, and the stained glass window. *Women and Therapy, 19*(4), 27–35.

Silvera, M. (1991). Man royals and sodomites: Some thoughts on the invisibility of Afro-Caribbean lesbians. In M. Silvera (Ed.), *Piece of my heart: A lesbian of color anthology* (pp. 14–26). Toronto, Ontario: Sister Vision Press.

Smith, A. (1997). Cultural diversity and the coming out process: Implications for clinical practice. In B. Greene (Ed.), *Ethnic and cultural diversity among lesbians and gay men* (pp. 279–300). Thousand Oaks, CA: Sage.

Smith, B. (1982). Toward a Black feminist criticism. In G. Hull, P. Scott, & B. Smith (Eds.), *All the women are White, all the blacks are men, but some of us are brave* (pp. 157–175). Old Westbury, NY: Feminist Press.

Tafoya, T., & Rowell, R. (1988). Counseling Native American lesbians and gays. In M. Shernoff & W. A. Scott (Eds.), *The sourcebook on lesbian/gay health care* (2nd ed., pp. 63–67). Washington, DC: National Lesbian and Gay Health Foundation.

Taylor, A. T. (1983). Conceptions of masculinity and femininity as a basis for stereotypes of male and female homosexuals. *Journal of Homosexuality, 9,* 37–53.

Thompson, C. (1987). Racism or neuroticism? An entangled dilemma for the Black middle-class patient. *Journal of the American Academy of Psychoanalysis, 15*(3), 395–405.

Thompson, C. (1989). Psychoanalytic psychotherapy with inner-city patients. *Journal of Contemporary Psychotherapy, 19*(2), 137–148.

Walters, K. (1996). Negotiating conflicts in allegiances among lesbians and gays of color: Reconciling divided selves and communities. In G. Mallon (Ed.), *Foundations of social work practice with lesbian and gay persons* (pp. 47–75). New York: Harrington Park Press.

Weatherford, R.J., & Weatherford, C. B. (1999). *Somebody's knocking at your door: AIDS and the African American church.* New York: Haworth Press.

Wekker, G. (1993). Mati-ism and Black lesbianism: Two idealtypical expressions of female homosexuality in Black communities of the diaspora. *Journal of Homosexuality, 24*(3-4), 11–24.

West, C. (1993). *Race matters.* New York: Vintage Books.

West, C. M. (1995). Mammy, Sapphire, and Jezebel: Historical images of Black women and their implications for psychotherapy. *Psychotherapy, 32*(3), 458–466.

West, C. (1999). Cornel West on heterosexism and transformation. In E. Brandt (Ed.), *Dangerous liaisons: Blacks, gays, and the struggle for equality* (pp. 290–305). New York: New Press.

Whitley, E. B. Jr. (1987). The relation of sex role orientation to heterosexual attitudes toward homosexuality. *Sex Roles, 17,* 103–113.

Wildman, S. (1996). *Privilege revealed: How invisible preference undermines America.* New York: New York University Press.

Wyatt, G., Strayer, R., & Lobitz, W. C. (1976). Issues in the treatment of sexually dysfunctioning couples of African American descent. *Psychotherapy, 13,* 44–50.

## CHAPTER 6

# The Courage to Hear

## *African American Women's Memories of Racial Trauma*

### JESSICA HENDERSON DANIEL

This chapter focuses on understanding racism as a reality-based and repetitive trauma in the lives of African American women. By concentrating on African American women's memories of racial trauma, this chapter explores the following issues: the usefulness of feminist-psychodynamic practice and theory for Black women; racial silence in psychotherapy; distorted images of African American women as a form of trauma; and specific traumatic racial memories. Finally, the notion of "legend ladies" is introduced.

Other chapters in this volume have discussed the absence of African American women's voices in the construction of psychodynamic and feminist therapies. Most theoretical approaches to psychotherapy with African American women are both androcentric and ethnocentric and have failed to acknowledge the importance of the role of race in the lives of African American women (Spelman, 1988). Effective treatment strategies must consider both environmental and intrapsychic factors, as well as their interactions, if therapists are to fully and accurately appreciate the behaviors and struggles of African American women. Many of their life experiences and life memories can be directly linked to race and racism. Similarly, the psychological literature puts forth a perception of trauma that is not inclusive. This perception of trauma fails to take racism into account as a locus of traumatic experiences for African American women.

## THE CHALLENGE OF RACIAL SILENCE: THERAPISTS AND AFRICAN AMERICAN WOMEN

African American women come to psychotherapy with a range of issues including those that evolve from racial incidents and traumatic circumstances. In psychodynamic therapy, memories are critical resources for understanding the etiology of current affective states and behavior. The need to manage and negotiate racial barriers is an important part of the life narratives of African American women (Greene, 1994b). The provision of services at the emotionally laden intersection of trauma, race, and gender can be problematic when therapists have limited knowledge about the various life contexts of African American women. Limited conceptualizations of the kinds of events that may constitute trauma, and limited perceptions of what kinds of people may be victims of trauma, are problematic in psychotherapy. More inclusive concepts of trauma are necessary if therapists who treat African Americans are to be able to correctly identify many of their race-related experiences as traumatic. Racial segregation, both legal and de facto, has effectively limited the level and nature of the contact between African American and European American people so that many European American therapists are not familiar with the life contexts of their African American clients. Inherent in this racial distancing is a racial hierarchy that has required African Americans to understand European Americans for their own survival and protection, while European Americans have not had to do the same.

Therapists who have some familiarity with the impact of race on the lives of African American women are more prepared to hear, explore, and validate their narratives. Equally important, they are better able to discriminate between contexts where race is a critical issue and where it is not (Greene, 1994a). Therapists who collude consciously or unconsciously with their patients in avoiding disclosure of life experiences with racial content or who deny the existence of racism will impede the healing process.

Detailed history taking, that is, recording the patient's specific memories, is essential in therapy. Both the interview process and the actual data collected may reflect the wide variability in training, theoretical orientation, and life experiences of the therapists. Training institutions that continue to marginalize, distort, and exclude African American history and psychosocial experiences produce mental health professionals who lack knowledge about African Americans and other people of color. Graduate and professional school course curricula and training programs vary in their approaches to teaching about racial groups, from total omission of the topic to a single course specific to racial issues. Generally, instructional materials about the impact of race are not integrated into non-race-specific courses. The inclusion in syllabi of isolated research studies and theoretical papers that focus on African American populations without placing them in racial contexts could result in the misinterpretation of data and the miseducation of students. The content of therapists' instruction and training often communicates tacit permission to avoid the topic of race. Even when trauma is placed in a sociopolitical context, race can be excluded from the analysis or discussed "in a stereotype," as it is in the highly acclaimed book *Trauma and Recovery* (Herman, 1992). No discussion of racism as a psychological trauma or of the affiliative civil rights movement is included in the book (Daniel, 1994). Several commentaries elaborate on the issues of exclusion and the interpretation of trauma in racial contexts (Dines, 1995; Garcia, 1995; Melendez, 1995; Sanchez & Nuttall,1995; Wilkins, 1995).

Therapists' avoidance of issues related to race and racism is an understandable, although not an acceptable, practice. In a classic article, Tatum (1992) identifies three major reasons for resistance to talking about race. First, Tatum observes that the topic has been historically taboo, especially in racially mixed company. Many individuals in our culture, particularly Whites, recall that when they were children and noticed that people differed in skin color or hair texture, they were silenced by adults if they voiced their observations. The adults appeared anxious about the children's observations of racial differences. Such reactions communicated that something was "wrong" with speaking about these often very apparent differences among people. For people of color, their first experiences around race are often negative and emotionally painful, for example, being targets of racial epitaphs and being subjected to social exclusion.

The second reason Tatum (1992) cites is that discussions about race question the validity of the belief that the United States is a meritocracy. In a true meritocracy, by definition, people get what they work for, earn, and deserve. Those who do well are presumed to have earned their privileged positions and those who are socially disadvantaged are presumed to deserve their ill-status at the bottom. White individuals may feel discomfort, pain, and guilt after hearing about life experiences that reveal racial discrimination. Acknowledging the existence of racial discrimination and racial hierarchies challenges the myth of the meritocracy. When White Americans realize that they benefit from the privilege of white skin, at the expense of others who are denied those privileges, their personal sense of self-worth may be threatened (McIntosh, 1989).

Finally, Tatum (1992) notes as a third reason for the avoidance of talk about race that racism in the United States is not restricted to the activities of overtly racist organizations, like the Ku Klux Klan (KKK) with its cross burnings and lynchings. Racism is also expressed in subtle, but equally troubling, individual everyday acts. The acknowledgment of personal as opposed to institutional racism and the personal responsibility for eliminating racism in the United States may be difficult for some persons to process (Holzman, 1995).

Some therapists may neglect to pursue their clients' racially based experiences because they believe that racism no longer exists. Others may believe that African Americans are overly sensitive about race and habitually use racism as an excuse for not succeeding to the same degree as others (both European

Americans and other persons of color). Yet others may fear that a discussion about racism may prompt the African American to become angry or even violent (Grier & Cobbs, 1968).

Some African American therapists avoid the subject of race because they fear that the patient's narratives may evoke painful memories for them. Others may believe that African Americans can and should be able to accommodate a certain (undefined) level of racism without complaining about it. These beliefs are reflected in comments like "Things used to be a lot worse," "At least people are not being lynched like in the past," and "Folks don't use the 'n' word in your face . . . for the most part." These comments suggest that because racism is not as obvious in public forums or not as routinely and overtly vicious as it used to be, that it should be a lot easier to negotiate, less dangerous, and less painful (Lipsky, 1987).

For some therapists, racial silence may reflect a lack of awareness of race as a part of their life experiences. They may feel that the salience or lack thereof in their own lives is generalizable to other people, even other people who are members of different ethnic groups. This is a common ethnocentric perspective. The salience of race as an important social characteristic is an inevitable part of living in the United States. In her groundbreaking work, Frankenberg (1993) documents the existence of racial themes in the lives of White women in this country, including women raised in all-White communities. Her analysis examines the complexity of White people's "thinking through race" on many levels simultaneously, including race, race difference, racism and its impact, and the self in a racially positioned society.

African American patients may seek to "protect" themselves or the therapist by self-censoring, that is, by withholding the disclosure of certain memories. Black-on-Black traumas may be easier for some therapists to hear since they are consistent with distorted and demeaning cultural images of Blacks (Riggs, 1987, 1991). Some African American patients may refuse to reveal such traumas, however, because they believe that by doing so they may reinforce the European American therapist's negative stereotypes concerning the Black race. Traumatic experiences with White perpetrators and Black victims or with Black perpetrators and White victims are also difficult to disclose. Neither Blacks nor Whites may feel comfortable discussing such events as interracial relationships, especially negative ones, in mixed company. White therapists may wish to avoid feeling guilty or ashamed or angry; Black patients may seek either to protect their White therapists from such feelings to guard against damaging the therapeutic alliance or to hide their own hurt and negative feelings. A critical consequence may be that questions about traumatic memories related to race may never be asked and those topics never explored in therapy.

Therapists and patients may differ in their capacity and willingness to discuss racial issues. If both deny race as a possible factor in their lives, then memories regarding race and racism will be excluded by mutual consent from the therapy hour. It is helpful if the therapist assumes a "valuing differences" position. This position implies a receptivity to issues related to race and provides the African American patient with a "protective" mode to preserve the relationship. In this way, the therapist can create a supportive context that allows racial memories to emerge.

Guthrie (1995) provides an evocative example of a racial memory. Carol, an African American woman, recalled an incident that took place when she was 5 years old. Her best friend, Sharon, a Jewish girl, was about to have a birthday party. Carol was not invited. When she confronted Sharon about her exclusion, Sharon was unable to answer her. "Instead, she rubbed her right thumb on the skin of her left forearm just below the elbow. Then Carol understood. Her skin was black and because of that she could not attend the party." This incident had psychological sequelae for Carol that endured into her adulthood. Another therapist, the mother of an African American girl, told a similar story recently at a professional conference. This time the year was 1995 and the 9-year-old girls were African American and European American. Such race-based, traumatic memories and their cumulative effects are very painful "microaggressions" (Pierce, 1988).

The issue of African women and their hair is an important example of context when discussing racial issues. At a professional symposium on women, I heard a prominent White female scholar make the statement that all Black women wear their hair straight because "they want to be White and hate their blackness." Sitting at the same table was a Black woman scholar with straight hair. The White woman's assumption was outrageously ethnocentric, and could be regarded as a racialized assault on a fellow professional. The perceived intent was to silence the Black woman scholar with straight hair, that is, to score a scholarly knockout. Despite this assault, the Black woman scholar took the opportunity to point out that one cannot determine the politics or the stage of racial identity of a Black woman by her hairstyle alone. Although the Black woman responded quickly and appropriately to her attacker, the disparaging personal statement that was made about her hair, in an open professional forum, constituted a form of racial assault. Once the generalization was made, she was forced to negotiate it on both conscious and unconscious levels. The Black scholar could have added that some Black women have naturally straight hair because of mixed European American and Native American ancestry.

Current (1990s) events that include race as a dominant theme have prompted some African American women patients to speak more openly about the impact of race in their lives. Informal reports by African American therapists suggest that the Clarence Thomas–Anita Hill U.S. Senate hearing, the Rodney King beating incident, the trial of the Los Angeles police officers who beat King and the subsequent riots, the O. J. Simpson trial and verdict, and the "Million Man March" have all been introduced into therapy sessions by African American women patients. Therapy offered a place for some African

American women to process their feelings about these complex events. Such discussions provided an opportunity for therapists to explore patients' perceptions of the reactions European Americans had to African Americans and themselves in particular, and the meaning of the events for them personally and for the African American community at large. For some women, these events helped to surface memories of personal, familial, and community racial trauma and other forms of trauma.

Besides the above issues related to racial silence in therapy, some Black women who have been raised as "race women" rather than as "gender women" may struggle with another kind of racial silence. Gender silence for African American women (Crenshaw, 1992; Daniel, 1995) has meant that those African American women who have been traumatized by African American men have remained silent rather than involve the authorities (police, judicial, and penal systems) associated with racism toward African Americans. To have filed charges would have incurred the personal risk of being accused of racial disloyalty for placing an African American man in places where he would be vulnerable to racial abuse. The Clarence Thomas–Anita Hill Senate hearing, for example, triggered memories of silenced personal trauma and family secrets of sexual victimization. Such silence may have been "for the good of the race," but was bad for the individual females. The traumatic memories stimulated by the hearing were twofold: the initial victimization and then the denial of it.

Finally, the different constructions of African American women by the mental health community (which will be discussed more fully below) generally do not allow African American women to be recognized as victims of sexual trauma. The historical social constructions of African American women and the reconstructions (Daniel, 1995) that emerged from the Thomas–Hill hearing suggested that many Whites only view a Black woman as a "real" victim when she has first been deraced, that is, regarded as a White woman. Thus the state of being deraced, not really being Black, becomes the condition for being recognized as a victim. This adds another layer of trauma to an already complex picture. It is traumatic to deny or to diminish one's identity to be recognized, yet many Black women have memories of such demands and their compliance, often as silence, as a survival mechanism.

## IMAGE DISTORTION AS TRAUMA

The social constructions of African American women have been woven into the fabric of American society for hundreds of years. Marlon Riggs's classic film documentaries *Ethnic Notions* (1987) and *Color Adjustment* (1991) are critical resources for understanding the importance of image-making. *Ethnic Notions* chronicles 150 years of negative images of African Americans in popular culture up to the television age. *Color Adjustment* examines the impact of television on the images of African Americans in America, placing television shows in the sociopolitical contexts of the eras in which they were created. The images of African Americans are painfully negative or absent.

In the media the physical features of African Americans have been distorted to make them appear grotesque. Examples are "fright hair," unkempt hair standing up straight on top of the head as though the person had been electrocuted; grossly elongated thick lips; enlarged eyes; and the portrayal of African American children as more animal than human. Stereotypic characters were further distorted, as in the Mammy, who was depicted as cruel to her own children while kind to White children. Cartoons were particularly damaging in their portrayal of African Americans because they used humor effectively to mask rabid racism. Such visual images were (and are) a source of psychological trauma for Blacks. They taught some African Americans to hate those physical characteristics that were distorted and ridiculed. The intended results were self-hatred for African Americans and a sense of superiority for European Americans.

How have African American women been depicted in America? According to the motion picture and television industries, Black women are maids who are more loyal to their White employers and their families than to their own families (i.e., the Mammy image). Black women are sexually available, loose, and immoral (i.e., the Jezebel image). Black women are demanding, self-sufficient, and demeaning of Black men, as seen in the notoriously stereotypic TV program *Amos 'n Andy*, (i.e., the Sapphire image). Black women are the mothers of the criminals who terrorize good people and themselves are financial parasites (i.e., the Welfare Queen image). Or she is the very light-skinned African American woman who is often portrayed as "passing for White" and living in fear that her secret will be discovered (i.e., the Tragic Mulatto image). In a more recent image, she is the "super African American woman," in the persona of Claire Huxtable on the *Bill Cosby Show*, a popular television program of the 1980s. She manages a home without any domestic help, holds a high-powered job, and somehow manages to be always glamorous (Ward, 1993).

Each of these images is related to the relative value of the African American woman in a racist society. The Mammy, who is in effect a functionary, that is, primarily valued by her functioning in the lives of the White people she serves, may be the only woman of some value (Daniel, 1995). The other images are not valuable, and, one may infer, not worthy of sympathy as victims. Even the Claire Huxtable image would not necessarily generate sympathy. Any woman who is that accomplished, it is presumed, can take care of herself and everyone else (i.e., she is an "upgraded Sapphire").

The reconstructions of African American women that emerged from the Thomas–Hill hearings (Crenshaw, 1992; Daniel, 1995; Lubiano, 1992; McKay, 1992; Painter, 1992) are problematic. The first image is that of the mentally unstable woman, to raise issues is to disturb the status quo; one must be mentally ill to do so. The "mentally ill" complainer is easily dismissed or ignored, and her complaints can be labeled as trivial, irrelevant, and lacking merit. The second image is that of the Affirmative Action person, a more modern and successful cousin of the "Welfare Queen." Both are the recipients of unmerited compensation. The third image is the strange African American woman who is responsible for the oddness in the African American family. Her achievements are cited as the cause for the disproportionate number of African American men who have "failed" to achieve. Usually single, she is seen as having taken a place that should be occupied by an African American man. She, rather than a racist society, is blamed for the plight of the African American man and the African American family. The final image is that of the deraced woman, that is, an individual who is seen as just a woman. In American society, the emblematic woman is European American. It is in that image that the African American woman can be a victim.

Memories of the distorted images of African American women are a source of racial trauma for African American women. Therapists practicing today were raised with a steady viewing of these distorted images, which in turn became their "reality" of what African Americans are. Current reruns of old movies and old television series perpetuate these negative images. The constructions and reconstructions of the African American woman have also effectively limited not only society's perceptions of the African American women as victims, but also some Black women's perceptions of the legitimacy of their own victimizing experiences. Denial of the victim state compounds the trauma. The position presented in this chapter is that race is related to the experience of trauma, not only as a source of trauma, but as a force shaping its acknowledgment and its outcomes.

## EXAMPLES OF TRAUMATIC RACIAL MEMORIES

Current conceptions of trauma focus primarily on child abuse (physical and sexual) and domestic violence. For the past 2 decades, the recognition of child abuse and domestic violence in patient populations has been included in education and training for mental health professionals. While these sources of trauma have been a part of some African American women's experience, other sources of trauma also exist for African American women that derive from living in a racist society.

To hear the traumatic racial memories of African American women, therapists must expand their cognitive and affective lenses to include the real racialized lives of African American women. If permitted to talk about race, what might African American women reveal in therapy? Giving therapists examples of racial memories might increase the possibility of race being allowed into the therapy hour, that is, therapists' fear of listening to memories of racial trauma may decrease. The result could be that racial memories, both traumatic and positive, would no longer be effectively excluded by patient and therapist. Most of the remainder of this chapter focuses on historical and contemporaneous racial trauma in the lives of African American women.

This section discusses sexual trauma, violence (actual and threatened) and trauma, law enforcement and judicial trauma, medical trauma, educational trauma, economic trauma (in employment and housing), and trauma associated with social activism. The traumas are varied. Some will reflect personal experiences, but others will constitute trauma as a function of witnessing events involving kin, friends, and community members. Some will be trauma engendered by media presentations. However, others will be prompted by listening to family narratives and community folklore, and some by reading fictive and nonfictive depictions of African American women's lives.

Greene (1995a) writes:

> My parents are "survivors" of an American "holocaust," the Mississippi and Georgia of the late 1920s through the late 1940s. For those unfamiliar with the racism of the rural south, my father's walk to school would include passing a tree whose branches held "strange fruit." "Strange fruit" was the term made famous by the Billie Holiday classic of the same name, calling up the macabre images of the work of Southern lynch mobs. Strange fruits were the dead bodies of Black men hanging by the neck, often castrated and visibly disfigured. (p. 303)

"The American holocaust" refers to the trauma heaped upon African American individuals because of slavery, segregation, and ongoing racism. The intersection of history and racial trauma in the lives of African American women is littered with many untold stories. Just as the descendants of the European Holocaust associated with World War II have needed to process the trauma of its Holocaust survivors, so do the descendants and survivors of the American holocaust (Gump, 1997).

Current incidents that are reminders of the reality of the American holocaust of racism often trigger patients' memories and disclosures of racial trauma. Take, for example, the Susan Smith case in South Carolina, in which a mother falsely identified the kidnapper of her children as a "Black man" when she in fact had murdered them herself; a recent lawsuit related to the burning of an all-Black town in Florida in the 1920s; the apology of a White man to the family of a Black man who had been framed for a murder and then killed by the same White men; the recent passage of legislation in Mississippi that finally outlawed slavery; and the burning of more than 100 Black churches. All these events have been *recent* racial news items. In the exploration of patients' feelings about these emotionally laden news items, memories of personal racial traumas surfaced and their disclosures allowed important therapeutic work to continue. These incidents provided important opportunities for therapists to help their African American patients understand their current interactions with European Americans, and explore how prior experiences may continually affect their current relationships. Additionally, these experiences have affected their sense of power and belonging in predominantly racist contexts, and impacted their problem-solving strategies.

## Sexual Trauma

For readers, fiction written by African American women can provide insight into trauma and its effects. For others, the narration's merit is in its literary style and content. Such a response can reduce African American women's trauma to being an interesting story at best and an entertainment at worst. Walker (1982), Cooper (1987), and Petry (1946) are just a few of the African American female writers whose African American women characters are sexually assaulted by White men. Several of these stories illustrate the reality that African American women who worked as domestics were especially vulnerable to the sexual advances of White male employers, a continuation of practices from the era of slavery (Giddings, 1984). Wade-Gayles (1993), in her autobiography, remembers being warned to run away from White men who would cruise through her community seeking sex from African American females of any age.

In her autobiographical play, *From the Mississippi Delta*, Endesha Ida Mae Holland (1993) depicts her rape at age 11 by a White man. She had been hired as a babysitter in the home of the family. The mother literally led this child to her husband's bed. As a young woman, African American, and poor, Ms. Holland was powerless to defend herself from this sexual assault that had a profound impact on her life. In the play, her character remarks that she stopped being a child that day. The year was 1955. Other now-adult Endesha Ida Mae Hollands have suffered similar sexual traumas as children and adolescents.

For African American women who work with White men, experiences and perceptions of White men as sexual predators who do not have to be accountable for their behavior toward African American female victims can be very problematic. These perceptions are reinforced when White men continue some form of this behavior and abuse of power, for example, sexual harassment, sexualized jokes, and displays of distorted images of African American women. The women's resulting feeling of anger, disgust, and victimization can be intensified by childhood racial memories.

## Violence (Actual and Threatened) and Trauma

Physical and psychological violence, both actual and threatened, have been directed at African American people for centuries. Painter (1995), in an essay entitled "Soul Murder and Slavery," documents extensive violence toward

African slaves. Racial violence continues even today. The recent pattern of burning Black churches exemplifies attempts to intimidate the African American community. Historically, burnings, beatings, and lynching have been the primary tools of "White on Black" violence in the United States.

In my practice, I have listened to patients' memories of persons being secreted out of the African American community in the dead of the night to save them from angry Whites. Any reason—fabricated transgressions, anger, or even the desire to be entertained—was sufficient cause for deadly force against African Americans. While the KKK is most associated with such actions, participants have not been limited to members of the Klan. Abuses have been perpetrated by law enforcement officers, the very arm of society charged with the prevention of such activities and the protection of all citizens.

Especially in the Jim Crow South, in KKK-like enclaves in other sections of the United States, and in urban centers, racial violence has been an ever-present threat to African American families. Patricia Williams (1991) writes about an incident in the late 1950s when her family was traveling through the South and their car was stopped by the police. As her parents were being questioned, one police officer pointed a gun directly at her head while she sat in the back seat of the car. Under these circumstances, African American parents were powerless to protect their children from trauma, thereby compounding their own trauma.

The clinical and literary narratives of African American women reveal the realities of persecution based on race, including the murder of their fathers and brothers by racists and African American men being falsely accused of crimes committed by Whites. In my clinical work, I have found that most of these stories are related in muted tones. Patients often report that when they have attempted to retrieve details of violent events in the family history, older family members appeared very uneasy about even recounting such events in their lives. At times, it has required considerable effort and much persuasion to retrieve the missing pieces of a traumatic event in the family history. In some families, the fates of the murdered persons are withheld from the younger generation to protect them from painful stories. In other cases, the stories are told to the young people to warn them about the danger associated with angry Whites. The reality is that many African American children grow up with an inescapable sense that being in the company of Whites is very dangerous because of their race and that they cannot count on protection from the larger, that is, White, society when they are in danger. Such perceptions can result in a sense of physical and psychological vulnerability and a state of hypervigilance, the feeling of never being able to let down one's guard when in the company of Whites. Psychological consequences of past and current racial violence clearly affect issues of trust and respect in interracial relationships today.

## Law Enforcement and Judicial Trauma

Most African Americans do not view the savage beating of Rodney King by Los Angeles police as an anomaly in the treatment of African American men by law enforcement personnel. In the African American community stories abound of individuals being harassed by the police, for example, being stopped because they were considered suspicious just for being African American. To decrease the likelihood of police brutality, African American parents expend considerable energy trying to persuade their children, especially their sons, to be very cooperative and even docile when stopped by the police. The Rodney King beating reminded many African American individuals of police brutality they themselves had experienced, witnessed, or heard about from kin and friends. These memories are often accompanied by feelings of intense anger at law enforcement officials' refusal to recognize that most African Americans are not criminals. For example, Williams (1991) relates an incident that occurred at a Miami-area diner in the 1970s in which a police officer and an eight-member SWAT team converged on three African American women after one refused to pay for a glass of sour milk. Intimidation and excessive use of force by the police continue to create a siege state for African Americans in this country.

The judicial system has also been the site of trauma for African American women. Race is a major determinant of treatment in the courts. Reports of disrespect toward African Americans and demeaning lectures by judges are all part of the story of being an African American woman in court. Anger, anxiety, and avoidance of the judicial system may be consequences of memories of actual experiences or stories related about abuses involving African Americans in the judicial system. Therapists who treat African American women who have been or are involved in the judicial system (as either plaintiff or defendant, in civil or criminal court) need to be sensitive to these issues and their consequences.

## Medical Trauma

Many African American women experience medical institutions and their staff as hostile and threatening. Although some African American women feel that they will be adequately treated by the health professionals, others have been traumatized by acts of medical omission and commission. Reproduction issues have been a major concern for African American women. In contrast to the slavery era, when Black births contributed to the economy as merchandise and labor, the emphasis now is on decreasing the number of births to single women in the African American community. The issue of involuntary sterilization has been a concern, especially for women who are welfare recipients.

The disproportionate and at times inappropriate use of African Americans for medical research is also a concern. The Tuskegee Study is one of the most flagrant examples of medical abuse in the name of science in the history of the United States. In 1932, 400 African American males in Macon County, Alabama, were denied treatment for syphilis in a study conducted by the U.S. Public Health Service. The researchers misrepresented the study to the men, who were falsely led to believe that they were the recipients of medical care. While the study involved men, they had wives who were also affected by their illnesses and who also were not treated. The revelation of this 40-year study only confirmed the suspicions of many African Americans regarding racism and lack of integrity in the field of medicine. The syphilis could have been treated with antibiotics. The descendants of this study are living today. Minimal compensation was provided to the survivors and their relatives by the federal government. The small amount of the settlement was a message that African American lives have little value.

Traumatic medical memories include the loss of relatives who died enroute to distant sites seeking medical care, having been denied access to nearby "White-only" medical facilities. Women recall the era when some White physicians would not treat African Americans. African American physicians were routinely denied hospital privileges. Health care options were limited. Simultaneously, White physicians would treat African Americans, but only on certain days of the week and if they entered the building through the back door. Separate and unequal medical wards based on racial segregation are also in the memory banks of many African Americans today. Medical care and indignity thus have been merged in memories. Experiences including premature discharge from the hospital, inappropriate medication, poor care, and neglect in the hospital have been reported. Complaints abound of no information, conflicting information, and rude treatment by the care providers. Many African Americans continue to feel that they do not have access to the same level of care provided to Whites. The act of seeking services at health facilities can be experienced as being placed at risk for psychological abuse and inadequate medical care.

## Trauma in Educational Settings

The image of African Americans as intellectually inferior was needed to justify slavery despite the reality that the plantation system depended on the intelligence, resourcefulness, and skills of slaves. To keep slaves "in their place," teaching slaves to read was illegal. Scientific racism practiced in support of the sociopolitical system "documented" the inherent inferiority of Blacks (Greene, 1995b). In the Jim Crow era, segregated housing patterns generated segregated schools in the North and in the South. The schools for African American children were consistently housed in inferior structures;

teachers were provided with outdated and inadequate teaching materials. Consequently, in the United States, the overwhelming majority of African Americans have not received the same quality of education as Whites. Residual thinking about the alleged limited intellectual capacity continues to undermine the educational experiences of many African American children and adults.

Publications such as Jacoby and Glauberman's *The Bell Curve Debate* (1995), which offer empirical and theoretical analyses to counter arguments about African American inferiority, have been limited in effectiveness to redress this long-standing perspective. In the late 1960s and early 1970s, well-intentioned educational programs were developed for the "culturally deprived." Unfortunately, this term conveyed the message of inferiority and must be regarded as a particularly distressing and demeaning label given the appropriation of African American culture, in the form of music, language, and style, by Whites in this country (hooks, 1992). Unfortunately, some educators treated the children as though they were culturally deprived or at best culturally disadvantaged. The latter term was only a little less insulting. Learning in a context of presumed cultural deprivation and disadvantage was a challenge for African American children, teacher aids, and other African American adults (parents and professionals) associated with the programs. The ambivalence experienced by those who were aware of the implications of the labels made for less-than-ideal work settings. Therefore, in some places, countering internalized racism became an unspoken part of the curriculum.

Currently successful African American women who attended first desegregated and later integrated schools as children have memories of placement in remedial classes. Elementary-school memories with Black girls in the "black bird" reading group and White girls in the "blue bird" reading group are still vivid and painful. Assertive and persistent Black mothers were sometimes successful in rescuing their daughters from low and remedial groups. African American women proudly recall being placed in the high groups after such maternal actions. For the African American young woman, school became a daily battleground to prove to an embittered teacher that her mother had been right, that is, that she belonged in the high group, the honors class, or the advanced placement class.

Even today, academically gifted African American students may avoid honors and advanced placement classes because of the hostility of White teachers and professors. Sometimes abuse appears in the form of racist examination questions and class examples (Williams, 1991). When African American students protest, the response is often that they are being "too sensitive" or that the examples have been used for years and no one has ever objected before. African American women's memories of trauma in educational settings can have an impact on confidence in their intellectual skills. Even if African American women feel smart enough, they frequently dread the added burden of having to be twice as good as Whites in order for their skills and accomplishments to be recognized.

## Economic Trauma (Employment and Housing)

Cose's *The Rage of a Privileged Class* (1993) identified 12 "demons" experienced by African American middle-class persons who work in integrated job settings: inability to fit in, exclusion from the club, shattered hopes, faint praises, perception of failure, coping fatigue, pigeonholing, identity troubles, self-censorship, silence, mendacity, and guilt by association. Many examples are provided to illustrate daily racial trauma experienced by those who have "made it in White America." Being successful offers little if any protection from racial trauma. African Americans employed in lower level jobs are often targets of more overt racial trauma. Work has been the primary war zone of racial trauma for African American women.

Housing is another site of racial trauma and stress for Black women. In the United States, segregated housing is the normative pattern. Moving into integrated communities can be the beginning of racially motivated harassment that may result in the family opting to move out for safety reasons, both physical and psychological. These incidents have occurred and continue to occur across the United States. Loan officers continue to practice discrimination that perpetuates segregation in housing. African Americans have difficulty in securing bank loans, especially when they seek housing in a predominantly White community for those who persist in seeking a mortgage, the experience can be degrading and difficult, not to mention potentially unsuccessful.

## Traumas Associated with Social Activism

African Americans who have been active with civil rights initiatives have suffered from the assaults of Whites who seek to stop such activities. History documents the bombing of the homes of civil rights workers in the 1960s. Relatives are living today of those who were murdered and wounded for daring to challenge a racist society. The memories of the deceased's relatives are alive in the family narratives. Viewing public assaults on African American women has been traumatic for many Black women in this country. Examples are Dr. Joycelyn Elders, the former surgeon general of the United States, who was called the "condom queen," and Professor Lani Guinier, a presidential nominee, who was called the "quota queen." Except in the entertainment world, whenever the term "queen" is bestowed on an African American woman by the White press, it has a pejorative meaning. The intelligent, vocal, active, and thinking African American woman is an easy target for abuse and ridicule. Witness how political cartoonists distorted Lani Guinier's hair to make it look like "fright hair."

## LEGEND LADIES AND THE LEGACY OF LIBERATION

Talking about race in the African American community has been therapeutic, especially when individuals have shared how they have dealt and continue to deal with racist remarks and behaviors. Silence about racism leads to limited ways to "manage racism" and to potential internalized racism, that is, self-blame and self-hate. Discussions that acknowledge the existence of racism do not yield problems. Rather, they create solutions and something just as important: hope. Older African American women who tell their stories about racism and racists are critical community resources. They are "legend ladies" who speak about "managing racism" and accurately label racism as wrong. Their stories provide proof that some individuals have survived racists by using their wits and their faith. The legend ladies wisely point out that today's racism is just a version of the old racism. Initially, African American women may not recall the legend ladies in their lives—trying to find the headline "legend ladies" such as Harriet Tubman, Sojourner Truth, Ida B. Wells, or Mary McLeod Bethune (Giddings, 1984). Most African American communities have legend ladies who are identified as the catalysts for a range of changes in their communities. Once African American women identify these women, they can begin to remember and pursue the legend ladies' stories.

Using wisdom often cloaked in humor, the legend ladies' stories tell of triumph and the preservation of self-respect. Armed with these stories and drawing on the strength of the legend ladies, African American women can fast-forward their thoughts into the current era and better manage today's racism.

## SUMMARY: USING MEMORIES OF RACIAL
## TRAUMA IN THERAPY

Toni Morrison (1992a) states that it is problematic to be less than honest about the past. The truth is that race matters in the lives of African American women. It may be related to trauma and their response to trauma. To deny this reality in psychotherapy is effectively to limit the memories that African American women will reveal in treatment. Therapists who have been provided with examples of racial trauma may be more willing to create a therapeutic milieu that will welcome uncensored memories of African American women that include racial trauma. Discussing racial trauma in the therapeutic hour also gives the African American woman client a reality check. Excluding racial trauma from their therapy work is usual for many African Americans, because of the belief that there is nothing to be done. Clients also fail to bring racial trauma to the therapy hour because of the "victim" nature of their response. Contemporary racial trauma is of the unobtrusive type, very subtle, and often clients blame themselves for their circumstance. Whether the client is experiencing anxiety, depression, or posttraumatic stress disorder–like symptoms, it is important for the therapist to help clients make connections to the experiences in their lives and not have them believe it is something within themselves that is at fault. Working through the resistance that might interfere with acknowledging the trauma associated with racially degrading experiences is necessary for the therapist. It is also an opportunity for the therapist to strengthen the therapeutic alliance with African American women clients because of the empathy needed to hear and understand these narratives. Another added benefit of strengthening the therapeutic alliance is giving the client permission to take care of herself and to receive nurturing, which is very difficult for some African American women to do. Typically, they nurture everyone else. The strength and resiliency necessary for that role is often not enough to protect her from the cumulative effect of racial memories or racial trauma.

A therapeutic environment that will allow for the processing of a range of traumas can contribute to the healing process for African American women patients. This form of narrative therapy is appropriate in both individual and group modalities. This intervention is a valuable tool for therapists whatever their theoretical orientation. However, for the therapist working from a psychodynamic perspective, it allows the therapist to understand both the inside and the outside effects of racism and how the African American woman client has understood and responded to that racism.

Perhaps in the future therapists will be more open to exploring the role of race in the lives of their White patients as well. Therapy can be a place of liberation for all who seek services. Informed therapists do not require that patients check their race, gender, class, sexual orientation, or trauma at the door before they enter the therapy room.

## REFERENCES

Cooper, J. C. (1987). Redwinged blackbirds. In J. C. Cooper, *Some soul to keep* (pp. 66–95). New York: St. Martin's Press.

Cose, E. (1993). *The rage of a privileged class.* New York: HarperCollins.

Crenshaw, K. (1992). Whose story is it anyway? Feminist and antiracist appropriations of Anita Hill. In T. Morrison (Ed.), *Race-ing, justice, en-gendering power* (pp. 402–440). New York: Pantheon Books.

Daniel, J. (1994). Exclusion and emphasis reframed as a matter of ethics. *Ethics and Behavior, 4*(3), 229–235.

Daniel, J. (1995). The discourse on Thomas vs. Hill: A resource for perspectives on the Black woman and sexual trauma. *Journal of Feminist Family Therapy, 7*(1–2), 103–117.

Dines, G. (1995). A feminist sociologist responds to Daniel's "exclusion and emphasis reframed as a matter of ethics." *Ethics and Behavior, 5*(4), 369–391.

Frankenberg, R. (1993). *White women, race matters*. Minneapolis, MN: University of Minnesota Press.

Garcia, M. (1995). Responsibility versus defensiveness: Inclusion of ethnicity in the conceptualization of theory. *Ethics and Behavior, 5*(4), 373–375.

Giddings, P. (1984). *When and where I enter*. New York: Bantam Books.

Greene, B. (1994a). Diversity and difference: The issue of race in feminist therapy. In M. P. Mirkin (Ed.), *Women in context* (pp. 333–351). New York: Guilford Press.

Greene, B. (1994b). African American women. In L. Comas-Díaz & B. Greene (Eds.), *Women of color: Integrating ethnic and gender identities in psychotherapy* (pp. 10–29). New York: Guilford Press.

Greene, B. (1995a). An African American perspective in racism and anti-Semitism within feminist organizations. In J. Adelman & G. Enguidanos (Eds.), *Racism in the lives of women* (pp. 303–313). New York: Haworth Press.

Greene, B. (1995b). Institutional racism in the mental health professions. In J. Adleman & G. Enguidanos (Eds.), *Racism in the lives of women* (pp. 113–126). New York: Haworth Press.

Grier, W., & Cobbs, P. (1968). *Black rage*. New York: Basic Books.

Gump, J. (1997). *Rage and sorrow in the African American family: Sequelae of slavery and an American trauma*. Paper presented at the Miniconvention on Racism at the annual meeting of the American Psychological Association, Chicago.

Guthrie, P. (1995). Racism in academia: A case study. In J. Adleman & G. Enguidanos (Eds.), *Racism in the lives of women* (pp. 44–54). New York: Haworth Press.

Herman, J. (1992). *Trauma and recovery*. New York: Basic Books.

Holland, E. (1993). *From the Mississippi Delta*. Boston: Huntington Theatre.

Holzman, C. (1995). Rethinking the role of guilt and shame in White women's antiracism work. In J. Adelman & G. Enguidanos (Eds.), *Racism in the lives of women: Theory, testimony and guides to practice* (pp. 325–332). New York: Haworth Press.

hooks, b. (1992). *Black looks*. Boston: South End Press.

Jacoby, R., & Glauberman, N. (Eds.). (1995). *The bell curve debate*. New York: Random House.

Lipsky, S. (1987). Internalized racism. *Black Re-emergence, 2*, 1–17.

Lubiano, W. (1992). Black ladies, welfare queens, and state minstrels: Ideological war by narrative means. In T. Morrison (Ed.), *Race-ing, justice, en-gendering power* (pp. 323–363). New York: Pantheon Books.

McIntosh, P. (1989, July–August). White privilege: Unpacking the invisible knapsack. *Peace and Freedom*, pp. 10–12.

McKay, N. (1992). Remembering Anita Hill and Clarence Thomas: What really happened when one Black woman spoke out. In T. Morrison (Ed.), *Race-ing, justice, en-gendering power* (pp. 269–289). New York: Pantheon Books.

Melendez, M. (1995). Blind spots and clinical training. *Ethics and Behavior, 5*(4), 359–367.

Morrison, T. (1992a). *A conversation with Toni Morrison* [Videotape]. (Available from California Newsreel, 149 Ninth St./420, San Francisco, CA 94103)

Painter, N. (1992). Hill, Thomas, and the use of racial stereotype. In T. Morrison (Ed.), *Race-ing, justice, en-gendering justice* (pp. 200–214). New York: Pantheon Books.

Painter, N. (1995). Soul murder and slavery: Toward a fully loaded cost accounting. In L. Kerber, A. Kessler-Harris, & K. Sklar (Eds.), *U.S. history as women's history* (pp. 125–146). Chapel Hill, NC: University of North Carolina Press.

Petry, A. (1946). *The street.* Boston: Beacon Press.

Pierce, C. M. (1988). Stress in the workplace. In A. F. Comer-Edwards & J. Spurlock (Eds.), *Black middle class families in crisis* (pp. 27–33). New York: Brunner-Mazel.

Riggs, M. (1987). *Ethnic notions* [Video documentary]. (Available from California Newsreel, 149 Ninth St./420, San Francisco, CA 94103)

Riggs, M. (1991). *Color adjustment* [Video documentary]. (Available from California Newsreel, 149 Ninth St./420, San Francisco, CA 94103)

Sanchez, W., & Nuttall, E. (1995). It's about time. *Behavior and Ethics, 5*(4), 355–357.

Spelman, E. (1988). *Inessential woman.* Boston: Beacon Press.

Tatum, B. D. (1992). Talking about racism, learning about racism: The application of racial identity development theory in the classroom. *Harvard Educational Review, 62*(1), 1–24.

Wade-Gayles, G. (1993). *Pushed back to strength.* Boston: Beacon.

Walker, A. (1982). *The color purple.* New York: Harcourt Brace Jovanovich.

Ward, K. (Producer). (1993). *From Aunt Jemima to Claire Huxtable: Images of African American women on screen* [Videotape]. (Available from Links, Inc., Boston, MA)

Wilkins, S. (1995). Response to Herman and Daniel. *Ethics and Behavior, 5*(4), 377–378.

Williams, P. (1991). *The alchemy of race and rights.* Cambridge, MA: Harvard University Press.

## CHAPTER 7

# The African American Supervisor
## Racial Transference and Countertransference in Interracial Psychotherapy Supervision

### MICHELE OWENS-PATTERSON

In recent years a focus on multicultural competency and the delivery of mental health services has emerged. It is partially due to the changing demographic face of America, where more than 50% of the population of the United States will be people of color shortly after the year 2050 (Cravatta et al., 1997). Moreover, these demographic changes will impact the non-Caucasian clinicians trained to deliver mental health services, and to interpret and reinterpret traditional theory and clinical practices for the benefit of a more varied racial and ethnic patient group.

As an increasing number of people of color have entered the ranks of mental health practitioners, the configuration of treatment dyads (and triads) has changed. Traditionally, White clinicians have treated most patients of any color (Bradshaw, 1982). With the entry of greater numbers of therapists who are people of color, patients have begun to be treated by persons of a wider range of ethnic backgrounds. Furthermore, as African American clinicians credentialed in the 1970s through the 1980s matured in their careers, the complexion of senior clinicians, teachers, and supervisors changed. Thus, the potential in treatment for a variety of dynamic interactions and unconscious responses will develop in response to this experience of difference. The examination of this inter- and intraethnic experience in supervision is the focus of this chapter.

## COUNTERTRANSFERENCE IN INTERRACIAL SUPERVISION

The therapeutic process in the ethnically mixed therapeutic dyad can take on a particularly strong character by virtue of the many permutations of transference resistance, countertransference, and counterresistance that might occur. This process is further complicated when the supervisor–supervisee dyad is interracial (or interethnic) and specifically when the supervisor and patient share the same ethnic background. The particular combination of African American supervisor/White therapist/African American patient will be considered here as a paradigm for the discussion of issues in supervision and treatment where interracial (interethnic) treatment situations exist. It is particularly useful as an illustration of the impact of racial/ethnic differences on the way psychotherapy is conducted and of the kind and quality of parallel processes that the interracial (interethnic) triad can elicit in the supervisory space.

Until recently little had been written about the phenomenon of mixed-race supervisor–supervisee dyads. There are many reasons for this situation. First, it may be difficult for many senior clinicians to be objective about their own difficulties in this area. To develop an appropriate awareness of these issues requires a level of self-analysis that makes most people feel uncomfortable. Many trained clinicians have undergone a self-analysis via the psychotherapy that was a part of their professional development. However, such analysis rarely includes issues of race, ethnicity, and the hierarchies of social power and disadvantage that accompany those human distinctions. Before the inclusion of greater numbers of therapists of African American descent in the discipline, such dyads were extremely rare, and thus, easy to ignore. When the supervisor and the supervisee are White and the patient is African American, the same issues are not elicited. Because of the difficulties associated with these explorations, there may be both conscious and unconscious motivation, between supervisors and supervisees, to distance themselves from the kind of material necessary to develop greater insight in this area. Cook (1994) views racial identity development as an integral aspect of both the therapeutic and the supervisory relationship that should be recognized and discussed in supervision.

Another problem is the paucity of formal didactic training in this area. Where it exists, multicultural analyses are often relegated to one course in the curriculum, if covered at all. Minimal treatment of this material sends a message to trainees about the unimportance of considering these matters.

Some earlier papers on the topic focused more on the relationship between the European American supervisor and the foreign trainee (Miller, 1972; Muslin & Val, 1980). Here the issue of the supervisory resistance to the formation of an alliance with the therapist/trainee is highlighted and discussed as the potential for failure to empathize with the supervisee and to "see the patient through his eyes" (Muslin & Val, 1980, p. 547). The problems encountered by the foreign student when he or she is unable to perceive the supervisor as an ally are also examined. This failure occurs as part of a mutual inability and/or resistance to acknowledging differences and examining their meaning. Consequently, the process of emotional learning is blocked as the supervisor fails to empathize and identify with the supervisee's need to secure mirroring, reward, and leadership.

While these ideas have some application to the triadic relationship we are considering here, they do not address the particular forces that are in play when the therapist is the representative of the mainstream or dominant group. Other scenarios where the supervisor is White do not challenge the normative power relationship and the essential question of who is "in charge." When the supervisor is White and the supervisee and patient are both African American, the White supervisor's belief in his or her own normalcy, superiority, or essential "rightness" is assumed, and with that assumption the supervisee's and patient's "difference" may in fact be confirmed. When the supervisor and the patient are African American and the supervisee is White, the supervisee may experience his or her racial/ethnic difference more profoundly because as a supervisee he or she is not, in this triad, the person with power. In my view, the power differential, that is, who has it and who does not, can perpetuate the status quo or elicit greater intensity in these relationships.

Other cross-cultural literature reflects the more frequent pairing of the African American patient with the White therapist (Bradshaw, 1982). This literature seems to fall into three categories. The first category addresses and discusses the reality-based problems that arise in these treatment situations (Sattler, 1970). Differences between therapist and patient in terms of expectations regarding treatment, problems establishing rapport, and misinterpretations due to language barriers and ethnocentrism are highlighted. Additionally, issues such as the differential meanings of the structure of therapy and the values inherent in the various psychotherapeutic approaches are explored (Gardner, 1971; Sue & Sue 1977; Vontress, 1971).

The second category of writings explores the impact of these racially mixed dyads in more classical ways by addressing transferences, countertransferences, and resistances (Holmes, 1992; Schacter & Butts, 1968; Waite, 1968). Gardner (1971) and others (Cavenar & Spaulding, 1978; Curry, 1964; Fischer, 1971; Grier, 1967) have observed that the presence of racial differences can often serve to elicit transferential material earlier and more powerfully than it might otherwise occur. This is particularly the case when the therapist is African American and the client is White, given the richness of meaning of "African American-ness" in this society. However, writers such as Grier (1967) and Waite (1968) emphasize the importance of being able to separate the reality issue from its particular meaning and interpretation for the individual patient. They cite the danger involved in the therapist's overemphasis on the exigencies of a racist society.

The third category of work analyzes the various cultural identifications, ethnic/racial identifications, and gender issues in the supervisory relationship

(Comas-Díaz & Jacobsen, 1987; Cook, 1994; Cook & Hargrove, 1997; Greene, 1985; Holloway, 1998).

Traditionally, the psychotherapy literature (Banks, Berenson, & Carkhuff, 1967; Dorfman & Kleiner, 1962) has not consistently supported the hypotheses of investigators who posit that significant differences exist for the delivery of mental health services when patients are faced with a clinician who is "other" than they (and vice versa). However, a growing body of research does support this notion. Findings have surfaced revealing differential performance of patients on test measures, differential responses in experimental exploration, and differences in depth and length of treatment by clinicians (Sattler, 1970). We are left with the question of how these issues are further complicated when the supervisor, therapist, and patient form a triad in which racial and ethnic difference (and sameness) is a prominent feature. Furthermore, how might the therapist and the supervisor, in their relationship, explore the impact of these differences such that they may maximally help the patient in integrating the reality of the difference with its individual internal meaning for the patient?

Using the paradigm of the African American supervisor, the White therapist/supervisee, and the African American patient, this chapter discusses potential areas of countertransference, resistance, and counterresistance. This paradigm has the potential for a particularly intense experience in the confrontation of the color difference (both in therapy and in supervision) because of the powerful symbolic associations of African American-ness and Whiteness, and the powerful meaning and affect of race and racism in the United States. Symbolic associations to African American-ness might include ideations that range from exoticism, emotional abandon, and exaggerated sexual prowess to ignorance, laziness, and savagery. However, other racial combinations within this triad will be addressed to highlight the potential for similar countertransference issues and all of the projections that come with them.

## COMMON ASPECTS OF SUPERVISORY COUNTERTRANSFERENCE

It is of paramount importance that African American supervisors are aware of their own feelings and beliefs about White therapists treating people of color. The supervisor's own personal history and relationships with White people, as well as what has transpired in his or her own training and clinical experience, can influence the countertransferential feelings aroused in the supervisory space. While typically this topic is not broached in open and ongoing ways with White colleagues and supervisors, it is also an important issue for the White supervisor and the White supervisee to explore. Often such a question is not consciously considered because the circumstance of White therapists treating African American patients is so common that it is experienced as normative.

However, until White clinicians explore their own feelings and beliefs about White therapists treating patients of color, they cannot begin to explore the many unconscious feelings and assumptions likely to exist in their work with African American patients.

For example, I observed a young, White, female psychology intern speak with great ease of her disdain for her African American patients to an African American peer! The ease with which she could express her contempt for African American patients to someone who shared a major locus of identity with them highlights the importance of routinely exploring this material in supervision. The young woman worked in an inner-city private hospital. The catchment area of the facility was inhabited predominantly by African American and Latino patients who were also poor. She complained that her patients were the most "disgusting and disturbed" patients she had ever seen and observed that she longed for the time when she could practice privately in another area. Clearly her feelings, fears, and insecurities in treating people of color who were urban and poor raised intense feelings within her. By their very nature these negative feelings toward her patients, as a group, surely influenced the therapeutic interaction and the quality of the care she delivered to them.

The fact that she could so easily and openly express these negative feelings to an African American colleague is also revealing. Besides demonstrating her obliviousness to the inappropriateness of the content of her comments, it also displays a crude insensitivity to her African American colleague. If she could be this oblivious to a colleague's feelings, how insensitive would she be to the feelings of her patients? It is difficult to believe that someone could maintain this attitude if she were being monitored and her work analyzed effectively either in supervision or in her own therapy. Her comments do not merely convey her personal contempt of and hostility toward people of color, they reveal that this young woman had been denied the opportunity to understand herself in another, less familiar way such that her work with these and other patients might be free of distortions and bring out the best in them both.

The African American supervisor's personal feelings about White persons must also be explored and evaluated for optimum supervision to occur. Frequently, for supervisors of color, these attitudes and feelings are compartmentalized. Most African American clinicians at this level have felt some compatibility with their White peers and/or have learned to project this compatibility. At times the compatibility and congruence are disrupted, often at the end of the workday, so that the full impact of any differences is not felt. Thus, the African American clinician may go home to an experience that reflects more accurately how he or she is "other" than the clinicians with whom he or she is compatible during the day.

This can also occur in the treatment room where the African American supervisor has felt the need to filter selectively, refine, or reject what he or she has learned in ethnocentrically biased training to provide more culturally competent/sensitive treatment to African American patients. Frequently, however, the breaks in sameness and congruence are not confronted. This failure to confront these issues occurs because African American and White clinicians have learned how to interact with each other as professionals and as friends, while ignoring the limitations of interactions that do not address these issues directly. Ignoring the incongruities in their relationships as colleagues often seems necessary to preserve their alliance as colleagues. This can reverberate for the White supervisee such that the supervision proceeds without any recognition of the feelings about the members of the other cultural group. Thus, for example, a White supervisee may struggle to apply a prevailing clinical viewpoint or theoretical framework to a treatment case. If the supervisor has not confronted feelings about White persons and their frequent misconceptions about her cultural group, it may be difficult for her to accept her own adjustments to classical theory as legitimate modifications to traditional approaches. If this occurs, the supervisor may be reluctant to fully share his or her thinking with fledgling clinicians, particularly if they are White. While this has implications for the treatment of the patient, it also leaves the supervisor limited in his or her ability to help supervisees to think more creatively and to explore the potential limitations of traditional theories whose cultural sensitivity is often limited.

African American supervisors must also address their personal feelings and perceptions concerning their roles in supervision. Does the clinician see him- or herself as an agent of change in which he or she will bring something different and special to his or her role as supervisor? Perhaps the supervisor perceives him- or herself to be an instrument of the institution that employs him or her or the product of a mandated requirement for diversity. The perception of one's role in supervision is likely to have an impact on the supervisor's response to the trainee as well as to the material presented, particularly if this perception has not been examined by the supervisor.

This is not to say that the supervisor must deny the presence of certain political realities (requirements for American Psychological Association approval and other forms of certification) and the role of those realities in the hiring of African American supervisors. At times, the presence of supervisors of color in institutions is required as part of a larger mandate. This mandate may include requirements for accreditation, funding purposes, political correctness, or the like. African American clinicians are justified in acknowledging the role that their racial classification is playing under these circumstances. Acknowledging the presence of these realities, and the ways that they can affect your own and others' understanding of what you do and why you are there, is important. Feelings about these matters are often "in the air," with the tension that accompanies them, even if they remain unspoken. It is when they are unspoken that they are most dangerous. However, this creates a particular context for both the supervisor's and the supervisee's perceptions of the supervisory process. If African American supervisors have concerns that their position or employment has more to do with race than with a recognition and appreciation of their skills and ability, there is a heightened potential for these concerns to interfere with the process within the supervision dyad. One possibility is that the African American supervisor might identify with the perceived inferior status of the African American patient. Meanwhile, the White trainee might project inferior status onto the African American patient and supervisor. The projection of these feelings into the supervisory space might also affect the White trainee's perception of his or her own status and/or the quality or usefulness of the supervision he or she is receiving. The White trainee may feel devalued by being assigned to a supervisor whom he or she perceives to belong to a devalued group.

A salient example of the variety of dilemmas confronting African American supervisors is reflected in the following experience of a young African American female supervisor, newly assigned to her supervisory duties. During one of her own supervision meetings, Dr. L was told that she was to "make friends with Ms. K," who was the supervising nurse on the psychiatric unit where Dr. L worked. Dr. L was taken aback by this request and wondered what role this expectation played among the reasons for her promotion to supervisor. Dr. L understood that Ms. K was generally viewed as a strong, assertive, sometimes strident and "difficult" middle-aged African American woman. Dr. L wondered if her new role as supervisor was to render Ms. K more manageable and/or assist in rendering her less "difficult" for other staff to deal with. This in turn led Dr. L to question how she herself was perceived. Was she viewed as a more docile and manageable African American woman from whom her White peers could expect a minimal amount of challenge and/or conflict? What did all of this mean with respect to expectations of how she would supervise both her African American and White subordinates? Was she to avoid controversial or difficult aspects of material her trainees presented? Perhaps she was to ensure the docility of any African American trainees while making certain that her White trainees were not made anxious by aspects of her own or their patients' personalities. Finally, she was left wondering if her concerns, questions, and suspicions about this matter were out of proportion to the realistic magnitude of this request.

Wherever the "truth" of the matter lies, this particular context and the person of the African American supervisor create a new and often unexplored range of possibilities. For African American supervisors, these are significant questions to explore in their understanding of their perception of the supervisory role. To the extent that African American supervisors explore their own feelings, attitudes, and perceptions in this area, it is likely that they can help their supervisees to explore their own feelings as well. Additionally, the impact for both the African American supervisor and the White trainee on how the supervision and the treatment are proceeding can be examined in the richest of fashions when such issues are viewed as essential aspects of the development of the supervisee's cultural and therefore clinical competence.

The experience of the African American supervisor's own supervision is an essential component in the progression of supervision in the mixed triad. The quality and content of the supervisor's supervision, as well as his or her own feelings about how successfully racial/ethnic/cultural issues were addressed in his or her own supervision, typically play an important role in how supervisors currently display their own expertise. The supervisor may have experienced some disappointment due to his or her own supervisor's limitations in this area. As a result, he or she might be prone to attempt to supervise differently, almost in protest to the guidance or lack thereof that he or she experienced in developing skills in cultural competence.

The failure to examine and bring to the surface one's own feelings in this regard can encourage a more active and directive approach toward supervision with less regard for the patient or the supervisee. To ensure that general cultural issues are addressed, a sense of curiosity about the uniqueness of the patient and the supervisee may be lost. What is needed instead is a working through of one's own personal experience of what was lacking in one's own supervision and its impact so that the formulation of a more relevant supervisory experience can occur.

The African American clinician may feel a pull to identify with the patient of color for a variety of reasons. For example, there is often the sense that as another African American person or person of color, one is intrinsically better able to understand and therefore care for an African American patient. However, this belief may in fact reflect the unconscious striving of the African American clinician to take care of him- or herself indirectly by caring for someone with whom he or she identifies. This is of particular import in cases where supervisors see themselves as providers of an alternative to what typically has been available to patients of color, that is, as an alternative to the White, culturally limited, and perhaps even racist clinician. There may be a greater potential for these feelings to be elicited in African American supervisors if they have concerns about how African American patients have been historically ill-treated by mental health professionals, a result of cultural incompetence and ethnocentrism in psychology. Such feelings may also have a greater chance of being elicited if African American supervisors feel themselves to have been personally affected by this history of ill treatment. In such cases, African American supervisors may minimize or ignore the presence of psychopathology out of some unconscious concern that African American patients have been inappropriately overrepresented among persons diagnosed with more serious mental illnesses. There may even be a belief that such diagnoses are always a function of racist thinking. While there is an element of truth in these beliefs, this kind of behavior may ignore the presence of pathology in a patient where it is indeed present, and of course precludes assisting him.

The potential for the occurrence of a parallel process between the supervisor–supervisee and the therapist–patient also exists. White therapists/

supervisees may become anxious about the potential for their own unconscious racial attitudes to leak out into the dyad if they discern that the African American supervisor has concerns about unfairness in the diagnosis and treatment of African American patients. When this occurs, the White supervisee is likely to avoid any direct discussion of these issues. While his or her anxiety may serve to alert the student to the impact of these issues in the therapy, it might also interfere with his or her accurate use of these observations and assessment of the patient. The fear of propagating stereotypical evaluations of African Americans' behavior and inner emotional lives may prevent the delivery of necessary levels of care.

The African American supervisor may also feel compelled to make generalizations about all patients of color based on his or her personal experience. Such supervisors may have an unexamined belief that the experiences that are common to people who face societal discrimination because of their race create a certain universal internal experience that is easily recognized by African Americans. This can interfere with the ability to hear how the individual patient has responded to these issues in his or her own unique way.

For example, an African American supervisor recalled a therapy consultation she had conducted in which the patient, a young African American man, had entered the corporate workforce after finishing college. The patient described feeling a sense of "culture shock" in the new environment with pressure to "mingle" more frequently with coworkers than to affiliate primarily with a more traditional group of his friends. The African American supervisor presumed to feel a sense of recognition of similar circumstances in which the supervisor once felt a pressure to mix with her White counterparts in lieu of establishing close ties to members of her own racial group. She noted later that the look of recognition must have registered fully in her facial expression and nods of understanding, for the patient (to her surprise) shook his head to show "No" and said, "And it's not pressure by my White colleagues. . . . It's pressure by the Blacks here to stick together, eat lunch together, to socialize together after work." He explained that this was foreign to his experience as he had always attended integrated schools, had many White friends, and felt comfortable with a more diverse experience than his current African American peers did.

This story exemplifies how the assumption of common experience can obscure the true communication of the patient. For the African American supervisor, it is necessary to avoid suggesting or imposing these interpretations on the supervisee without allowing for the curiosity, free exploration, and examination of the supervisee's experience with the patient. When the African American supervisor fails to do this, it may unintentionally give the White therapist/supervisee permission to generalize about patients from whom he or she differs. This in turn may represent a means of avoiding any sense of curiosity, ignorance, or anxiety about the experience of the difference. The many permutations of the extent and impact of the therapist/supervisee's ignorance on the therapy are avoided through these generalizations. The White therapist/supervisee's understanding of the patient is now blocked, just as the supervisor's understanding of the therapist/supervisee has been blocked. When this occurs, some cultural issues may be superficially addressed and some differences between therapist and patient noted, but typically it is not apparent to the supervisor and therapist that despite appearances, a substantive analysis of issues of difference has been avoided.

For some African American supervisor/clinicians, there may be a need to avoid identification with the African American patient. This is often a function of the supervisor's own internalized racism. In these cases, the wish to deny or avoid feelings about the impact of race, culture, and racism in one's own life and training may be present (Comas-Díaz & Jacobsen, 1991; Schacter & Butts, 1968). These supervisors may have a tendency to minimize or deny the impact of these variables in the lives of patients, to deny essentially that the patient's race or ethnicity is of any significance in understanding the patient. To avoid being influenced by the consideration of racial or cultural factors, the African American supervisor may bend over backward to understand the patient in more narrow, traditional ways.

Such supervisory behavior may mask negative feelings toward one's own racial group. These may result in a tendency to classify those African American patients the supervisor finds "most embarrassing" or hated as incurable, severely disturbed, lacking the capacity for insight, of low or inadequate intelligence, and so on (Bradshaw, 1982; Calnek, 1970). Additionally, the supervisor may view the patient's material as less worthy of examination and certainly of lesser interest. In more extreme cases, the supervisor may propagate damaging stereotypes concerning how African Americans feel and think. These maneuvers, whether conscious or unconscious, serve to create distance between the self of the supervisor as a person of color and the patient as a person of color. The African American supervisor's need to distance from African Americans and other people of color may unwittingly provide the White therapist/supervisee with a comfort zone from which he or she may feel free to pathologize the African American patient's experience. This can result in the White therapist's distancing from the patient, just as the African American supervisor has distanced him- or herself from the patient's material in the supervision process.

## CULTURAL STEREOTYPES IN SUPERVISION

The issue of power is a most salient feature of institutional racism. Power colors the nature and quality of interracial interaction and influences the expectation and understanding of various groups in relation to each other. Power is also an issue that influences the impact, understanding, and expectations of patients and clinicians within the therapeutic process. Though rarely discussed directly in clinical circles, the issue of power is obvious. Our abilities to diagnose, select treatments, recommend treatment settings, determine custody outcomes, render judgments of mental competence, and so on, are areas in which we have the power to significantly affect the lives of others.

However, there are other venues in which the issue of power is struggled with and felt. Power impacts the supervisory process, where the supervisor's power to assess the therapist's efficacy, to guide his or her performance and influence patient outcomes is ever present. In the interracial triad, the impact of power and its meaning for all parties is present on at least three levels: (1) within the context of race relations and their associated hierarchies in the United States, (2) within the broader context of clinical practice, and (3) within the context of the supervisory process. The paradigm we are considering here reverses the typical power relationship in which the supervisor is White. Here, the power position is occupied by an African American supervisor (someone with less societal power and advantage) while the therapist/supervisee is White (and has more societal power and advantage). For both parties, there exists the potential to respond in a manner that will maintain the more familiar power relationship. This can occur because of a need to avoid anxiety about the differences. In this paradigm, the difference has particular meaning. The meaning of the racial difference and the reversal of the normative power arrangement are directly connected to issues of power. Acknowledging the differential of power within the room, in a configuration that is not familiar to the White supervisee and perhaps not familiar to many African American supervisors, requires a simultaneous acknowledgment of why this arrangement is atypical. The specialness of this arrangement derives from the reality of racism and discrimination on a broader societal level that usually results in the White person in the dyad occupying the position of conferred expertise, knowledge, and power. Here, the need to avoid anxiety about the difference between African American supervisor and White supervisee frequently results in the denial that issues of power (as they relate to race, status, and therapy) are present in the therapeutic space just as they are present in the outside world.

For the supervisor, this may emerge as an inability to allow oneself to supervise truly the therapist/supervisee or to require that the supervisee acknowledge the supervisor fully in this role. Actions that deemphasize the status of the supervisor as a powerful figure may become impediments to the supervisory process and to the supervisee's growth. Thus, resistances to supervision may be ignored and the supervisee's own expertise may be exaggerated or assumed. This prevents the opening up of the supervision to the very issues of power, status, and hierarchy that the African American patient may experience with his White therapist. Consequently, these issues may be suppressed, ignored, or misjudged by the therapist in the therapy to the detriment of the patient's treatment. Instead, what is needed is the opportunity to explore the assumptions about power that may indeed surface. These include the assumption of Whiteness as a basic underpinning of power and as an entitlement to it. An earnest exploration as well as a direct confrontation of how, when, and why these issues surface in the therapeutic (and supervisory) space is necessary.

Related to this issue is the assumption of "underdog" status for the African American patient. Both the supervisor and the therapist might be vulnerable to some variation of this belief and may perform from this perspective if they fail to become aware of it. For the supervisor, what may occur is a tendency to overextend the boundaries of the treatment or to ignore genuine resistances by the patient. This may be due to an emphasis on the patient's "underdog" status as an automatic justification for much of what the patient experiences and for how the patient behaves. Additionally, the inappropriate response by the supervisee to this perceived status of this patient may likewise be ignored. All this may foreclose a deeper understanding for supervisees and interfere with their ability to discern how these beliefs become a part of their countertransferential response and their clinical work in general.

If supervisors are unaware of their own feelings in this area, they may have trouble hearing this theme when it emerges for supervisees. Does the supervisee perceive the patient (and him- or herself) as the underdog, and if so, how does this feel? Does the therapist/supervisee blame or denigrate the patient? If so, is the therapist/supervisee unduly frustrated by the patient's failure to use the therapy to pull up his or her bootstraps and move on? Perhaps the therapist/supervisee feels impressed by or envious of the patient's ability to navigate through life while oppressed and as such misses the particularly painful aspects of the patient's survival efforts or the defenses employed to negotiate his or her struggle. This may reflect a romanticizing of the patient's struggle. It is problematic because it obscures the high price that many patients pay for survival. There is an opportunity here for the supervisor to help the therapist/supervisee to expand his or her understanding of the range of feelings, general psychological impact, and countertransferential potential engendered by such issues.

This dilemma was exemplified in the supervision of a White therapist/supervisee who sought to advocate for an African American patient to receive a computer in her home. This patient was severely disturbed with developmental delays and had become obsessed with the desire of having a computer in her home. The therapist saw this desire as a positive attempt by the patient to gain some mastery in a world that she felt to be overwhelming. Without arguing the merits of such a move, the African American supervisor attempted to assist the supervisee in exploring his concurrent tenacity about the patient's need to obtain a computer, with an eye toward any surfacing countertransferential material. The therapist could not appreciate the concerns of the treatment team for a patient they felt might be too limited (both personally and in terms of support) to utilize a computer on her own toward the ends she hoped for. The therapist also failed to recall that a feature of this patient's behavior when frustrated by her limitations was to throw heavy appliances (televisions, stereos, etc.), thereby destroying them. What did he suppose made these less salient considerations than the fact that this patient hoped to master a computer and become a "technologist"? Was there something about this patient that led him to advocate so strongly in this way? With encouragement, it emerged that the supervisee felt that giving this patient a computer would give the patient a chance in a world in which her chances were severely limited. He further described a sense that the patient's emotional and cognitive problems were exacerbated by the fact that she was African American, and that while she might improve psychologically, her "triple underdog" status made it necessary for "someone" (i.e., the therapist) to advocate for her. Further exploration revealed a strong degree of guilt and anxiety over any failure to support the patient's wishes. For this therapist, challenging the patient's wishes or plans was equated with harboring the belief that the patient was "down on the bottom where she belongs." This was discussed at length in supervision and examined as the therapist's attempt to mitigate his own guilt and as such was a response to the therapist's needs, not the patient's needs. The therapist needed to avoid feeling like the "overdog oppressor" and sought to do so by attempting to rescue the patient and compensate for past societal disadvantage.

This therapist could recognize the potential for a patient's discernment of this attitude and the possibility that he could be experienced by the patient as patronizing, insincere, and in collusion with her need to deny her own difficulties. Instead of having a real sense of hope, the anxiety expressed by this patient might represent anxiety about the therapist's ultimate belief that the patient requires rescue. Here, the patient may feel that a rescue is employed because the therapist believes that the patient is incapable of achieving any mastery on her own.

## HISTORICAL INFLUENCES

A strong stereotypic and symbolic figure in American life that is pregnant with symbolism for this country is that of the "mammy." Because there is an appropriate element of nurturance in the psychotherapy relationship, and in the relationship between clinical supervisor and supervisee, this symbolic relationship might be easily revived between the African American female supervisor and her White supervisee. We can think of it as the "mammy complex" or, for those in more urban areas in the 1990s, the "nanny complex."

Historically, in the realm of symbolic icons in the United States, the mammy figure symbolizes the idealized, nurturant, all-giving, and all-forgiving mother who is narcissistically used for one's own gratification (Thomas & Sillen, 1972). There is no consequence for this, nor is there any criticism for those who use her in this way. She provides a sense of loving indulgence and requires nothing back for herself. While many may consider this a stereotype of an earlier historical period, one need only examine the ongoing involvement of African American women in domestic work and childcare for White families to see that such symbolic figures are alive and well in American households today. The image of the mammy is present in an American society that experiences little discomfort in viewing African American women as if their most salient identities are as unselfish providers of nurturance and domestic assistance.

In this context, it would not be unusual for a White clinician to respond to a person of color, particularly a female, as the idealized, yet demeaned, nurturing, uncritical caretaker and mother substitute. Such an internal response can call forth wishes for gratification of one's needs for nurturing. The combination of an African American supervisor and an African American patient has the potential to bring this fantasized, wished-for relationship into the life of the therapy by the supervisee. Similarly, the African American female supervisor may find herself enacting her own feelings about this historical interaction between African Americans and Whites in this country. This presents the potential for an overinvestment in nurturing and giving, such that the supervisee's gratification needs are often met without any understanding of their existence or impact on the therapy, the patient, or the supervisee.

Resentment or disdain for this stereotypical role can serve as a backdrop for a struggle between supervisor and supervisee. In this scenario, the African American supervisor may act out her need to minimize gratifications so that she can avoid feeling narcissistically used while fundamentally disrespected. Meanwhile, the supervisee may be struggling with realistic and idiosyncratic wishes for gratification through his or her professional development in the supervision.

Related to this stereotype, but also separate from it, are sexual stereotypes, which are powerful facilitators of transference and countertransference. Grier (1967) describes patients who are also inclined to sexualize the racial factor to "intensify the process of sexualization" (p. 1589). Given the strong racial mythology and animalistic sexual stereotypes associated with the sexuality of African Americans and other peoples of color, it may be very tempting for the supervisee to introduce countertransferential material into the therapy and supervision that reenact relationships based on this racial and sexual mythology. This countertransference may also appear in the supervisee's resistance to learning with an African American supervisor whom he or she experiences as more inclined to animalistic abandon than to rational thought.

An example of these dynamics is illustrated by a young White male supervisee who consistently complimented his African American female supervisor's hair, clothing, jewelry, and the like during supervision. The supervisor was aware of her own subjective discomfort with these compliments and began to explore the meanings of this behavior, both internally and with the supervisee. She recognized that for her it raised concerns about being taken seriously in her professional role. Furthermore, she felt objectified. She related this behavior to male–female dynamics in general and to the historical interactions between White males and African American females in particular. She wondered if the supervisee felt more emboldened by an unconscious and historical pattern in which African American women were responded to as denigrated objects of possession and mere vehicles for the expression of White male urges.

She attempted to understand this phenomenon with the supervisee. She wondered if sexualizing the relationship served to help him manage the unfamiliar—an African American female supervisor/authority figure—in a way that felt familiar and did not threaten him. She further expressed curiosity about whether and in what ways the supervisee might reduce the treatment of his African American patients to elements with which he is most familiar to maintain his own level of comfort during their treatment.

While these explorations were awkward and difficult at first, they opened up for both supervisee and supervisor an understanding of how "difference" is experienced and surfaces in treatment. Other areas of potential exploration include the pull for oedipal competition when the supervisor is an African American male (Grier, 1967).

Genetic stereotypes may also influence the dynamics and the paradigmatic triad. One such stereotype is that African Americans are less intelligent than Whites (Jenkins, 1995). While many White clinicians are too sophisticated to actually voice or openly acknowledge such a belief, it is one that deserves our attention. If such beliefs are present, they can contribute to the supervisee's tendency to minimize or be suspicious of the supervisor's ability to help, teach, or demonstrate. When these attitudes are used in the service of resistance to the change in the more common and familiar power relationship (of White supervisor–African American supervisee), they can obscure the White or African American supervisee's anxieties about his or her own ignorance in treating others.

An example of this phenomenon is the case of a young, White, male supervisee who was being supervised by an African American female clinician. This supervisee often stressed his enrollment in a prestigious graduate program and talked of having worked with a prominent, much published clinician in the field. While his supervisor recognized the anxiety underlying this behavior, she began to question other aspects of the supervisee's need to appear learned and expert. She explored with the supervisee the possibility that this need to be an expert was also expressed in his treatment of clients. While this was a difficult exploration, it pointed out for both of them the influence of unconscious stereotypical beliefs about the hierarchy of authority, knowledge, information, and competence in mixed racial encounters. Furthermore, it brought to the surface the supervisee's countertransferential reactions to patient responses he found to be challenging of this hierarchy and, by inference, his self-perception of competence. He responded to patients' responses that challenged what he believed was his rightful hierarchical position by rendering diagnoses consistent with the presence of pathology. This revealed his tendency to characterize patients who did not respond in ways that he was comfortable and familiar with as further evidence of their pathology. What could now be considered was the very real possibility that the therapist might himself be ignorant in ways he had yet to discover. Furthermore, he might be taught through the "otherness" of both supervisor and patient and such a phenomenon could be growth-enhancing to patient and therapist alike.

## ADDITIONAL CONCERNS FOR OTHER INTERETHNIC/RACIAL TRIADIC COMBINATIONS

In addition to the paradigm discussed above, other racial combinations present challenges to the treatment process. The White therapist and supervisor treating the patient of color may harbor an unconscious sense that they form an appropriate hierarchy of power. White supervisors may feel that they have a sufficient understanding of the other ethnic group by virtue of their experience, which is deemed normative, and by whatever their exposure may have been, even if it is limited. However, if they have not examined their own feelings about treatment of the "other," they will be unable to assist trainees in fully confronting this aspect of the therapy. The failure to examine one's own Whiteness as a racial lens that colors one's perceptions, as well as the powerful impact of that whiteness on a person of color, will prevent any suggestion that the White supervisee attempt this understanding as a tool in broadening his or her multicultural competence.

The supervisor's failure to acknowledge his or her own ignorance of other cultures may grow out of an unconscious discomfort or guilt about this ignorance. The supervisee then stands to become caught between his or her own ignorance and the supervisor's failure to acknowledge that ignorance as an issue that may impinge on the treatment. Such a situation encourages a scenario in which the White supervisor's misinterpretations of the "other," his or her ignorance and discomfort, result in compensatory efforts to restore his or her sense of being knowledgeable, competent, and "on top" of the therapy case. The wish for gratification of these needs can be conveyed to the supervisee and expressed by him or her in therapy in counterproductive ways. The heightened desire to remove the sense of difference interferes with the free and open exploration in the supervisory space.

In the early years of my career, several student clinicians met in a peer supervision group. One member, a wealthy White female therapist, openly described her treatment of a lower class woman of Caribbean descent whom she experienced as sarcastic and cynical in her presentation. A discussion ensued in which the group examined and hypothesized about the behavior and interaction described. One member of the group, an African American female, noted that she had a similar sense with a couple of Caribbean patients whom she was seeing. She raised the question of whether this behavior might have some particular cultural basis or meaning. The treating clinician replied curtly, saying, "If it is cultural, then it is a cultural pathology." This response served to immediately cut off for that group any potential to explore the impact of both culture and difference in the therapy for both patient and therapist. The assumption here was that the cultural difference between patient and therapist is pathological when viewed from the therapist's own personal sense of normalcy. This response further suggests that such a foreclosure also existed in this therapist's attempt to conduct treatment with this patient, thus rendering it ineffective. This exemplifies the way in which differences that make a dominant group therapist uncomfortable can be categorized as pathological and then dismissed.

Such an example also speaks to the issues that might surface when the therapist and the patient are African American and the supervisor is White. The potential for an identification and an alliance based on the therapist's and the patient's experienced sense of likeness can arouse the White supervisor's anxiety. This anxiety might catalyze the need for the White supervisor to reinforce his or her sense of the rightful balance of power in which he or she is the all-knowing teacher and source of influence. Subtle efforts to negate or undermine the development of any African American on African American alliance have been known to result.

In a clinic serving a large African American and Caribbean population, a rather striking, stylish, well-to-do Caribbean female therapist/supervisee was met with disdain by a White senior clinician and supervisor. The supervisor told another African American trainee that "they [patients] have trouble with Ms. X," insinuating that her African American patients had difficulty relating to her. A more likely interpretation of this comment suggests that the supervisor was feeling anxiety and hostility aroused by the trainee's identity outside the stereotype (held by this supervisor) of the lower class, less educated, help-seeking African American patient. It was the latter with whom the supervisor seemed to be more familiar and to feel more competent. Although the Caribbean supervisee was different in many ways from the patient population with whom the White supervisor had become familiar, she (the supervisee) was also "similar" to the patients in ways her supervisor might never be. She was, in the final analysis, an African-descended woman from the Caribbean, just like many of the clinic's patients.

The issue here seemed more related to the White supervisor's need to negate any likeness between African American therapist and patient and to ignore differences (and the feelings aroused by them) between supervisor and therapist. Issues of class, race, and power were also beyond the supervisor's awareness, resulting in less culturally competent supervision. The supervisor's need to alleviate her anxieties about the "otherness" of the trainee and her patient remained unexplored and unavailable as material with which she might assist herself in supervising multiculturally.

## SUMMARY AND CONCLUSIONS

What lessons can be gleaned from the exploration of mixed racial triads and their impact on clinical supervision and psychotherapy? Clearly, there is a wealth of considerations for both the supervisor and the supervisee in opening up the discussion of patient work in a more competent, multiculturally sensitive way. This discussion has raised some possible scenarios and attempted to expand understandings of the potential for transference, countertransference, resistances, and counterresistances.

What we as clinicians and supervisors must begin to do is to conceptualize an alliance between student and teacher in which the exploration of differences and sameness is an underlying tenet of the notion of a successful supervisory experience. This requires the supervisor's ability and willingness to accept, understand, and experience what the supervisee has experienced while recognizing the potent emotional and psychological content of issues of culture and "otherness." To the extent that the supervisor can do this in a respectful, nondeprecatory manner, the supervisee can develop a better sense of him- or herself in his or her clinical role vis-à-vis these issues. Only then can we hope to foster an exploration of these issues that is frank, uninhibited, and fully open to our curiosity rather than marked by our guilt and anxiety.

Inhibitions, anxieties, and countertransferential responses are more likely to be observed and positively explored in an atmosphere where supervisors have accepted and embraced their own needs for exploration in this area. This learning alliance is more likely to be circumvented when the supervisor experiences the supervisee as too dissimilar to him- or herself (and vice versa) to warrant such exploration. However, in such cases the work to be done in developing multicultural competency is to understand together what this block means in the supervisory relationship. It would be necessary to explore what it reflects about the self-centeredness of one's own sense of cultural identity and the assumptions, projections, and resistances about that of the "other." In such a way this process can be modeled and used in the treatment of the culturally "other" patient. Additionally, this can facilitate the understanding and confrontation of culturally determined transferential behavior (Myers, 1988; Remington & DaCosta, 1989; Varghese, 1983).

In attempting to maintain an awareness of racially motivated therapeutic behavior, supervisors and supervisees alike can systematically examine their own clinical interventions to assess them on several dimensions. Calnek (1970) urges examining one's level of personal involvement in the therapeutic process, one's ability to conceptualize what is "normal" in another culture, and one's capacity to avoid pathologizing ethnic folkways. He also points to the need to recognize the strengths and the cultural lifestyles of others and the ability to explore and distinguish (and help the patient to do so) between racial issues as a defense/resistance and racism and racial barriers as realistic obstacles.

In addition to the above, it is imperative that the therapist be able to help the patient explore the racial/ethnic/cultural experience as an internalized part of his or her intrapsychic world. This point assumes that each individual possesses a unique internalization of ethnically/racially/culturally tinged experience. As such, it negates the notion of a universal experience and therefore augments the number of possibilities that exist at the juncture of personal and cultural experience.

Some might choose to argue this point to dilute the sense of the widespread impact of culture, ethnicity, and race on psychological experience. However, it would appear that the opposite is the case. That the impact is present, powerful, and widely spread is fully the point. How each person in his or her individual way creates a social and internal reality as a result is the puzzle we can only address with a full multicultural perspective. We can only activate this perspective when we are willing to examine closely, fully, and painfully what this juncture of personal and cultural experience has created in each of us. When we are successful, we can truly deliver culturally sensitive service to patients and assist them in developing deeper, richer understandings of themselves, their lives, their relationships, and their therapy. As supervisors, we can give clinical supervisees the model and the opportunity to develop themselves and understand the "other" through this examination. In this way, supervisors can become the preparers of the most effective tool of all in the delivery of culturally sensitive psychodynamic psychotherapy: the multiculturally competent clinician.

## REFERENCES

Banks, G., Berenson, B. G., & Carkhuff, R. R. (1967). The effects of counselor race and training upon counseling process with Negro clients in initial interviews. *Journal of Clinical Psychology, 23,* 70–72.

Bradshaw, W. H. Jr. (1982). Supervision in Black and White: Race as a factor in supervision. In M. Blumenfield (Ed.), *Applied supervision in psychotherapy* (pp. 200–220). New York: Grune & Stratton.

Calnek, M. (1970). Racial factors in the countertransference: The Black therapist and the Black client. *American Journal of Orthopsychiatry, 40*(1), 39–46.

Cavenar, J., & Spaulding, J. G. (1978). When the psychotherapist is Black. *American Journal of Psychiatry, 135,* 1084–1087.

Comas-Díaz. L., & Jacobsen, F. M. (1987). Ethnocultural identification in psychotherapy. *Psychiatry, 50,* 232–241.

Comas-Díaz, L., & Jacobsen, F. M. (1991). Ethnocultural transference and countertransference in the therapeutic dyad. *American Journal of Orthopsychiatry, 61*(3), 392–402.

Cook, D. A. (1994). Racial identity in supervision. *Counselor Education and Supervision, 34,* 132–141.

Cook, D. A., & Hargrove, L. P. (1997). The supervisory experience. In C. E. Thompson & R. Carter (Eds.), *Racial identity theory* (pp. 83–95). Mahwah, NJ: Erlbaum.

Cravatta, M., Crispell, D., Dortch, S., Edmondson, B., Kate, N., & Klein, M. (1997). What if . . . ? *American Demographics, 12,* 1–11.

Curry, A. (1964). Myth, transference, and the Black psychotherapist. *Psychoanalytic Review, 51*(4), 7–14.

Dorfman, E., & Kleiner, R. J. (1962). Race of examiner and patient in psychiatric diagnosis and recommendations. *Journal of Consulting Psychology, 26,* 393–398.

Fischer, N. (1971). An interracial analysis: Transference and countertransference significance. *Journal of the American Psychoanalytic Association, 19,* 736–745.

Gardner, L. (1971). The therapeutic relationship under varying conditions of race. *Psychotherapy: Theory, Research, and Practice, 8*(1), 78–87.

Greene, B. A. (1985). Considerations in the treatment of Black patients by White therapists. *Psychotherapy, 22,* 389–393.

Grier, W. (1967). When the therapist is Negro: Some effects of the treatment process. *American Journal of Psychiatry, 123*(12), 1587–1592.

Holloway, E. (1998). The supervisory relationship: The influence of individual and developmental differences. In J. M. Bernard & R. K. Goodyear (Eds.), *Fundamentals of clinical supervision* (pp. 34–60). Boston: Allyn & Bacon.

Holmes, D. E. (1992). Race and transference in psychoanalysis and psychotherapy. *International Journal of Psychoanalysis, 73,* 1–11.

Jenkins, A. H. (1995). *The psychology of the Afro-American: A humanistic approach.* New York: Pergamon Press.

Miller, M. H. (1972). The foreign resident as a disappointed person. *Psychiatry, 34,* 252–260.

Muslin, H., & Val, E. (1980). Supervision and self-esteem in psychiatric teaching. *American Journal of Psychotherapy, 34,* 545–555.

Myers, W. A. (1988). Some issues involved in the supervision of interracial and transcultural treatment. In J. M. Ross & W. A. Myers (Eds.), *New concepts in psychoanalysis and psychotherapy* (pp. 140–148). Washington, DC: American Psychiatric Press.

Remington, G., & DaCosta, G. (1989). Ethnocultural factors in resident supervision: Black supervisor and White supervisees. *American Journal of Psychotherapy, 43,* 398–404.

Sattler, J. (1970). Racial experimenter effects in experimentation, testing, interviewing, and psychotherapy. *Psychology Bulletin, 73,* 137–160.

Schacter, J. S., & Butts, H. F. (1968). Transference and countertransference significance. *Journal of the American Psychoanalytic Association, 19,* 736–745.

Sue, D. W., & Sue, D. (1977). Barriers to effective cross-cultural counseling. *Journal of Counseling Psychology, 24*(5), 420–429.

Thomas, A., & Sillen, S. (1972). *Racism and psychiatry.* New York: Bruner/Mazel.

Varghese, F. I. (1983). The racially different psychiatrist: Implications for psycho-therapy. *Australian and New Zealand Journal of Psychiatry, 17,* 329–333.

Vontress, C. (1971). Racial differences: Impediments to rapport. *Journal of Counseling Psychology, 18*(1), 7–13.

Waite, R. (1968). The Negro patient and clinical theory. *Journal of Consulting and Clinical Psychology, 32*(4), 427–433.

CHAPTER 8

# Hair Texture, Length, and Style as a Metaphor in the African American Mother–Daughter Relationship
## Considerations in Psychodynamic Psychotherapy

BEVERLY GREENE
JUDITH C. WHITE
LISA WHITTEN

Sensitivities about hair have many complex determinants and may be symbolic of a woman's feelings about other aspects of herself. This may be true of all women. However it may be intensified for African American women because the history of American racism has included a conspicuous devaluation of African physical features and the establishment of beauty standards based on idealized depictions of White women's physical features (Hall, 1995; Martin, 1964; Neal & Wilson, 1989). We are aware that many African American men also experience conflicts about their hair texture that can be damaging to their self-esteem. Nonetheless, physical beauty is a more powerful social variable for women than for men (Greene, 1990, 1994, 1997; Hill-Collins, 1991; Rich & Cash, 1993). In this context the dominant culture's toxic messages about African American's physical features may be more intensely felt by African American women than by men (Greene, 1996, 1997). Modifications in psychodynamic theory and technique provide useful ways of understanding and exploring this material in psychotherapy (Greene, 1997).

This chapter focuses on the metaphorical meaning and significance of hair in the context of the relationship between African American mothers and their daughters, and the symbolic significance of hair texture, length, and style in the psyche of African American women. We pay particular attention to the many historical antecedents and contemporary determinants of these factors, as well as to their significance as a rich source of information about a client's feelings about herself in the psychotherapeutic inquiry. Integrated understandings of psychodynamic theory and feminist psychotherapy theory serve as the lens through which we understand this phenomenon.

We are aware that many of the conflicts we discuss also exist for other Black women of African descent. But our comments in this chapter are based primarily on our observations of Black women of African descent who are born and raised in the United States. It is this group that we refer to as "African American women." We use the word *Black* to describe a more general group of persons that can include Black persons of African descent born and raised in Africa or the Caribbean, in addition to those raised in the United States.

## THE METAPHORICAL SIGNIFICANCE OF HAIR IN WOMEN'S LIVES

As feelings and attitudes about hair texture, length, and style have many complex psychodynamic determinants, these feelings may be symbolic of a woman's sensitivities about other aspects of herself. This assumption is accurate in varying degrees for all women, but it may be intensified for African American women because the history of racism has included a devaluation of African physical features, body types, facial features, and hair textures. Simply put, beauty standards for American women are based on idealized and not realistic depictions of White women's physical features (Greene, 1994, 1997; Hill-Collins, 1991; Neal & Wilson, 1989; Okazawa-Rey, Robinson, & Ward, 1987; Robinson, 1998). In one of the earliest publications on race and standards of beauty, Martin (1964) observed that both American Whites and other Americans employ a common standard when judging beauty in the female face that considers Caucasian features to be more attractive than "Negroid" features. While these standards are out of reach even for many White women, they are wholly unattainable for a much larger group of African American women (Greene, 1994). African American women in the United States form a large group of consumers who spend millions of dollars per year on hair care products, permanents, and artificial hair (Adams, 1996; hooks, 1988; Robinson, 1998). This large and flourishing hair care products industry is predicated on and actively promotes a variety of perceptions—of questionable validity—held by the members of the dominant culture and by many African American men and women about themselves. The essence of many of these erroneous perceptions is that physical features characteristic of or associated with people of African descent are unattractive, unfeminine, or ugly; that they diminish one's worth; and that they should be cosmetically or even surgically eradicated. The corollary of these perceptions is that to be attractive and feminine one must approximate the American beauty standard in which White women are depicted as the ideal (Greene, 1990; Hall, 1995; Hill-Collins, 1991; hooks, 1988; Martin, 1994; Robinson, 1998).

A woman's feelings about her hair are often symbolic of her conscious and unconscious internalized feelings about herself, her racial identity, and significant others (Berg, 1936; Hall, 1995). As such, inquiries about a client's hair and her feelings about it may represent a rich source of information about how the client regards herself (Berg, 1936). Many of these feelings and attitudes may not be consciously available and known to her, but their influence may be evident in her behavior and attitudes. These feelings deserve exploration and often surface readily with gentle probing by the therapist. Furthermore, the exploration of these feelings may serve as a catalyst for the investigation of other central issues. Feelings about hair texture and styles may also reflect intergenerational attitudes and conflicts in African American families. For example, mothers who experienced conflict about their own hair while growing up are likely, both consciously and unconsciously, to transmit these feelings to a daughter. Hair may also become the repository of split-off feelings about the self. We hasten to add that the presence or absence of natural hairstyles, the use of hair-straightening combs, or the employment of chemicals alone does not tell you how a woman truly feels about her hair, the adequacy of her physical appearance, or her ethnic identity. Weathers (1991) states that you may not assume that a Black woman hates either herself or her heritage simply because she straightens or perms her hair. Weathers views the process of straightening hair as something that is as much a part of African American hair culture as is the decision to wear hair naturally tightly curled or "unaltered." The heterogeneity of African American women as a group means that there are many individual variations and permutations of choices, feelings, conflicts, and resolutions about this issue. Jones (1994) observes that just as hair can be a source of pain in African American women's lives, it also can be an expression of self-love and adornment.

Any African American woman's feelings or attitudes about her hair will have been shaped to some degree by the history of racism in our society and its derivatives, and will reflect the complex nature of African Americans' connections to both African and American cultures (Greene, 1994, 1996; Hall, 1995; hooks, 1988; Robinson, 1998). However, it will also represent a woman's individual adaptation to the realities of racism, sexism, and heterosexism as they interact with her family dynamics, individual personality dynamics, realistic social and/or occupational demands at that particular point in time, contemporary styles and attitudes about them, and both the chronological and psychological developmental stage in her life (Cash & Duncan, 1984; Jenkins & Atkins, 1990; Leeds, 1994; Mack & Rainey, 1990). Weathers (1991) writes:

"Our hair's style is ever present in a variety of decisions, for example, keeping a job, pleasing a male partner, rebelling against the status quo, or bonding with other African American women in various hair rituals whether they be cornrowing or hot comb pressing" (p. 58). Weathers used ethnography and the African American oral tradition to document the hair experiences of a group of 16 young African American women at Vassar College. She concluded that there is a distinct "hair culture" among African Americans and among African American women in particular. She also determined that a range of complex and convoluted factors influence African American women's aesthetic choices, and that these factors are directly related to the social, political, and economic location of African American women in society. Hair styling, Weathers concludes, is a powerful vehicle for self-expression for African American women and also represents resistance to the exploitation they have suffered in overt and subtle ways.

In our clinical experience, the sociocultural context of racism and sexism facilitates the development of conflicted feelings about hair texture and length in African American women. The mere presence of such conflicts in some form is quite common, but they may assume pathological proportions in some individuals. Hence, it is not simply their presence that is pathological, but the role they play in undermining feelings of self-esteem and worth in the woman who holds them (Hall, 1995).

## HISTORICAL AND CONTEMPORARY CONTRIBUTIONS

Hair texture and length among African American women are issues that have failed to receive significant attention in the psychological literature. In many instances conflicts and feelings about hair have been taboo topics that African American women have been reluctant to reveal or discuss outside of their immediate social circles. Because of the dominant culture's ignorance about many of these issues, they have often been completely overlooked as important sources of inquiry in clinical work. Many factors may contribute to their higher level of visibility today. African American women form a more visible presence as consumers of psychological services than they have in the past. The recent increase in the numbers of African American clients, psychologists, and clinicians may have contributed to a greater willingness to talk about these issues and may give them greater prominence (Greene, 1996).

In one of the earlier references to the issue of hair texture and beauty standards in the African American community, Grier and Cobbs (1980) discuss the rejection of "Black" hair as one of the many ways that "Black" women's bodies are devalued. They describe the daily, arduous task of grooming "Black" girls' hair as well as the perceived need to do so. They also note that this strenuous grooming does not transform the child into a "beauty" by the dominant culture's standards, but is presumed to be required just to make her "acceptable" or minimally presentable. They further suggest that many African American girls reach the subconscious conclusion that "if mother has to inflict such pain on me to bring me just to the level of acceptability, then I must have been ugly indeed before the combing"(p. 43). Grier and Cobbs suggest further that "the implications and regularity and torture involved suggest that it is of vital importance that the child not be seen in her natural state" (p. 43).

Black literature is full of references to hair. For example, James Baldwin (1964) wrote:

> One's hair was always being attacked with hard brushes and combs and Vaseline: it was shameful to have nappy hair. One's legs were always greased so that one would not look "ashy" in the wintertime. One was always being scrubbed and polished, as though in the hope that a stain could thus be washed away. . . . The women were forever straightening and curling their hair . . . and using bleaching creams . . . yet it was clear that none of this effort would release one from the stigma and danger or being Negro; it merely increased the shame and rage. (p. 80)

Maya Angelou (1969) describes her own painful dilemma as a child:

> Wouldn't they be surprised when one day I woke out of my black, ugly dream, and my real hair, which was long and blond, would take the place of the kinky mass that Momma wouldn't let me straighten? . . . Then they would understand why I had never picked up a southern accent, or spoke the common slang, and why I had to be forced to eat pig's tails and snouts. Because I was really white and because a cruel fairy stepmother who was understandably jealous of my beauty, had turned me into a too big Negro girl, with nappy Black hair. (p. 2)

Gwendolyn Brooks (1972) writes:

> One of the first "world"-truths revealed to me when I at last became a member of SCHOOL was that, to be socially successful, a little girl must be Bright (of skin). It was better if your hair was curly too . . . or at least Good Grade (Good Grade implied, usually, no involvement with the Hot Comb). (p. 37)

Kim Green (1993), a freelance journalist, notes:

> I grew up mad at my hair because it wasn't pretty like the swinging manes of the white children who surrounded me. It was short and petrified. It stayed where I put it and even where I didn't. It refused to move with me and fought against me. (p. 38)

It is very difficult, although not impossible, for any Black woman to escape the negative messages from the dominant culture about her hair. Regardless of the particular texture of any woman's hair, the large majority of Black women struggle with negative feelings about their hair, and spend a great deal of time, money, and energy attempting to change it. Boyd-Franklin (1991) writes that many Black women in group psychotherapies report anger, pain, resentment, and confusion about various aspects of their bodies and physical appearance. Appearance, Boyd-Franklin (1989) observes, can become a toxic issue or secret in the family. When the toxic secret is acted out in families, it may take the form of scapegoating certain family members, embarrassment, and the projection of negative (or positive) characteristics based on the presence or absence of certain physical features. Consistent with Boyd-Franklin's (1989) observations, skin color and hair textures, whether lighter or darker, straight or nappy, can be revealing of secrets about paternity, just as they can be idealized or devalued. Hall (1995) observes that concerns about the adequacy of their hair represents one of a constellation of concerns that Black women may express that may be better understood as representations of body-image problems. Black women with shorter kinkier hair textures are often disparaged and devalued by both the dominant culture and segments of the Black community as less feminine and less attractive than their counterparts. This phenomenon is perhaps more familiar to readers than its corollary. Indeed, many Black women with distinctly short hairstyles are stigmatized as lesbians.

Given the pronounced homophobia in both the African American community and the dominant culture, the inference that something about a woman's physical stature or appearance makes her look like a lesbian is intended to be insulting and suggests that the behavior or characteristic should be avoided. It is often incorrectly assumed that African American women who are lesbians either want to look like men, are inherently unattractive, or are less involved in concerns about their physical appearance than their heterosexual counterparts. Overall there is an assumption that a lesbian is less concerned about approaching the dominant culture's female beauty standard. Based on our clinical and personal experience, these views are not supported. In many ways Black lesbians face a double stigma because their attractiveness, worth, and femininity are demeaned even more than those features of heterosexual women. Conversely, there may be pressure to assiduously avoid conforming to female beauty standards within some lesbian communities while simultaneously feeling pressured to conform to these standards by the Black community. Whether or not the woman in question is closeted may also influence her concerns about her physical appearance. Furthermore, there is scarcely any empirical research with large numbers of Black lesbians: most empirically derived observations in this realm are based on overwhelmingly White samples.

Black women with long and straighter hair textures historically have been idealized by some members of the Black community, deemed more acceptable by the dominant culture, and simultaneously accorded a higher level of social privilege in both communities. These preferences and values have their origins in the construction of racial myths required to rationalize the pervasive ill-treatment of African slaves, indeed, the institution of slavery itself. In this context, Africans were defined as the uncivilized other, the devalued and despised, or opposite of all things European and desirable (Hill-Collins, 1991; Robinson, 1998).

Preferences for lighter skin color and straighter hair textures among African Americans continue in some fashion today, although they are less overt than they were prior to the 1960s. The civil rights and Black power movements of that era gave rise to the increasing desire to be more affirmative of Africa and African cultural derivatives. In this period the slogan "Black is beautiful" encapsulated the desire to embrace African characteristics and African cultural derivatives. In some circles it even represented a repudiation of anything associated with European culture and style. It was in this context that the "natural" or "Afro" hairdo gained increasing popularity among African Americans. The afro hairstyle introduced what Robinson (1998) describes as the notion of hairstyle as a political statement and a kind of tension that linked one's hairstyle with embracing one's African heritage. Looking as "Black" as possible was associated with higher status in Black communities. Conversely, attempts to emulate European styles were regarded as a rejection of one's heritage and resulted in lesser status. Hence, in this social context, acknowledging a preference for straight hair or lighter skin color was presumed to represent self-loathing. Elements of this judgment persist in some form in many Black communities today.

Nonetheless, while many African American men and women are more cautious today about openly expressing a preference or wish for straighter hair textures and lighter skin colors, this caution does not mean that people no longer have such desires. In some ways, this may make these preferences harder to identify and requires the therapist to be more proactive in trying to elicit this material. We are not suggesting that Black women whose hair textures fall along the spectrum between these extremes are immune to painful ridicule and scorn—quite the contrary. Few Black women socialized in the United States, regardless of their hair texture, escape the confusing conundrum of experiencing external pressure from family, peers, and/or society to have hair textures and styles that result in privileges within the Black community and the dominant culture, and of wishing for or even attempting to have them without estranging themselves from other segments of the Black community (Hill-Collins, 1991; Martin, 1964; Neal & Wilson, 1989; Weathers, 1991).

Black women whose hair textures fall at either of the extreme ends of the hair texture and length spectrum may elicit more intense reactions of varying sorts and for a variety of reasons. For example, Black women with straighter hair textures, while privileged in the dominant culture, may face a high degree of ridicule, contempt, and estrangement in segments of the Black community that is deeply painful for them. They may also become objects of envy from family members and/or peers and face the task of managing the resentment that follows (Boyd-Franklin, 1989; Greene, 1990, 1996; Hill-Collins, 1991). It would be a mistake to assume that the privileges obtained in the dominant culture, and in some segments of the Black community, compensate for estrangement from other Black peers.

African Americans who idealize the dominant culture's beauty standard, particularly when that standard includes an explicit devaluation of other expressions of beauty, express their own internalized racism. Okazawa-Rey, Robinson, and Ward (1987) observe that when Black women "despise and degrade" other Black women for having dark skin (and/or nappy/kinky hair textures), their behavior represents identification with their oppressor. Similarly, when Black women "turn against" other Black women for their light skin or straighter hair textures, their behavior often represents their own subconscious frustration and envy. Okazawa-Rey and colleagues (1987) suggest that the negative feelings that African American women direct at one another would be better directed at race and gender oppression in society. It is those forms of oppression that reduce Black women's worth, and to some extent the worth of all women, to the single measure of their physical beauty/femininity.

Having straighter hair textures may garner privileges but it is not experienced without ambivalence if it estranges one from the Black community (Hill-Collins, 1991). This must be understood when engaging Black women in clinical work. The mere possession of a characteristic will not necessarily tell you how the individual feels about either the characteristic or the treatment derived as a result of that characteristic. Furthermore, the meaning attributed to being at either extreme (straighter versus kinky hair textures) of the hair texture spectrum may vary depending on what part of the country the individual comes from.

G is a 30-year-old African American woman who presented in therapy with symptoms of depression, anxiety, and compulsive behavior. She talked at length about her experiences as a light-skinned woman with shoulder-length hair. In the urban Northeast she was admired for these attributes. However, when she moved to Louisiana to attend a historically Black college, she found that these same attributes were hardly noticed. She remarked that this required a considerable adjustment for her, as she went from being considered special to being regarded as average. G also observed that she was glad that her therapist wore her hair natural because it reminded her of her mother, who wore her hair in locks.

The degree to which a woman's appearance differs from that of her peers and community is an important factor in how she regards her own appearance. For example, a Black woman showed photographs from her trip to Greece to her family. She had recently cut her hair (which had been below her shoulders at one point) very short, and her fair skin was quite tanned in the photos. After a few minutes, her father interrupted and said, "Has anybody seen my daughter? She has light skin and long hair." This serves to further illustrate the great value placed on light skin and long hair in some families and the anxiety created when this image is even temporarily disrupted.

Generally, when hair texture and length are idealized and prized, or disparaged and devalued, it accrues a power to define an individual beyond its realistic significance and magnitude. This occurs as hair per se comes to eclipse the realistic attributes and character of a person and is used to define what that person is or to predict what she can or should become.

## AFRICAN AMERICAN MOTHERS AND DAUGHTERS: THE HAIR WARS

How an African American mother feels about herself may be reflected in her attitudes and care not only of her own hair but also in her attitudes toward and care of her daughter's hair. They may even be generalized and reflect her attitudes and feelings about her daughter altogether. This relationship can lay the groundwork for long-standing, deeply rooted feelings in African American daughters about their hair, sexuality, self-image, femininity, racial identity, personal value, and adequacy. The nature of this relationship is not always problematic (Jones, 1994; Powers, 1994). For some African American mothers, concerns about the adequacy of their daughter's hair and demeanor reflect more basic and practical concerns. These concerns are often about how their daughter's acceptance by the dominant culture as well as the African American community will be facilitated or undermined by her physical appearance. Such concerns may also reflect mothers' anxieties about how their parenting skills will be perceived by others. Simply stated, mothers are held accountable in our society for the appearance, social decorum, and socialization of their children. The child who is deemed unkempt may be seen as a negative reflection of her mother's adequacy as a mother and a caretaker. Conversely, mothers are reinforced for "working" on their daughter's hair when it is complimented. Thus, the focus on hair and hair care in the African American community is perpetuated as an essential element of grooming and as an indication that a child, especially a female child, is loved and valued or conversely, ignored and neglected by her caretakers (Weathers, 1991).

Hair is not necessarily an inevitable source of conflict between all African American mothers and their daughters. However, we have frequently observed that it is a significant source of conflict in many African American mother–daughter relationships. Acknowledgment of such conflicts, however, is not routinely forthcoming or obvious. This material may not be readily available for therapeutic inquiry if the therapist does not take the time to raise specific relevant questions. In this discussion, we assert that when hair or control over hair care or hairstyle is or has been a source of conflict between an African American mother and her daughter, it may have deeper meaning and thus would warrant therapeutic exploration. Who is in control of whom, what is being controlled, and so on, are important considerations. The conflicts expressed around hair care and control may be symbolic of more unconscious struggles between the two and it may also reflect specific characterological issues in each individual that are acted out in the relationship around hair.

## PSYCHODYNAMIC AND HISTORICAL SIGNIFICANCE OF HAIR

Hair is an overdetermined object of unconscious projections about a person's feelings about their relative attractiveness, self-worth, worthiness, or general adequacy. As physical appearance and attractiveness are more salient social variables for women than for men, and are often seen as the major determinant in calculating a woman's social value or status, women experience greater overt distress and unconscious conflict about their hair and its relationship to their attractiveness (Berg, 1936; Greene, 1990, 1996, 1997; Hall, 1995; Synnott, 1987; West, 1995).

Hair, unlike skin color, height, weight, body build, and to some extent facial features (nose and lip shape) is somewhat malleable and therefore easier to alter or control (Synnott, 1987). A mother can spend several hours working on her daughter's hair and see visible, tangible results. In this instance she may feel that she has a direct positive impact on something in a world where so many of her actions and efforts, as an African American and as a woman, are met with resistance and result in failure. Hair grows, it can be cut in various shapes, its texture can be changed, and it can be styled in many different configurations. When hair is cut, it grows back; when it is chemically altered, it resumes its natural state when the chemicals are removed, the treated hair is cut off, or the hair grows out. Hair is a physical characteristic that can be controlled to a greater degree than other physical characteristics. Indeed, *control* is a word frequently used by African American mothers to describe their aim where their daughters' hair is concerned. Hooks (1988) observes that Black women are conditioned to believe that their hair is a part of their bodies that must be "controlled." It also suggests a more generalized perception that the hair of African Americans in its natural state is "out of control," or unmanageable. We may ask in this context what it means for hair to be "out of control" and why such intense, negative feelings are often associated with this perception.

Control is an important issue for African Americans, who as visible ethnic minorities in a racist country often have little control over events and circumstances that have great import in their lives. The need to exercise control over some aspect of one's destiny may be displaced onto hair because it can be controlled in ways that other aspects of one's life cannot.

If we assume that hair in and of itself has no power and does nothing, we may ask: Why is its control so important? What will it do if it is out of control? In this context we may suggest that in some mother–daughter dyads the need to control something other than hair is operative, however unconsciously, and expressed via the conflict about or intensity of feelings surrounding the mother's concerns about her daughter's hair texture and style.

Feared impulses may be displaced onto hair. Sometimes serious conflicts about hair erupt between mothers and daughters during the adolescent period that have not been observed prior to this period. Two normal aspects of adolescence include the child's burgeoning sexuality and overt interest in matters sexual and the adolescent's desire to be freer of parental control. A natural struggle emerges between most parents and their children around these issues. However, a parent who has difficulty with her daughter's burgeoning sexuality, an event that is out of her control, may displace her anxieties and concerns about this issue onto characteristics and behaviors that are less significant but are "controllable." She may seek to control other aspects of her daughter's behaviors and comportment in ways that are excessive and sometimes unduly rigid. When great tension and conflict is organized around control of the daughter's hair, the therapist would be wise to ask what kinds of things in the daughter's life are either out of the parent's control or are perceived to be that would be alarming to her.

One of the negative ethnic stereotypes used to stigmatize African Americans is that they lack impulse control in a variety of areas, but particularly in the modulation of sexuality and aggression (Greene, 1990; Grier & Cobbs, 1980; Hill-Collins, 1991). Overt expressions of sexuality or aggression are deemed negative in cultures dominated by Western Christian religiosity (Greene, 1996, 1997; Hill-Collins, 1991). Stereotyped as violent, bestial, sexually promiscuous, and "uncivilized" by the dominant culture, African Americans who have internalized such stereotypes may unconsciously seek ways of managing or disproving them.

## TRANSFORMATION, TREAT, OR TORTURE?: VISITING THE HAIRDRESSER

Robinson (1998) writes that the demand for professional hair care in the African American community steadily grew after Emancipation. Doing hair in one's home or in a beauty shop became a viable way of making a living for many African American women. In her examination of hair and beauty culture,

Robinson observes that the hair care business became one of the most "established categories of African American entrepreneurs." Indeed, Madame (Sarah) C. J. Walker, an African American woman, was the first female self-made American millionaire. Although her enterprise sold many personal and hair care products, most of her money derived from the design and sale of a metal comb with wide teeth used to straighten kinky hair. This "hot comb" was heated and then passed through the hair to alter its texture, pressing or straightening the hair. "Going back" was the term used to describe what happens when kinky/nappy hair is pressed or straightened and then comes into contact with water or humidity. Going back means that the hair returns to its original nappy state, much to the consternation of the woman who attempts to maintain a hairstyle that requires straight hair. Green (1993) writes about the despair many Black women feel when they attempt to maintain straight hair despite the realities of weather conditions that will reverse hours of "pressing" in moments: "Rain has ruined dates, outdoor concerts, and good vibes. I'm a slave to rain; it decides whether I go or don't and if I go, whether I'll stay" (p. 38).

Women's beauty shops also became gathering places where "gender bonding" could occur in ways that provided an important social function for African American women and where the female child's first visit was often a "coming of age ritual" (hooks, 1988; Robinson, 1998). To be able to pay to get one's hair professionally "done" was and continues to be a sign of status for some women. Going to the beauty shop is a way of allowing oneself to be personally attended to and cared for. This is not difficult to understand. Where their hair was concerned, not all women had negative experiences. For some women, having their mother or other caretaker comb, wash, and groom their hair is remembered as a ritual that left them feeling nurtured.

Despite the important social function of beauty parlors and the role of many hairdressers as "wise women" whose advice is sought out, many women have had extremely negative experiences in beauty parlors. When viewed as a whole, such experiences raise additional questions about the dynamics of this process. We suggest that the intense conflict around hair texture and length that most African Americans experience may be manifested in the damage done by some hair care specialists to Black women's hair. Determinants of this behavior among hair stylists may be both conscious and unconscious. Many women report that when they request a trim or haircut they are routinely subjected to the removal of significantly more hair than requested, usually to their dismay. For example, W requested the operator to *trim* her shoulder-length hair. The male operator proceeded to cut off 3 inches of hair. On seeing the shock on his customer's face, the operator laughed and retorted, "I'll put it in a bag for your husband if you want me to." Others report the "careless" use of toxic chemicals in permanents that left them with scalp burns and lost patches of hair. Green (1993) recalls such experiences:

> Then, of course, there were the days when lazy hairstylists or their new assistants would carelessly rinse my head of the devilish lye, and it would leave scars and burns that marred my scalp for weeks, which frantically itched and reminded me of the power and pain of living the lye. . . . I would scratch my head so hard that patches of hair would give up and throw themselves to the ground in silent protest. . . . Those were my first days of true rage. (p. 38)

In another example, L went to a beautician for a mild permanent that would have allowed her to wear her natural hairdo and straighten it if she desired. The female operator applied the perm and combed it vigorously. When the chemicals were washed out L discovered that her hair was lying flat on her head, which indicated that too much of the chemical had been used, or that it was left in her hair for too long a period of time. This made it impossible for her to wear her hair in a natural hairstyle until the treated hair completely grew out. The operator sarcastically responded to L's shock by telling her "I guess you won't be wearing your natural anymore."

These examples reflect behavior that is laced with hostility toward Black female customers. We wonder if such behavior is a manifestation of the operator's conflict about his or her own hair or his/her negative feelings about women, particularly Black women. Despite these occurrences, this is not a one-sided issue.

Many hairdressers and other operators in the hair care industry lament their struggles with consumers who demand that they use dangerous or ill-advised products or methods to achieve a particular hairstyle. They report that they often explain the considerable risks associated with the use of many procedures or products (particularly the use of chemical permanents on top of hair dyes or other chemical treatments). They also point out the likelihood of an outcome that does not resemble what a magazine advertisement or package promises, and the potential for serious damage to hair and scalp if the product is used. In spite of their attempts to provide honest information about the limitations and dangers of such products, they report finding themselves the targets of angry consumers who are driven, often with a sense of desperation, to achieve a certain outcome that they will do anything to get. If the hair care professional still refuses to undertake the procedure, they may face more resentment as well as a loss of business. Lois Dennis (personal communication, May 23, 1996), a 30-year veteran of the hair stylist industry, reports that such occurrences became so frequent that she instituted a policy that requires consumers to sign the equivalent of an informed consent agreement. In this document, the consumer attests that she has been warned of the risks of the procedure and the possibility of its failure to provide the desired look, and agrees that it is being performed at her insistence, against the operator's professional advice. Dennis and her colleagues marvel at the intense sense of urgency and the desperation of many women to have long, straight, idealized hairstyles that are simply inconsistent with their natural hair. The use of other strategies, such as weaves, braids, and wigs to transform or hide one's natural hair also attests to the extent and expense many African American women are willing to go to in the interest of achieving a desired style. The notion that their own hair is "good enough" is quite foreign to many of them.

## IMPLICATIONS FOR PARENTS

Attitudes about hair texture and length are put into place very early in life. Because hair care is such a major part of the grooming process for African American girls, mothers, fathers, and other loved and trusted figures must be particularly sensitive to these issues from the very beginning. For example:

> A babysitter exclaimed "Look at those eyes! Look at that hair!" as 3-year-old Jennifer entered the house. She has hazel eyes and sandy hair that reaches below her shoulders. Camille, who has dark brown eyes and short nappy hair, and who is the babysitter's primary charge, quietly listened to her exclamations. The babysitter had never complimented her hair or eyes. This could have contributed to Camille's preoccupation with long hair, and her devaluation of her own short locks.

In this scenario, Jennifer is at much at risk as Camille, albeit in different ways. Jennifer could grow up to assume that her physical attributes are the most important aspects of her personhood.

It is crucial for parents to question, explore, and challenge themselves regarding their own attitudes about hair while they work toward building positive attitudes about hair in their children. Without a doubt, mothers, who are usually charged with the responsibility of grooming their children's hair, can easily transmit their own conflicts about hair to their daughters. Such conflicts may be transmitted in subtle and unconscious or overt and mean-spirited ways.

Parents as well as other caretakers could benefit from ideas and suggestions on how to manage these issues. Hopson-Powell and Hopson (1990) offer some suggestions about the management of skin color conflicts that are also useful in the management of conflicts about hair texture. They suggest that it is key to reinforce in little girls' minds that they are "good enough" just as they are and that radical means are not required to make them look acceptable. Short thick hair should be admired for its thickness, texture, and healthiness. This requires taking the time to compliment girls on the attractiveness of their existing features and characteristics and emphasizing their assets and strengths. They will learn to value and cherish themselves if they are taught to focus on their strengths more than their shortcomings. Clearly, this has implications for other aspects of their person outside of their physical appearance. Physical appearance per se must be delinked from worthiness and one's value as a human being. This is difficult to accomplish in a society that bombards children with the opposite message, and where people are often rewarded or punished for the presence or absence of certain physical characteristics. Still, over time, change can occur and these values can be imparted. Overall, children must learn to establish their own standard rather than comparing themselves to other girls/women, whether real, advertised, or imagined.

One of the authors has a godchild with short nappy hair. Whenever she sees her she tells her, "You have such pretty, nappy hair." It is important that boys hear these kinds of communications too, since pleasing men is often the object of what heterosexual women do with their hair. Weathers (1991) observes that if African American women want their men's biases to change, they must consider how they may be reinforcing those biases.

Parents can mitigate the negative effects of the stigma associated with nappy hair textures and short hair. They may do so by being self-conscious about what they communicate to their male and female children about physical characteristics, such as who is considered attractive among friends and family members, and what makes them attractive. African American parents may need to give their children more positive feedback about their appearance than their White counterparts, to buffer the negative messages their children receive from the dominant culture. Whitten (1994) suggests the following comments as examples of affirmative responses to a child's hair or appearance that reinforce natural qualities:

> I just love the way your hair sparkles when its just been washed!
> Your hair is so nice and fluffy!
> I really admire how you take care of your hair.
> Lets think of some new ways we can style your hair.
> Its fun to try new hairstyles, isn't it? Your hair is so easy to style!
> Your hair smells so fresh!
> Here are some pictures of some girls in Africa with nice hair, just like yours!
> Our ancestors in Africa used to braid their hair like this. When we do it, it's a way for us to carry on their traditions.

Making positive comments about a child's hair is certainly a good thing, but such comments may not reach the depth of inadequacy or envy that some children may experience about their hair. It is important that parents do not respond to a child's unhappiness about her hair or other physical characteristics with anger or a dismissal of her feelings. It is important to respond empathically so that the child can feel that her feelings, even if unpopular to the parent, are being heard and accepted. This makes it important to have additional responses in our repertoire such as:

> Sometimes people want to be like other people.
> Sometimes its hard to be happy with ourselves the way we are.
> I'm glad you're sharing your feelings with me. . . . Can we talk about this some more?

> It sounds like you're not feeling too happy with yourself right now.

When the child has spoken about his/her feelings in some depth, parents can work on developing problem-solving strategies, such as:

> I wonder what we could do together to find some new hairstyles that you might like?
> I wonder what we can do to help you feel better about your hair?

Parents can look for images of other children that are similar to their own children to post around the child's room. Pictures of the child him- or herself should also be displayed and admired. When children admire the hair or features of other children that are different from their own, parents can say:

> Yes, she does have pretty long hair. Many kinds of hair are pretty. I like your hair because it is so thick and healthy (because it's such a pretty color, because it's so soft, because it's so fluffy, etc.).

Comments that degrade, minimize, or criticize the natural characteristics of a child's hair (texture, length) should be scrupulously avoided, as they are often much more painful and keenly felt than they appear to be. Such comments can often have a negative effect on a Black girl's sense of the adequacy of her physical appearance during childhood, which can carry over into the rest of her life. Furthermore, healthy children must learn to establish their own personal standards rather than comparing themselves to other women or girls, real, idealized, or imagined.

## CASE EXAMPLE

Our hair, as with any part of our body, can be symbolic of intrapsychic conflict at any level of psychosexual development, pregenital as well as oedipal (Berg, 1973). Exploration of a patient's feelings about and experiences around hair can reveal intrapsychic conflicts and illustrate the transference. As we as clinicians come to understand the patient's experience of hair care in the context of the mother–child interaction, we will gain a deeper appreciation of transference dynamics.

Kaye is a 41-year-old African American woman who has been in combined psychoanalytically oriented psychotherapy, with individual therapy twice a week and group therapy once a week. She has been in individual psychotherapy for the past 9 years; group was added during the 4th year of treatment.

Kaye entered therapy complaining of headaches. She is from a two-parent working-class African American family with six offspring. Kaye is the third eldest child. Kaye and her two older siblings were born one right after the other, giving her mother little physical and emotional respite between pregnancies.

Although Kaye is 41, she appears to be significantly younger. Recently, she remarked that she dresses like a teenager. She almost always wears a blouse with a sweater, jeans, and sneakers. Her factory coworkers have told her that she dresses like a welfare client. Her clothing is often frayed and shabby, even though she could afford to buy new clothing. She told her therapist that she wears such clothing in an attempt to conceal her body.

For the entire course of therapy, she has worn her hair in one style, medium length and tightly curled, a hairstyle she has been told is outdated. Although Kaye goes to a professional hairdresser every 2 weeks to have her hair straightened with a hot comb, pressed, and curled, her hair frequently looks unkempt. Her unkempt appearance is a result of her self-acknowledged habit of playing with her hair and then not combing it before going out in public.

At the time she entered therapy, Kaye and two of her siblings were still living at home. She describes her mother as being angry and complaining. Kaye feels that her older sister is her mother's favorite. Her mother experienced Kaye as "never doing anything right." She presents her father as a shadowy figure, working long hours and spending little time at home. When at home, he barely speaks. When Kaye was in her late 20s she decided to move into her own apartment. Her parents told her they were afraid she could not care for herself if she lived alone, and actively discouraged her from moving out of the family home. With both of her parents, Kaye has maintained a silently angry dependent relationship. Furious with her parents both for not supporting her attempts to be independent and not nurturing her at home, Kaye withdrew from the family, preferring to spend time alone in her room, sleeping and watching television.

The following vignettes from sessions are presented to illustrate Kaye's experience with her hair, how these experiences highlight her intrapsychic conflicts, and how they are manifested in the transference.

THERAPIST: [I drew attention to her hair—all askew. During the course of our relationship her hair was consistently poorly groomed, motivating me to bring this to her attention.]

KAYE: Well, I know. I guess I could brush it before I leave the job but I don't carry a brush. I have a comb on the job. I look in the mirror and I see how messy it looks and I just leave it.

THERAPIST: What are you communicating to people by having it this way?

KAYE: It looks like I don't care.

THERAPIST: What more about that?

KAYE: I don't know. I didn't do much with it. I don't know how to explain it.

THERAPIST: It's hard for you to talk with me about not caring for your hair?

KAYE: I was never that conscious about my looks and when it came to my hair . . . I just don't care. Maybe I figure it is not going to change things. It's just part of being depressed. Someone asked me about that. I wouldn't comb it . . . after leaving the gym. It's similar to how I handle my clothes . . . I wear the same clothes. It's a similar pattern to how I have my hair. [The way she experiences her hair is symbolic of how depressed and inadequate she feels.]

THERAPIST: You are feeling hopeless. Caring about your hair is not going to change things. What about being depressed?

KAYE: Well, I guess I don't care. It's part of being depressed. Maybe, if I took care of my clothes . . . I would take care of my hair. Well, I have stopped wearing the ragged sweaters. . . . I didn't care about my clothes—so my hair goes, too.

Although Kaye cites her progress, that is, not wearing ragged sweaters anymore, she quickly moves away from it.

KAYE: Well, I'm not happy and I know it relates to what happened when I was younger. I regret not doing more, feeling I should have done things when I was younger. It's depressing!

Kaye continued to speak about depressing aspects of herself: eating fattening foods, not going to the gym, and dressing like a teenager.

THERAPIST: You said your feelings of unhappiness relate to what happened when you were younger. In the past you have talked about not feeling cared about as a child. Who took care of your hair when you were younger?

KAYE: My mother braided my hair every day and it did look nice. In junior high school, I didn't know what to do with it. I picked the simplest style.

THERAPIST: I think we could learn more about your relationship with your mother if we talk about your interaction with her when she did your hair. Describe the image of how your mother would take care of your hair, the way you do with dreams.

KAYE: I would be sitting on the floor. She would be on the couch. I would be sitting in between her legs. She would braid one part at a time . . . the left side, maybe. She would have a big braid at the top . . . one or two braids at the back. She would braid it so that all of the braids would be together [joined hands], the big braid would stick out.

THERAPIST: What were you in touch with/feeling/experiencing when she braided your hair?

KAYE: I didn't like the heat from the hot comb. I hate the fact that I had to straighten my hair.

The client continued to describe her dislike of the hair-grooming process and her sense of the inferiority of Black hair.

KAYE: I didn't like putting hair oil on it. Who would want to touch my hair? I wondered, What do White people think of my hair? We Black people don't have the options of doing different things with our hair unless we have good hair. In our family we talked a lot about "good hair" and "bad hair." When a baby was born we would wonder when the hair would start to get nappy. Nappy hair is a burden. When I would think about having children, I could not imagine myself doing their hair.

THERAPIST: Your feelings about your hair are strongly tied to your relationship with your mother?

KAYE: Maybe it's because I want her to take care of me. My mother still straightens my younger sister's hair and my sister is 38. I am proud of the fact that my mother doesn't do my hair.

She continued to discuss the ways her mother would discourage her and her sister from styling their hair in an updated way.

THERAPIST: You have talked a lot about what you disliked about the way in which your mother did your hair or how discouraging she was about your attempts to style your hair. However, you're saying your mother did care enough to braid your hair every day. [I wanted to highlight the nurturance that Kaye had received from her mother.]

Kaye: She braided my hair til I was 12.

THERAPIST: Did you feel comfortable when she braided your hair?

Kaye: Yes, I felt "new." I looked like a new person. Take braids out, grease it, put new ones in.

THERAPIST: Who would wash it?

KAYE: I don't remember. She probably did it. I know I didn't do it alone. It was not uncomfortable. *It was the most attention that I got from her.*

THERAPIST: What does that mean to you?

KAYE: Well, I wonder if she gave me attention in other ways, like when I was a baby, did she pick me up, play with me? I remember what you said about my sister coming right after me. And then my older sister was about 2 when I was born. I guess my older sister got more attention than me. My mother is friendly with my younger sister and with my nephew. I don't have that with my mother.

The following session, 2 days later:

KAYE: I want to continue with what we talked about on Wednesday. I would not have brought up the subject myself of my mother doing my hair. *It did make me think maybe I am not taking care of myself because I want my mother to do it.*

THERAPIST: What more about that?

KAYE: I guess I wonder why . . . I wanted my mother to take care of me more than my other brothers/sisters. Maybe it's from not getting . . . maybe I didn't get my full share compared to the others. D is not like that. If I did have children—girls—could [would] I do their hair right? Would I straighten their hair right? Would I burn it? Would I do anything right? Did I need more attention? [While she is talking, she is playing with her hair. Her left hand is stroking her hair, picking up strands of hair in hand and manipulating it between two fingers.] I was a year old when my sister was born.

Kaye was able to progressively move from discussing her experiences with her hair care to discussing her feelings about being depressed, to talking about her relationship with her mother, to now directly talking about deserving more nurturance from her mother. It is interesting to note Kaye's attention to the detail of how her hair was braided. She was also very animated when she described the experience of her mother braiding her hair. This is especially significant when compared to her overall lack of animation. It is possible that Kaye's hair-braiding experience was the most prolonged physical contact that Kaye experienced with her mother during her childhood years. We may wish to think about the hair braiding, washing, preparation, and so on, as a ritual that can further facilitate or disrupt attachment bonds between mother and child.

The vignette illustrates that while Kaye was talking about hair, the manifest content, the latent content was about a depressed woman who is still yearning for her mother and her therapist to take care of her. Her ragged sweaters and unkempt hair communicates her wish: Take care of me because I cannot care for myself.

## PSYCHOTHERAPEUTIC CONSIDERATIONS

Consistent with the appropriate interpretation of individual psychodynamics, no one interpretation of any behavior can be automatically generalized. The meaning of a particular hairstyle or feelings about it must be interpreted in the context of that specific individual's family and social history.

The therapist should understand that the emotional meanings of hair may be quite unique from patient to patient. For example, many clients may complain about the therapist's fee even though they spend a considerable amount of money on expensive hairstyles and their maintenance. In another example, a client who wished to save money to buy her own home traded hair care with a friend to save money.

An understanding of the emotional meanings of hair, especially the meanings of hair in the mother–daughter relationship and the family as a whole, may serve as a vehicle for identifying the developing transference dynamics. Emotional issues and conflicts about one's hair may be symbolic of conflicts at any stage of the psychosexual developmental process. Feelings about the self, particularly feelings of inferiority or shame, may be projected onto hair. The psychoanalytic techniques used in working with dream material may be particularly useful in helping constricted clients explore their early child–caretaker experiences about hair. The therapist should be prepared to see feelings of unexpected intensity from many clients during these inquiries. Furthermore, therapists must be aware of their own feelings about hair, beauty in general, and their role in the relationship with their own mother or caretakers. Therapists who have their own conflicts and anxieties about hair should be exploring these issues in their own therapy or supervision before exploring this material with clients.

African American families must mitigate unhealthy communications to their male and female children about hair. This means that we need to understand families within the context of a racist society and the patient's struggle with these issues in the context of ubiquitous racism. Many of the conflicts that we have discussed are a function of living in and managing a locus of social disadvantage and a falsely stigmatized identity (Greene, 1992). They do not occur outside of some context and should not be viewed as innate defects in the individuals who struggle with them—although they will certainly be colored by individual characterological dispositions. It must be noted that these issues arise in the context of societal pathologies, racism and sexism, and that these pathologies must be explicitly addressed as a part of the treatment process (Brown, 1994; Greene, 1992, 1994, 1996; hooks, 1988). Clients must be educated about the origins of hair-texture and skin-color preferences and their link to American racism and sexism. It is important that they understand where many of these ideas came from and how they have become toxic elements in the psyche of many African Americans.

Therapists must understand and communicate to clients that neutralizing the effects of these societal toxins requires much more energy and creativity on the part of African American families and parents than is required of their White counterparts, and therefore childrearing entails more work for African Americans (Greene, 1992). When parents' resources are overextended, they may not have the energy available to devote as much time to this process as is warranted. In these situations, therapists may need to devote some of the therapy process to this task. They may do this by sensitizing parents to these issues or directly addressing them in therapies with children.

Within the realms of self-image and sexual attractiveness for partners in relationships, hair may have a variety of meanings that are expressed in the dynamics of that relationship. Once again, hair may be given an emotional meaning and significance that is far greater than its realistic importance.

Male romantic partners may experience various feelings about their female partners that are expressed by touching or avoiding touching her hair (Cleage, 1993). Some women report that they have experienced subtle negative emotions in the sexual arena with partners who were not touching their hair because these women felt that their partners were repulsed by the texture of their natural hair. Conversely, a woman's hair may be so idealized that she correctly perceives that it, rather than her person, may be the focus of her partner's attraction. For example, D reported that her boyfriend would talk endlessly about her naturally straight, long hair and even bragged to his friends about her hair. She reported that he often made comments about how silky it was to touch, which he did frequently, and about how much he liked it when she wore it down on her shoulders. She reported that he made disparaging comments about other women with short, nappy hair and that she was criticized by him when she wore her hair styled up or curled. D felt that in many ways her hair was the real focus of his attention and that her boyfriend was really not interested in other aspects of her person. "It's as if my hair makes me what I am to him," she lamented angrily. "*I* am *not* my hair!"

Touching may be an expression of idealization of the hair, while not touching may express the partner's devaluation of the hair. In another example, F reported that when she casually mentioned to her boyfriend that she was considering wearing her hair in a natural style, he angrily challenged her about why she would want to do such a thing and announced that he would not touch her hair if she stopped straightening it.

Feelings about hair represent issues that frequently go unexplored in the treatment setting. Nevertheless, they are the repository for many intense feelings for Black women. Therefore, while it requires exploration, the inquiry must be sensitive, skillfully conducted, and always embedded in a strong therapeutic alliance. The conflicts and issues we discuss in this chapter should not be raised casually, out of mere curiosity or voyeurism. Clients may experience much shame in discussing experiences about hair or acknowledging the use of hair weaves, wigs, straighteners, and the like. Therapists need to appreciate this reality, proceed with caution, explore their clients' feelings about sharing the material, and consider the strength of the working alliance. Timing is important. The therapist must always consider the client's fragility and determine her emotional readiness to explore this issue. During the exploration of this material, periodically ask the client what is coming up for her. It is important to end the session early enough to allow the client to begin to process feelings that came up during the session and then help the client make the transition to the outside world.

It may be particularly important to raise this issue with clients who are clearly neglectful of or clearly overinvolved with hair care, or who exhibit frequent changes of hairstyles. When the client changes her hairstyle, this can be an opportunity for the therapist to explore what the change means for the client.

The therapist's own choice of hairstyle can affect the therapy process. Clients often have feelings about the therapist's hair and changes in the therapist's hairstyle. A client's inquiries about the therapist's hair can be used as an opportunity to raise questions about the client's feelings about her own hair. For example, a White, Jewish client praised her Black therapist's braided hairstyle. The therapist used this opportunity to talk to the client about her feelings of self-hatred, manifested in her aversion to men who looked "too Jewish." In another example, for some Black clients, the therapist's hairstyle can evoke a range of feelings that can positively or negatively affect the transference.

S was 29 years old when she began therapy. Her primary complaint was that she was preorgasmic. S was a very emotionally controlled woman who had great difficulty acknowledging or expressing anger or any other intense feelings. In the 2 years that she was in therapy the only time she was emotionally expressive was when she talked about her hair. In the middle of reciting her sexual history, S explained that she was never "girlfriend material" because of her extremely short hair. She cried as she described her experiences going to school wearing a wig, which the other children would often snatch off. Meanwhile, all three of her sisters had thick, shoulder-length hair. For much of her life she had to listen to her mother's friends offering her unsolicited advice about how to improve her hair. S reported that this "advice" was a source of great embarrassment to her.

W is a 40-year-old African American woman with dark skin and short nappy hair, which she wears straightened. She has been in therapy for 3 years and has talked at length about her conflicts about her hair. She often questioned whether or not she should continue to straighten her hair or instead cut it and wear it in a natural style. Her primary concerns centered around how other people would react, particularly the people in her family and men. She also observed that the therapist wore her hair natural and that this gave her the courage to do the same. Despite this, it took her almost a year to cut her hair and wear it in a natural hairstyle. More recently she has begun the process of locking her hair and is very happy with this decision. She reports feeling freer and acknowledges "This is *my* hair."

If the therapist has a strong reaction to a client's hairstyle, this may be a sign of deeper issues that the therapist needs to address. It may also represent some communication from the client to the therapist, for example, the client's attempt to distract the therapist. It would not be inappropriate to assume that a change in hairstyle to dreadlocks or braids indicates a point of positive cultural identification, but such a change might also have other meanings. For some women, it may represent their only way of having long hair, in a culture in which long hair of any texture is idealized as superior, sexier, or more feminine than shorter hairstyles.

In other cases, adolescents or young adult women may use hair as a vehicle for rebellion against parental figures. For example, the 16-year-old daughter of an afrocentric mother who was raised wearing natural hairstyles and taught that such styles were a positive reflection of her African heritage finally told her mother that she wanted to straighten her hair. Her mother was appalled and would not permit it. The ensuing struggle over hairstyle became problematic for them. In the therapist's work with the mother it became clear that the daughter was beginning to spend more time outside the home with her friends and was trying to define herself in ways that distinguished her from her family. In this case, separation–individuation issues were acted out around the struggles between mother and daughter about hair. In this same vein, for some clients, the choice of a particular hairstyle can represent identification with a certain family member just as it can represent the need to avoid such identification. While hair-care rituals between African American mothers and daughters may be tortuous experiences for some, these rituals may represent important opportunities for emotional bonding for other mothers and daughters. Some clients report that having their hair done was the only time they were ever touched by their mothers. Of that group, some recalled painfully that they were touched roughly, as if their mother begrudged them the contact or as if they were forcing their mother to undertake an unpleasant task. Other clients, however, reported that the care and attentiveness their mothers demonstrated during these rituals made them feel loved and valued and that they recalled those times with great fondness and affection.

When mothers or parenting figures are narcissistic, the child may be viewed as a competitor or as an extension of the parent, as if the child has no independent needs of her own. If her hair texture is markedly different, the mother may treat the child as if she is inferior. If, on the other hand, the mother envies her child's hair texture, she may respond to that child with hostility. In yet another scenario, if the parent does not know how to care for her daughter's hair and feels inadequate as a result, she may blame the child by treating her as if her hair is unmanageable or too difficult to make presentable. The latter is not an uncommon occurrence when a child is a person of color and the mother is White (i.e., when the child does not share the hair texture of the mother) as well as in cross-racial adoptions. It is important to help parents understand the nature of their own conflicts and feelings and the kind of conscious and unconscious messages they communicate to their daughters.

The therapist must be careful not to compliment a client on a change in her hairstyle before understanding how the client feels about the change and what brought it about. The therapist can say "I notice that you have changed your hairstyle" as a way of beginning such a discussion. This underscores the importance of understanding the multiple and varied meanings that hair holds symbolically for African American women, as well as its role in their relationships with their mothers (and other parenting figures) and later with romantic partners, as well as the development of their self-esteem and identity. These meanings are as diverse as African American women are diverse as a group.

Overall we are left with a range of questions that may help guide the therapeutic inquiry. Zarem (personal communication, September 25, 1999) observes that we must be aware of the importance of intergenerational information and poses a range of questions that assist in such an inquiry. For example, who is the client's mother? What was the mother's family of origin like and what values or conflicts has the mother unconsciously internalized? What was the nature of the sociopolitical environment in which the client's mother grew up? How do the issues in the family of origin interact with those in the African American community as well as in the dominant culture at that time in history? How does the client understand the nature of her mother's self and sexuality and how did the mother's experience become interwoven with that of her daughter? Similarly, who, as a woman, is the therapist to the client? What is the therapist's skin color, hair texture, and length like and what assumptions does the client make about its meaning that can be observed in the transference? Finally, what kinds of countertransferential issues are elicited in the therapist and what is their meaning?

## SUMMARY

In this chapter we have explored the varied symbolic and metaphorical meanings of hair texture, length, and style in both the psyches and the lives of African American women. This discussion reviews both the historical and contemporary sociocultural contexts of African Americans and their negative effects on the ways that African American women view their ethnic physical features. We have focused considerable attention on the historical and cultural contributions to the conflicts and tensions relating to hair that arise, between many African American mothers and their daughters, as well as to the important role that parenting figures play in mitigating the dominant culture's negative messages about African American features.

Our goal is to raise clinicians' level of awareness about a potentially rich source of inquiry in psychotherapy that has been virtually ignored in the psychological literature. The absence of an exploration of these issues stands in stark contrast to the degree to which they are routinely discussed by African American women within their families and with their peers.

It is important for clinicians to give this material greater consideration in therapies with African American women as it is likely that most have been affected by them in some way. To the extent that hair texture, length, and style feature prominently among their clients' concerns, therapists must be competent to explore and sensitively respond to such material. In our experience, psychodynamic techniques can be very helpful in conducting these inquiries if they are approached in a way that is sensitive to the unique position of African American women in a racist, sexist, and heterosexist society. Any approach must include an explicit understanding and consideration of the sociopolitical context of African American women's feelings about their hair.

Alice Walker (1988) writes of her experiences with hair in "Oppressed Hair Puts a Ceiling on the Brain":

> Eventually I knew precisely what hair wanted; it wanted to grow, to be itself, to attract lint, if that was its destiny, but to be left alone by anyone, including me, who did not love it as it was. (p. 73)

## ACKNOWLEDGMENTS

The authors wish to thank Lois Dennis, Lawrence Greene, Monica Pierrepointe, and Dr. Sara Zarem for their helpful comments and discussions during the preparation of this chapter.

## REFERENCES

Adams, M. V. (1996). *The multicultural imagination: Race, color, and the unconscious.* New York: Routledge.

Angelou, M. (1969). *I know why the caged bird sings.* New York: Bantam Books.

Baldwin, J. (1964). *Nobody knows my name: More notes of a native son.* New York: Vintage International Books.

Berg, C. (1936). The unconscious significance of hair. *International Journal of Psychoanalysis,17,* 73–88.

Boyd-Franklin, N. (1989). *Black families in therapy: A multisystems approach.* New York: Guilford Press.

Boyd-Franklin, N. (1991). Recurrent themes in the treatment of African American women in group psychotherapy. *Women and Therapy, 11,* 25–40.

Brooks, G. (1972). *Report from Part I: The autobiography of Gwendolyn Brooks.* Detroit, MI: Broadside Press.

Brown, L. S. (1994). *Subversive dialogues: Theory in feminist therapy.* New York: Basic Books.

Cash, T. F., & Duncan, N. C. (1984). Physical attractiveness stereotyping among Black American college students. *Journal of Social Psychology, 122,* 71–77.

Cleage, P. (1993). Hairpeace. *African American Review, 27*(1), 37–41.

Green, K. (1993, June). The pain of living the lye. *Essence,* 38.

Greene, B. (1990). Sturdy bridges: The role of African American mothers in the socialization of African American children. *Women and Therapy, 10,* 205–225.

Greene, B. (1992). Racial socialization as a tool in psychotherapy with African American children. In L. Vargas & J. Koss-Chioino (Eds.), *Working with culture: Psychotherapeutic interventions with ethnic minority children and adolescents* (pp. 63–81). San Francisco: Jossey-Bass.

Greene, B. (1994). African American women: Derivatives of racism and sexism in psychotherapy. In E. Toback & B. Rosoff (Eds.), *Genes and gender series: Vol. 7. Challenging racism and sexism: Alternatives to genetic explanations* (pp. 122–139). New York: Feminist Press.

Greene, B. (1996). Psychotherapy with African American women: Considering diverse identities and societal barriers. *Annals of the New York Academy of Sciences:* Women and mental health, *789,* 191–210.

Greene, B. (1997, June). Psychotherapy with African American women: Integrating feminist and psychodynamic models. *Journal of Smith College Studies in Social Work, 67*(3), 299–322.

Grier, W., & Cobbs, P. (1980). *Black rage* (2nd ed.). New York: Basic Books.

Hall, C. I. (1995). Beauty is in the soul of the beholder: Psychological implications of beauty and African American women. *Cultural Diversity and Mental Health, 1*(2),125–137.

Hill-Collins, P. (1991). *Black feminist thought.* New York: Routledge.

hooks, b. (1988, September). Straightening our hair. *Zeta,* 33–37.

Hopson-Powell, D., & Hopson, D. (1990). *Different and wonderful: Raising Black children in a race-conscious society.* Englewood, NJ: Prentice-Hall.

Jenkins, M. C., & Atkins, T. V. (1990). Perceptions of acceptable dress by corporate and noncorporate recruiters. *Journal of Human Behavior and Learning, 7*(1), 38–46.

Jones, L. (1994). *Bulletproof diva: Tales of race, sex, and hair.* New York: Doubleday.

Leeds, M. (1994). Young African American women and the language of beauty. In K. A. Callaghan (Ed.), *Ideals of feminine beauty* (pp. 147–159). Westport, CT: Greenwood Press.

Mack, D., & Rainey, D. (1990). Female applicants' grooming and personnel selection. *Journal of Social Behavior and Personality, 5,* 399–407.

Martin, J. G. (1964). Racial ethnocentrism and judgment of beauty. *Journal of Social Psychology, 63,* 59–63.

Neal, A., & Wilson, M. (1989). The role of skin color and features in the Black community: Implications for Black women and therapy. *Clinical Psychology Review, 9,* 323–333.

Okazawa-Rey, M., Robinson, T., & Ward, J. V. (1987, Spring–Summer). Black women and the politics of skin color and hair. *Women and Therapy, 6*(1–2), 89–102.

Powers, R. (1994, May–June). Bold type: Lisa Jones on race, sex, and hair. *Ms, 75.*

Rich, M. K., & Cash, T. F. (1993, July). The American image of beauty: Media representations of hair color for four decades. *Sex Roles, 29*(1–2), 113–124.

Robinson, L. C. (1998). Hair and beauty culture. In K. A. Appiah & H. L. Gates Jr. (Eds.), *Microsoft encarta africana: Comprehensive encyclopedia of Black history and culture* [CD-ROM]. Redmond, WA: Microsoft.

Synnott, A. (1987, September). Shame and glory: A sociology of hair. *British Journal of Sociology, 38*(3), 381–413.

Walker, A. (1988). Oppressed hair puts a ceiling on the brain. In A. Walker, *Living by the word: Selected writings, 1973–1987* (pp. 69–74). Orlando, FL: Harcourt Brace Jovanovich.

Weathers, N. R. (1991, Summer). Braided sculptures and smokin' combs: African American women's hair-culture. *Sage: A Scholarly Journal on Black Women, 8*(1), 58–61.

West, C. M. (1995). Mammy, Sapphire, and Jezebel: Historical images of Black women and their implications for psychotherapy. *Psychotherapy, 32*(3), 458–466.

Whitten, L. (1994, August). *African American women and attitudes about hair.* Paper presented at the 102nd annual meeting of the American Psychological Association, Los Angeles.

## CHAPTER 9

# Finding the Lost Part
## Identity and the Black/White Biracial Client

### KUMEA SHORTER-GOODEN

Developing a coherent identity is one of the central tasks of adolescence. For people of color in the United States, who live in a racist society, racial identity has been found to be a particularly important aspect of self-identification. Interestingly, while Erikson's (1968) concept of identity, or ego identity, derives from an ego psychoanalytic orientation, there has been little application of this concept to an understanding of psychoanalytic or psychodynamic therapy. How ego identity, and specifically ego racial identity, impacts the psychodynamic therapeutic process has rarely been examined. Moreover, little exploration has been done of the impact on psychological development and the therapeutic process when the client must wrestle not only with a singular racial identity (in the context of a racist society), but with a biracial identity in the context of a society that has little tolerance for biraciality or multiraciality.

The purpose of this chapter is to focus attention on Black/White biracial adolescent female clients and the psychodynamic psychotherapy process. I begin by providing a framework for thinking about the developmental process of these adolescents. This is followed by a detailed case study in which the therapeutic process will be the focus.

## THEORETICAL FRAMEWORK

What is the general context in which Black/White biracial adolescents in the United States live? The context is one in which interracial sexuality and marriage have long been taboo. Root (1992) reports that it was only in 1967 that a

U.S. Supreme Court ruling led to the repeal of laws against miscegenation in 14 states. Until then it was illegal in many parts of the country to marry a person of a different race. The offspring of interracial couplings challenged the status quo about race and race relations. Root states that "the presence of racially mixed persons defies the social order predicated upon race, blurs racial and ethnic group boundaries, and challenges generally accepted proscriptions and prescriptions regarding intergroup relations" (1992, p. 3). Of the varying racial groups, the "proscriptions and prescriptions" have been greatest with regards to African Americans and European Americans.

A few theorists and therapists have written about particular psychosocial issues that biracial people in the United States often contend with. Biracial people often wrestle with a sense of marginality, invisibility, or "otherness." The ambiguity of their racial status and the intolerance that many Americans have for an ambiguous or mixed racial heritage contribute to these feelings (Brown, 1990; Root, 1990). This sense of marginality may contribute to difficulty in establishing a sense of autonomy (Brown, 1990; Gibbs, 1987; Gibbs & Moskowitz-Sweet, 1991), and thus to an elevated sense of shame and increased vulnerability to assaults on self-esteem (Bowles, 1993; Gibbs, 1987), to excessive dependence on others' perceptions and definitions of oneself (Brown, 1990), and to difficulties separating and individuating from parents (Gibbs & Moskowitz-Sweet, 1991).

It is important to note, however, that while many biracial people may be challenged by a sense of marginality and "otherness," many others find their biraciality of minimal salience in their internal experience and in their experience of the world. Many Black/White biracial individuals grow up in African American communities, view themselves as African American, are viewed by others as African American, and establish an identity as African American (Miller, 1992). For them, being biracial—being half-White and half-Black—is not a salient part of their identity. For other Black/White biracial people, however, being biracial is a central issue that they must contend with. Whether or not being biracial is salient would seem to depend on the child's appearance, the parents' approach to and understanding of racial issues, the availability and involvement of the African American parent and extended family, and the racial composition of and level of racism in the community in which the child is raised. In other words, the very meaning and salience of biraciality has to do with the interaction between the person's inner world and the outer world of family, community, and society.

Erikson's (1968) theory of psychosocial development provides a framework for understanding this interplay between inner psychological processes and the larger social environment. In particular, Erikson's work on adolescent identity development highlights the importance, after early childhood, of the person's interaction with the environment in shaping the person's sense of self. For adolescents of color, Erikson points our attention to the broader sociocultural context in which youth develop and helps us to understand the impact of external societal racism on the adolescent's development of an internal identity.

Erikson (1968) coined the term *ego identity* to refer to a self-definition that is comprised of goals, values, and beliefs to which the person is committed and which provide a sense of continuity over time. The development of a coherent ego identity is seen as the major developmental task of adolescence and as a task that is important for the transition into a healthy adulthood. The development of an ego identity, often called simply "identity," is seen as important in the young person's separation–individuation from parental figures and in the development of the capacity for intimacy, and thus the development of a mature partnership of one's own. For Erikson, the development of an identity involves the exploration of different parts of oneself, the reworking of childhood identifications, and the integration of a sense of self that pulls together disparate pieces into a coherent whole and that makes sense for the person in her internal experience and in her interface with the larger world. The opposite of identity for Erikson is *identity confusion*, which is marked by a "split of self-images" (1968, p. 212) and the loss of a sense of coherence. Erikson felt that an optimal sense of identity is experienced as "psychosocial well-being" (1968, p. 165.)

Through empirical research, racial identity has been found to be an important, indeed, often central, component of identity for people of color (Parham, 1989; Phinney & Alipuria, 1990; Phinney & Tarver, 1988; Shorter-Gooden & Washington, 1996). Moreover, racial identity has been found to be positively related to emotional well-being (Parham & Helms, 1985a, 1985b; Phinney, 1989). In other words, for the person of color, developing a positive and coherent racial identity is an important adolescent developmental task that is likely foundational for the development of other aspects of one's identity. For the Black/White biracial youth, developing a positive racial identity is very important (Gibbs & Hines, 1992; Johnson, 1992), and yet, because of the complexity often associated with being biracial, this task may be particularly challenging.

## CLINICAL CASE EXAMPLE

The following case example of a Black/White biracial female client has been selected to illustrate the psychological functioning and treatment of a client who presented with identity issues and narcissistic pathology. In this case, I integrate an Eriksonian understanding of identity, as described above, with insights from self psychology (see Kohut, 1977). Self psychology provides an important and useful theoretical understanding of narcissistic disorders. Moreover, self psychology focuses our attention on "understanding the self as a cohesive whole" (Flanagan, 1996, p. 173), and the construct "self" in self psychology is similar in some regards to Erikson's construct of ego identity (Schamess, 1996). This case has been disguised and altered to protect the confidentiality of the client.

## Initial Sessions

S, a 22-year-old female, was referred to me by her mother, who was concerned about S's emotional well-being following the breakup of her relationship with her boyfriend of the past 2 years. S's mother phoned me initially, and then S herself called to set up her first appointment. S came to the appointment without her mother.

S appeared for the first session on time. She was an attractive young woman whose racial background was not obvious; she looked like she was part European American as well as part African and/or part Latino and/or part Asian. She seemed self-assured and serious, but not depressed. When asked about how she felt about coming to therapy, she indicated that she was unsure about it because she had never been in therapy before, but that she liked the way I sounded over the phone, and that this made it a little easier to come in. When asked about how she felt about seeing an African American therapist, she said that she had only considered seeing an African American therapist.

She indicated that she was distraught about the recent breakup of her relationship with R, a 30-year-old African American graduate student. She had wanted to marry R, but she felt that he "just wasn't ready." She was concerned about "how to have a successful relationship," and she indicated that she felt she had put her all into the relationship with R, and couldn't understand why it had not worked. About 6 weeks prior to her appointment with me, R had told her that he "needed some space" and he suggested that they spend less time together. She had tried to respect this request, by not calling him three times a day, which was her usual pattern, and by not spending all of her nonwork time with him, but she had difficulty holding to this plan. She felt increasingly anxious when she was not with him and she was fearful about the demise of the relationship, but she did not talk with R about her feelings. About a month later, R told S that he "couldn't do it anymore"; he wanted to break up. S reported all of this in a rather matter-of-fact manner with little affect.

S reported that since the breakup 2 weeks ago, she had been tearful and upset. She had called in sick to work a couple of days, but when she was at work she was able to function well. When she was not at work she spent most of her time at home with her mother, seemingly asking for advice and looking for support, or talking on the phone to one of several women friends. If her mother was not at home and if S could not reach a friend by phone, she felt very alone and sometimes became fearful and panicky.

The person whom S described to me seemed rather different than the one I was interacting with, who seemed very poised and independent (almost counterdependent), and who displayed little affect. In the first session, I felt like I was being kept at bay. S talked and carried the session along. She did not seem to want me to say much or to intercede. It was as if she needed to control the session in order to feel comfortable or safe.

I learned that she was employed as an administrative assistant in a computer sales and service company. She had graduated from a local college with a bachelor's degree 6 months previously, and had been working full time at this company since then. Throughout college S had lived at home with her mother and she continued to do so. Her mother was European American, in her late 40s, and an elementary school teacher. S had one younger brother who was away at an out-of-state college, but who spent most holidays and summers at home. S's father and mother had divorced when she was 15. Her father was an African American in his late 40s who worked for the post office. Her father had moved out of state and had remarried, and S had fairly limited contact with him. S reported that she had "a really good relationship" with her mother and that they were very close and talked a lot, but that her relationship with her father was somewhat strained, though it had been improving in the past few years.

S reported that she and R had met about 2 years earlier when she was a junior in college. He was a graduate student at the same college. The relationship had begun very quickly: within a couple of weeks she had a key to his off-campus apartment and was living much of the time with him, although she maintained her residence with her mother and kept most of her belongings at her mother's house. S talked about being very much in love with R. In the past 2 years, she seemed to have shaped her entire life around R and his world. She continued to attend classes full time and to do well academically, but she no longer spent time with other friends. In the evening after her classes and her part-time job, she often would go to R's apartment with groceries in hand and fix dinner for him. Sometimes he would arrive home from the library at 8 P.M., as they had agreed, but many times he arrived hours later. This hurt S but she rarely complained, and she continued to cook dinner for him several times a week, always spending her own limited money for groceries.

She seemed to have spent the relationship in a state of worry: worried about R's seeming interest in another student on campus, worried about whether she might say or do the wrong thing and alienate R, and, more generally, worried about R ending the relationship and leaving her. I commented that though this relationship had been a very important one in her life and very gratifying in many ways that I was struck by how difficult and painful it was for her even before the recent breakup.

In the second session S once again appeared poised and composed. I asked her how she felt after the last session, and she expressed concern that she may have seemed "disorganized" to me. S talked about her relationship with R, reviewing past events and reporting to me her conclusions about what had happened and why. She didn't seem to want my advice or my interpretation of what had happened. She talked with me in a rather reportorial fashion as if she were delivering a finished product to me rather than engaging with me in a process of exploration. Often she spoke of what "the Lord had told her to do" or how "God was having her deal with" the situation. I knew that these comments were based on her genuine Christian beliefs, but I experienced them, in part, as a defense, as a way of keeping me out; in other words, she dialogued with God but not with me.

Sitting with S, I felt bored and unneeded. It was difficult for me to feel genuinely connected to and interested in her. It seemed as if the function I was serving was to be physically present and to listen, but not to get involved.

At my request, at the next few sessions S talked more about her family history. She indicated that she had grown up in a well-integrated area that included substantial numbers of both African American and European American families. S felt that her mother was the responsible adult and parent in the family; her mother handled the family finances, family decision making, and most of the parenting responsibilities, but she was often "too busy" to notice what was going on with S and her brother. She described her father as "acting like the third child" in the family. He spent much of his nonwork time away from home, "hanging out with his friends." When he was around, S felt, he paid little attention to the rest of the family. At school, S was always a strong student, but she never felt like she fit in completely socially. She remembered being teased in elementary school for "looking like a White girl." She tended to be absent from school fairly often with a headache or stomachache. She acknowledged that when she stayed home from school she enjoyed the opportunity to be alone with her mother. S seemed to have a somewhat distant and competitive relationship with her brother, who was 3 years younger. While she did well in school, he excelled. While she was often "sick" and needing attention from her mother, he seemed to need little from his parents. S felt that both parents adored him.

The parents raised S and her brother as African Americans, rather than as European Americans, or as biracial. Most of S's friends from childhood through the present were African American. The mother, in particular, was active in buying Black dolls for S and finding children's books about African Americans for her daughter and son to read. The family belonged to a Black Protestant church, but only the children and their mother attended Sunday services and other events regularly. One got the sense that S's father was a peripheral figure in the family— relatively uninvolved, but humored, and tolerated.

S wasn't sure why her parents had divorced. She said that her father had often been publicly flirtatious with other women, but her mother had seemed to grin and bear it. S didn't know if her father had had affairs. Her mother, who seemed to handle her husband by being stoic and a martyr, initiated the separation and eventual divorce when S was 14. This was a difficult period for S not only because of the separation of her parents and her father's move out of the family home, but because she was wrestling with her social life as a teenager. She reported that around this time she began sleeping with boys and was "rather promiscuous." She felt that her parents were too preoccupied with their own difficulties to be aware of what was going on with her. She told me that she was "looking for love, looking for someone to care about her" and seemed to think that giving boys what they wanted sexually was the way to get this.

S reported that her relationship with R was her first relationship of more than 3 months' duration. While this relationship was highly sexual from its beginning, S felt that with R she had learned how to sustain and build a relationship over time and how to make a commitment. Because this relationship represented a victory on her part, she was particularly devastated by its ending.

S had majored in sociology. At the urging of a professor, she had briefly considered getting a master's degree in social work, but she had not yet made a decision about this career path when she became involved with R. After the relationship became serious, she decided not to pursue graduate studies right away. R was completing a graduate degree and would probably be relocating. S hoped to marry him and felt that there was no point in starting school and then moving and having to transfer. Moreover, she had more of an image of herself as a wife than as a social worker or career woman. She had received a couple of job offers upon graduation, and she had chosen the computer sales and service company because of its proximity to R's apartment.

She was overqualified for her position as an administrative assistant, but she seemed to be satisfied with the position and to be a very dedicated and hard worker. However, she sometimes expressed concerns to me about how she was viewed by her colleagues and her supervisor. She often wondered if a few of her colleagues were at times excluding her from important work-related conversations. The company was predominantly European American with a substantial number of Asian and Asian American employees. S was one of only a few employees of African ancestry.

## Clinical Formulation

After a few sessions my clinical formulation of S was as follows: I saw her as a young woman who was wrestling with narcissistic issues. She seemed to have gotten little emotional nurturance from her parents to help her develop a positive sense of self. Her father seemed immature. When S was a child, her mother seemed depressed and preoccupied, perhaps with her marital problems. S struggled with anxious feelings and low self-esteem. She seemed threatened by the notion that she might appear less than perfect and that she would be abandoned as a result of her imperfection. For example, in therapy, she was worried that she was too "disorganized." Thus she presented herself in therapy in a very "together" fashion; moreover, she didn't seem to want much from me, other than to be listened to and agreed with.

From a self psychology perspective, one might say that S was desperate for mirroring from others—to be seen as special and unique by others. In addition, she yearned to find safety and security in someone strong whom she could idealize. As a result, she seemed to have difficulty genuinely engaging with others in an adult fashion. She alternated between merging with and losing herself in others, on the one hand, and remaining distant and disengaged as a way to protect herself from injury to her sense of self, on the other hand.

As a middle adolescent, she had used sexuality as a way of feeling connected and cared about. As an older adolescent, she had ceased this behavior, but she continued to diminish herself in her romantic relationships. With R, she had essentially relinquished her identity to his. On the surface, the relationship with R had the potential to resolve (though perhaps not in the healthiest fashion) the adolescent identity questions of "Who am I?" and "What do I do with my life?" and to provide a transition to young adulthood. She had begun to center her identity around being R's girlfriend and his future wife. She had deferred work on career identity issues altogether; and she had decided to secure a job (a rather unchallenging one) that did not interfere too much with her relationship with R. Because of prevailing gender roles in this society, the fact that S was female had probably contributed to the ease with which she developed an identity centered around a male partner. The relationship with R also provided an opportunity for S to attempt to manage her feelings of abandonment by her father by merging with a substitute father figure. Thus, R's breakup with her left her adrift; she lost a person who provided a transition between childhood and adulthood, a person who served as a father surrogate, and a person who provided a solution to her adolescent identity struggles.

S had entered adolescence in a particularly vulnerable state. Though she felt "Black" and was connected to the African American community, as a biracial child who did not appear Black and who was teased at times, she never felt fully integrated with her African American peers. Her African American father's emotional immaturity and unavailability likely contributed to S's difficulty internalizing a sense of sureness around being Black. During adolescence S had done little exploration of her racial identity. It was hard for me to get a sense of what being African American meant to her or how being biracial figured into her sense of self. Her racial identity seemed unexplored and fragmented. And yet I got the sense that unconsciously Blackness and Whiteness were split for her. Blackness perhaps meant irresponsible, unavailable, and bad, whereas Whiteness meant responsible and good.

S had done little to separate and individuate from her mother and to develop a young adult sense of autonomy and competence. She was floundering in making the transition from adolescence to young adulthood. Her poorly integrated identity and her lack of a coherent sense of self contributed substantially to this difficulty.

## Middle Phase of Therapy

S and I continued to meet weekly. About once every 4 to 6 weeks, she would call to cancel the session at the last minute because she "needed to stay late to finish something at work" or because a friend of hers called and "needed her to help out with something." When I would raise the issue at the next meeting about her missing the session and whether there were other feelings that contributed to not coming to therapy, she would insist that there was no other meaning to her missed meetings. S continued to use the sessions to "report on" what was going on at work and how she felt about things with R, though as the weeks passed she mentioned R less and less.

One week she came in and reported that she had begun seeing J, whom she had met a couple of weeks earlier at a friend's house. What struck me was that she and J were already becoming fairly serious—S had begun to shape her life around his—and yet this was the first she had mentioned him to me. When I commented on this, in a somewhat typical fashion S said "Yeah" and then continued with her comments about this new relationship. J was a 26-year-old African American who worked full time in construction and who had attended community college off and on several years prior. S seemed to be excited by how beautiful J felt she was and how much he seemed to adore her. S was spending lots of time at his apartment, where he lived alone, and she was hoping to change her work schedule so that she could match her work hours to his.

S's periodic missed appointments were now due to "having to do something with J," and it was still difficult for her to talk about what else the missed appointments might mean. I was prepared for the likelihood that she would drop out of therapy altogether and was frustrated with my own inability to have an impact on her insight. I constantly had to remind myself that in some fundamental way S seemed connected to me and to the therapy; when asked, she admitted that she got a lot out of coming and talking to me.

The relationship with J seemed rather like the relationship with R. S enjoyed being admired and being special in his eyes. I sensed that J enjoyed having an attractive, devoted girlfriend who fit easily into his life and who did not ask for much. S spent most of her nonwork time at J's apartment; she stopped spending time with her mother or her other friends. For example, J did not attend church, so she stopped attending. They were in constant contact by pager, and they generally talked on the phone a couple of times a day from work. S seemed content with all of this, though occasionally she would allude to a fear that if she was not available for J all the time that he might "go back with his old girlfriend."

One pivotal session occurred during her seventh month of therapy, after she and J had been together about 4 months. In the middle of our session S's pager went off. She retrieved it from her purse, looked at the number on it, told me it was J paging her, and started to leave the session to return his call. I commented that I wondered what it meant that she needed to interrupt her own therapy to call J back right away. This comment seemed to surprise S, but she stayed in the session and did not call J back. S and I then talked about her anger at me for "stopping her" as well as what was behind her need to immediately respond to J's page. When she talked with J after the session, he was initially upset about the delay in her response, but after they discussed it he was okay. In the next session S and I continued to talk about this incident; she felt a sense of accomplishment for not having called J back right away and she felt reassured that he and she could handle the delay in contact.

This "pager incident" also marked her first discussion with J about the fact that she was in psychotherapy. Prior to that, she had told him she was staying late at work or that she "had to see a doctor." Moreover, she began for the first time to share concerns and problems that she had in the relationship with J with me. It was as if she was beginning to allow her relationship with me to become part of her relationship with him and vice versa. In other words, these two important areas of her life that had been kept separate were beginning to be integrated. She was beginning to integrate disparate parts of her identity—her sense of herself while with J was beginning to become part of her sense of herself while she was with me. Through this interaction with S, it became clearer to me just how much she needed to hide who she was in order to protect her fragile sense of self.

S's concerns about her relationship with J centered around her feeling that J might get involved with another woman, that she could not hold onto him, and that he would leave her. This was a source of tremendous anxiety for her. It led her to compulsively listen to his phone answering machine messages and to look through his mail in order "to find out what was really going on." J seemed to contribute to S's suspiciousness by spending time with old girlfriends, a number of whom were White, and by being surreptitious with phone calls from women friends. S's inability to trust J seemed to stem in part from his behavior but also from her difficulty trusting her own judgment and feelings. She was unsure of herself, so how could she tell if her relationship with J was solid? And for S, these concerns echoed issues in her mother's relationship with her father.

What made these issues even more complicated was that S had significant difficulty expressing any of her concerns to J or asking him for anything. Expressing her feelings would render her less than perfect in her own and in his eyes, and this seemed intolerable to her. She felt that if she shared her concerns—for example, about his friendships with former girlfriends—that he would become angry and leave her.

The fact that a number of J's women friends were White contributed to S's anxiety and distrust of J. When I encouraged S to talk more about what this meant to her, she revealed that she felt that she was physically attractive to men because of her European physical features—in other words, because her appearance was not very African. Although she felt threatened by the possibility that J might get involved with a woman of any ethnicity or appearance, she was particularly anxious about the possibility that he would get involved with a European American woman. S acknowledged that she felt that White women were as or more attractive than she was. This discussion, which was a painful one for S, helped her to get in touch with and begin to get freed up from her own internalized negative feelings about being Black. Although S's outward identification was as an African American woman, there were aspects of her blackness that she had been uncomfortable with and that she had devalued.

These discussions in the therapy about race led to S disclosing more about how race tinged different aspects of her life. For example, she disclosed that at work a number of her colleagues did not know what her ethnicity was, and she felt more comfortable with them not knowing. She never disclosed that she was part African American and part European American, or that she considered herself African American. When a colleague asked about where her boyfriend lived, S gave a vague response that would not flag that he resided in a largely African American area. S rationalized that her racial status and J's were "none of their business," but she also acknowledged feeling anxious about how she would be perceived by colleagues if they knew she were African American. She talked of "just wanting to fit in."

It seems that through talking about the impact of race on her day-to-day life, S was able to begin to look at herself and her personal relationship to blackness and to whiteness and to bring together in her consciousness and in her life two areas that had been relatively unexamined and rather compartmentalized. At my prodding she also began to talk about her thoughts and feelings about my racial identification. While she felt superficially comfortable with me as an African American person, she acknowledged that this surface comfort was combined with a tendency to distance herself.

I began to realize that my own feelings of distance from S paralleled her feelings of distance from most people, as well as her feelings of distance from being African American. I was "carrying" S's experience of superficial engagement with significant others and her experience of superficial engagement with her racial identity. Over time she and I began to see how this pattern with me was part of her life pattern: superficial connections with African Americans combined with a self-protective distancing. On the surface she had a Black identity, but underneath she had internalized negative views of blackness and was much more ambivalent. This resulted in her disengagement from those in the world whom she was closest to, which, of course, colluded with her narcissistic need to protect her fragile sense of self.

During this period S stopped her practice of canceling sessions periodically. We talked about the importance of the therapy as a time *for her*, when she could explore issues and concerns with less worry about what others might think. She began to see therapy as a gift to herself, as something that she deserved that took priority in her life. S seemed freer and more at ease in the sessions and less concerned about presenting a "together" facade to me. She continued to refer to her religious beliefs, but I no longer felt that her references to her religiosity were defensive, or a way of keeping me away from her. Thus, I began to feel less distanced by S. As I began to feel more visible in the therapy room, I found that my countertransference toward her became more positive.

With my support and encouragement, S began to take risks in her relationship with J and to share with him her feelings, concerns, and needs. Though J had difficulty initially with this change in their relationship, ultimately he was able to handle it: he did not retaliate or abandon her. As a result, S felt empowered to continue to find and express her voice. S was learning that she could be angry at me and that the therapy relationship would survive and that she could be angry at J and their relationship would survive. S began to feel less anxious and suspicious when she was away from J and she began to reconnect with women friends whom she had virtually ceased contact with since she had met J.

## Final Phase of Therapy

About a year and a half into the therapy, S began to consider and explore career possibilities. For several months she had talked about concerns about J's career motivation. For someone without a college degree, he had a fairly well-paying job, but she was concerned that being a construction worker was not a viable career in the long term. But she eventually moved from focusing on J to thinking about her own career identity and to making plans for her own occupational future. Over time, she realized that she was not happy in her administrative assistant position, nor was she interested in pursuing social work, which she had leaned toward while she was in college at the advice of a professor. As she encouraged J to go back to community college and to make career plans for his future, she began to seriously think about her own interests and her options and to consult others. She eventually decided she wanted to go to business school and pursue a career in finance.

S decided to terminate therapy after 22 months when she was about to reduce her work to part time and to begin business school. By the end of the therapy, S's relationship with J had continued and matured substantially. S had developed a clearer sense of her identity, of who she was as a person, of what she felt and what she needed, and of where she wanted her life to go. As a result, she did not feel the same emotional need to merge with a partner. She remained committed to the relationship with J, but was able to nurture and develop other relationships. In fact, her relationships with women friends seemed to deepen and become more intimate as a result of her growth. Notably, Erikson's theory

(1968) says that the development of genuine intimacy is contingent on the development of a sense of identity.

S was less anxious, more relaxed, and more able to be herself in a variety of situations. She was somewhat more secure with who she was racially, and she experienced greater comfort in both African American and non-African American settings. She was learning to integrate the different parts of herself; she was finding the lost parts.

## CONCLUSION

This clinical case example of a 22-year-old Black/White biracial female client illustrates the salience of issues of identity and racial identity, specifically, in this client's difficulties and in the unfolding of the treatment process. One striking element of this case is that since the client had been raised as African American, considered herself African American, and, in her personal and social life associated almost exclusively with African Americans, the identity issues related to her biraciality were not initially obvious. And yet her biraciality and how race impacted her were important issues and sources of pain for her that needed to be explored to free her up to develop an integrated sense of identity and to successfully move into young adulthood.

This case example points to the potent and complicated impact of societal values and messages on the sense of self of Black/White biracial persons. Moreover, this example highlights the value of culturally sensitive psychodynamic psychotherapy in helping clients of color rework and integrate racially devalued parts of themselves, and thus in facilitating the identity formation process and the transition to adulthood.

## REFERENCES

Bowles, D. D. (1993). Bi-racial identity: Children born to African-American and White couples. *Clinical Social Work Journal, 21*(4), 417–428.

Brown, P. M. (1990). Biracial identity and social marginality. *Child and Adolescent Social Work, 7*(4), 319–337.

Erikson, E. (1968). *Identity: Youth and crisis.* New York: Norton.

Flanagan, L. M. (1996). The theory of self psychology. In J. Berzoff, L. M. Flanagan, & P. Hertz (Eds.), *Inside out and outside in: Psychodynamic clinical theory and practice in contemporary multicultural contexts* (pp. 173–198). Northvale, NJ: Jason Aronson.

Gibbs, J. T. (1987). Identity and marginality: Issues in the treatment of biracial adolescents. *American Journal of Orthopsychiatry, 57*(2), 265–278.

Gibbs, J. T., & Hines, A. M. (1992). Negotiating ethnic identity: Issues for Black–White biracial adolescents. In M. P. P. Root (Ed.), *Racially mixed people in America* (pp. 223–238). Newbury Park, CA: Sage.

Gibbs, J. T., & Moskowitz-Sweet, G. (1991, December). Clinical and cultural issues in the treatment of biracial and bicultural adolescents. *Families in Society: The Journal of Contemporary Human Services*, 579–591.

Johnson, D. J. (1992). Developmental pathways: Toward an ecological theoretical formulation of race identity in Black–White biracial children. In M. P. P. Root (Ed.), *Racially mixed people in America* (pp. 37–49). Newbury Park, CA: Sage.

Kohut, H. (1977). *Restoration of the self*. New York: International Universities Press.

Miller, R. L. (1992). The human ecology of multiracial identity. In M. P. P. Root (Ed.), *Racially mixed people in America* (pp. 24–36). Newbury Park, CA: Sage.

Parham, T. A. (1989). Cycles of psychological nigrescence. *Counseling Psychologist*, *17*(2), 187–226.

Parham, T. A., & Helms, J. E. (1985a). Attitudes of racial identity and self-esteem of Black students: An exploratory investigation. *Journal of College Student Personnel*, *26*(2), 143–147.

Parham, T. A., & Helms, J. E. (1985b). Relation of racial attitudes to self-actualization and affective states of Black students. *Journal of Counseling Psychology*, *32*(3), 431–440.

Phinney, J. S. (1989). Stages of ethnic identity development in minority group adolescents. *Journal of Early Adolescence*, *9*(1–2), 34–49.

Phinney, J. S., & Alipuria, L. (1990). Ethnic identity in college students from four ethnic groups. *Journal of Adolescence*, *13*(2), 171–183.

Phinney, J. S., & Tarver, S. (1988). Ethnic identity search and commitment in Black and White eighth graders. *Journal of Early Adolescence*, *8*(3), 265–277.

Root, M. P. P. (1990). Resolving "other" status: Identity development of biracial individuals. In L. S. Brown & M. P. P. Root (Eds.), *Diversity and complexity in feminist therapy* (pp. 185–205). Binghamton, NY: Haworth Press.

Root, M. P. P. (1992). Within, between, and beyond race. In M. P. P. Root (Ed.), *Racially mixed people in America* (pp. 3–11). Newbury Park, CA: Sage.

Schamess, G. (1996). Ego psychology. In J. Berzoff, L. M. Flanagan, & P. Hertz (Eds.), *Inside out and outside in: Psychodynamic clinical theory and practice in contemporary multicultural contexts* (pp. 67–101). Northvale, NJ: Jason Aronson.

Shorter-Gooden, K., & Washington, N. C. (1996). Young, Black, and female: The challenge of weaving an identity. *Journal of Adolescence*, *19*, 465–475.

CHAPTER 10

# Psychoanalytic Group Psychotherapy with African American Women
## The Bad Mother in All-Female Groups

JUDITH C. WHITE

As an African American woman, I have maintained a lifelong interest in issues pertaining to my race and gender. As a clinical social worker, a psychoanalyst, and a psychotherapist, my professional life has focused on ways of integrating issues of race, ethnicity, and gender with psychoanalytic and psychodynamic thinking. My interest in issues of race and gender and most certainly group psychotherapy were very much influenced by my own family of origin. My family was a nuclear and extended family, which encompassed my parents, three siblings, six aunts, one uncle, and their respective spouses. One factor in my interest in leading all-female groups was rooted in being a developing young girl and then a maturing woman with six aunts. It is also quite possible that my desire to integrate men into the group paralleled my extended family's growth as my aunts married and brought men into the family. This describes how my own personal beginnings and the context of my development is reflected in my work. Understanding the role of our early life experiences and family dynamics in our current life decisions and relationships, what we seek to avoid, and what we seek to recapitulate exemplifies what the process of psychodynamic therapies seek to delineate.

This chapter explores the working-through process of the bad mother transference in combined individual and group treatment with all-female groups from an object relations perspective. Attention is paid to how the bad mother transference interacts with issues of race and ethnicity, and to ways of

208

healing the defensive splitting that gives rise to the bad mother transference. Karon and Widener (1995) cite the work of Melanie Klein (1930, 1948) in their definition of *splitting* as an unconscious defense mechanism that the patient is unable to integrate both the good and bad introjects (images) of mother and/ or of self. In relationships, when an individual engages in defensive splitting, the individual experiences other people and themselves as *either* all good *or* all bad. The realistic good and bad elements of both the self and others are not integrated and cannot be experienced simultaneously. Clinical vignettes are drawn from two groups in my private psychotherapy practice. Group 1, an interracial group, which began in 1984, was an all-female group. Men were integrated into the group beginning in 1991, the group's seventh year. Group 2 is an all-female group of African American women that began in 1992.

In a previous work (White, 1994), I explored the impact of race/ethnicity on transference and countertransference in combined individual/group therapy with an interracial group. Because individual psychodynamics can be cathected onto race, the group process elicits feelings about racial and ethnic differences with greater intensity than individual psychotherapy. Analyzing racial and ethnic issues can be challenging but can also be growth-enhancing in treatment. While the process of identifying conscious and unconscious feelings and thoughts can stimulate resistance and challenge the working alliance, working through those feelings can lead to a more rapid unfolding of core issues (White, 1994).

In my 1994 work, I make the following observations and generalizations about the treatment process of the interracial group. The group process in psychotherapy elicits feelings about a patient's own racial/ethnic group and feelings about different groups with greater intensity than individual therapy. When patients anticipate entering a multiethnic group they may produce more material about their own ethnicity as well as that of others. In group psychotherapy the repression and denial of racial/ethnic differences may be more difficult to maintain than they are in individual psychotherapy. In my clinical experience, when someone enters or leaves the group, racial and ethnic differences are elicited with greater intensity. There are two ways to measure the cohesiveness of a multiracial/multiethnic group. The first is the degree of freedom members experience to discuss feelings about the group they belong to as well as other groups (including stereotypes about each group). The second is the degree of freedom that members feel to express aggressive and loving feelings toward each other.

While African American women come to psychotherapy from diverse backgrounds and with a myriad of complaints, most of my patients are first-generation, college-educated or first-generation achievers, who at times are in conflict about seeking psychotherapy. Psychotherapy may be experienced by some African American women as culturally alien to their perception of ethnic identity and experience (Greene, 1996). Many have faced criticism from family members (especially their mothers) for seeking psychotherapy. One benefit of combined individual and group psychotherapy is that the group that includes other African American women can be an important source of validation for continuing in long-term psychoanalytically oriented psychotherapy.

Most African American women whom I have treated have indicated a preference for working with a therapist who was an African American woman. In fact, most patients discussed in this chapter have been privately referred. A few have often expressed over the telephone that they wanted to work with an African American psychotherapist and then asked if I was indeed "Black." (This often occurs even though I have been previously identified by the referral source as African American.) In the first session I always explore the patient's feelings and thoughts underlying this request (Greene, 1996; Smith, 1976). Patients have usually indicated a desire to work with an African American female because they assume that if the therapist's racial background parallels their own, they will be better understood (in a few cases patients had prior psychotherapy experiences with White clinicians). While I have acknowledged the importance of their wish to feel understood, I have also stated the importance of the patient telling her unique story.

My interest in working with all-female groups was a practical one. I had considerably more female patients than male ones. For me, there was no incompatibility between all-female groups and the psychoanalytic process. Bion's (1961) early groups consisted only of men. It surprised me when some of my colleagues—not all of them men—raised questions as to whether all-female groups could indeed be psychoanalytic. Colleagues expressed these objections to me at formal presentations or informally. The objections of these colleagues seem to center around the need for a group that would include both men and women so that group participants could practice interpersonal learning with both genders. Alonso (1987) spoke of her preference for mixed-gender groups because they "offer more options for working through personality traits that are gender linked" (p. 161). A few female colleagues felt that an all-female group would stimulate powerful countertransference feelings. It is also possible that colleagues were unconsciously threatened by the power suggested by an all-female group. Male colleagues may have feared the economic loss that might result from a proliferation of all-women groups.

As a practitioner, I have found combined psychoanalytically oriented individual and group treatment to be one of the most effective treatment modalities for promoting internal, intrapsychic development and interpersonal growth. The model of combined treatment that is described here involves individual and group treatment conducted by the same clinician in which group is added after the initial phase of individual treatment, during the working-through phase of individual treatment. The patient is seen simultaneously in individual and group treatment at least once a week. Caligor, Fieldsteel, and

Brok (1984) observe that when patients begin in psychodynamic psycho-therapy, it is in that setting that a working alliance is established; that psychodynamic understandings can be developed; and that the origins of the patient's behavior, embedded in that patient's unique history, can be explored. When this is accomplished, adding group therapy to the patient's individual analytic therapy allows the working-through process to be more realized. Insight promotes changes in behavior that are needed to modify entrenched characterological defenses. When we combine individual and group psychotherapy, that combination provides the patient with the opportunity for more varied and differentiated relationships (Caligor et al., 1984). Caligor and colleagues observe that the group process promotes the process of individuation, enhances the evolution of a stable sense of self, and fosters a more autonomous, self-determined connection with the therapist. Ultimately, the combination of individual and group therapy serves to more fully complete the developmental tasks that serve as the focus of analytic therapy.

A psychoanalytic object relations theoretical perspective is used throughout this chapter. The focus of this perspective is on how inner (intrapsychic) relationships between self and other shape a person's interpersonal relationships. Kibel (1993) observes that object relations theory is concerned primarily with internalized relationships. *Internalized relationships* may be seen as the psychic schemas about relationships between our mental representations of ourselves and others. These representations are called self images and object images and have their origins in early preverbal experiences. These images serve as foundations for later relationships, as they shape the quality and tone of future experiences. Internalized relationships and real relationships reciprocally influence one another; however, the dominant relationship, particularly when psychopathology is present, is usually based in the internal rather than the external (real) mental world (Kibel, 1993). The internal world shapes actual relationships in varied ways because feelings and fantasies, rooted in preverbal experiences, can produce distorted perceptions of real relationships. The purpose of the psychotherapy process is to change internal representations of external objects when those representations have been based on distortions. When those internal, mental distortions are corrected, therapy focuses on replacing them with more reality-based perceptions and actions (Kibel, 1993). Furthermore, Kibel states, object relations theory is particularly suited to group psychotherapy since it focuses on the use of interpersonal relationships as a method of inquiry and a tool for therapeutic change.

McWilliams and Stein (1987) cite Helen Durkin's (1954) *Group Therapy for Mothers of Disturbed Children* as a pioneering work that discussed the psychodynamics of women's groups led by women. Henrietta Glatzer's (1987) critique of McWilliams and Stein's (1987) article maintained that she and Durkin changed mothers' discussion groups into psychotherapy groups by focusing on each group member's transference as it arose.

McWilliams and Stein (1987) describe the devaluing transference of the woman leader that emerged in five all-female groups. The wish to devalue the female leader, that is, to project the member's sense of devaluation onto the leader, functions as a way of warding off the powerful preoedipal mother. McWilliams and Stein observe that Glatzer (1959, 1965), Durkin (1954), and Edwards (1984) are all analysts who have written most extensively about preoedipal processes in groups that are all female. In these groups, the negative transference, the bad mother, that emerged seemed intractable and unanalyzable. Glatzer (1987) maintained that McWilliams and Stein failed to analyze and work through the preoedipal resistance, and that the defensive structure of the members may have been too homogeneous, thereby contributing to the resistance in the group as a whole.

Anne Alonso's (1987) discussion of McWilliams and Stein's (1987) paper questioned whether the group members' behavior constituted a negative transference. She experienced the transference as both positive and negative. She wondered whether the leaders had inadequately accepted and honored the members' positive identifications. The leaders may have been frightened and made anxious by the group members' wish for erotic fusion with the leaders. Alonso observes that the groups' leaders may have had difficulty feeling and welcoming a homoerotic transference and instead focused on sadistic impulses, "thereby distorting the transferential field"(p. 161). Countertransference in these groups is always a problem, given the intensity of the yearnings and the universality of the "wicked witch" (p. 161) fantasies that are normative in new groups (and in group leaders). Alonso concludes by stating that she has stopped leading all-female groups and now leads mixed-gender groups because they allow "more options for working through personality traits that are gender linked" (p. 161).

This brief review of the literature suggests that there is a devaluing transference of the female leader in all-female groups and that its impact is important for all women who lead all-women groups to understand. In this phenomenon, female group members project their own feelings of inadequacy and sense of being devalued onto the female leader. This phenomenon may be more intense in all-Black female groups with a Black leader under specific circumstances. All-Black female groups whose members had more rejecting and greater separation experiences with their own mothers had more intense "bad mother" transferences with the therapist than groups whose members represented more varied experiences with their own mothers. The more chaotic and rejecting the early experience with the mother is, the more devalued a woman will feel. The more devalued she feels, the more likely she is to project that devaluation onto the group leader. We might speculate that the dominant culture's devaluation of Black women intensifies this phenomenon for Black women who were also devalued or rejected by their own mothers. This does not mean, however, that Black women are more likely to experience chaotic or rejecting relations with their mothers than White women. I suggest that it is advantageous to assemble women with a diverse mix of character pathologies when putting an all-female psychotherapy group together. This can serve to de-intensify the "bad mother" negative transference.

When there is an intense bad mother transference in the group, it may be difficult for the therapist to maintain the group. Some group members may find it intolerable to remain in the group when there is such a hostile and negative environment. Of those who leave, some may feel guilty about their participation in such intensely aggressive attacks on the group leader, who is a symbolic "mother." These patients may often leave treatment out of a fear of retaliation from the leader/mother.

Overall, there is support in the group psychotherapy literature, especially the classics (Durkin, 1954; Glatzer, 1974, 1987), maintaining that psychoanalytic work can be done in an all-female group.

There are certain commonalities that exist in all psychoanalytic groups irrespective of the race/ethnicity/gender of the membership. There are also differences that exist. The viability of an interracial group will depend largely on two factors. One factor is the degree to which the group leader understands how psychodynamics get cathected onto race. Another factor is the degree to which an African American clinician can generate referrals of White patients for a multicultural group and the degree to which a White clinician can stimulate referrals of African Americans and people of color for a multicultural group. The contributions of racial identity theorists (Helms, 1990) have enhanced our understanding of the developmental process of racial identity for both Blacks and Whites. These theories can be used to comprehend the group racial climate, "the conduciveness of the group's atmosphere to resolving intra- and interracial conflict and encouraging the development of positive racial identity development of group members regardless of their racial categorization" (Helms, 1990, p. 191), since at any one point in time group members can be at different levels of racial identity/awareness.

A homogeneous racial group of African American women in a psychoanalytically oriented therapy group will experience homogeneity in terms of race. However, diversity exists among them in terms of skin color, hair texture, class background, sexual orientation, diagnosis, and racial identity—among other things. These aspects of diversity within a racial group may stimulate as much emotional intensity as feelings of racial difference in an interracial group.

The concept of splitting is central to understanding the patient's experience of the group therapist (or the group, or a group member, or the self) as both a good mother and a bad mother. It offers a way of understanding the tendency of group members to idealize or devalue the group therapist. Melanie Klein has observed that in the paranoid–schizoid period of early infancy, infants project their own aggression onto a mothering figure who is then experienced as if she were "bad." Splitting is the defense mechanism employed to avoid the persecutory anxiety that results from the experience of one's own aggression. When splitting is employed, the ego fragments itself into separate parts: the idealized self (and object), and the bad self (and object) (Akhtar & Byrne, 1983).

When splitting is successful, aggressive impulses and concomitant persecutory anxieties are dispersed. The separation of "good" from "bad" experiences, perceptions, and emotions that we observe in patients is designed to avoid ambivalence and is a consequence of early defensive splitting. Akhtor and Byrne (1983) attribute this conceptualization of splitting and its origins to the work of Melanie Klein.

Patients who use extensive splitting see the world as being populated by "devils and angels" (Akhtar & Byrne, 1983, p. 1014). It is difficult for such individuals to accept the reality that there are human foibles in everyone, including themselves. To maintain an inner sense of "goodness" and to defend against vulnerability, the patient develops "the fantasy that the badness is out there and can be controlled" (Kibel, 1993, p. 167). This is the mechanism of projective identification. Hanna Segal (1973) describes *projective identification* as the process of splitting off parts of the self and internal objects. These unwanted parts of the self and internal objects are projected onto an external object (person) that "becomes possessed by, controlled and identified with the projected parts" (Kibel, 1993, p. 167). Object relations theorists understand patients in individual and group therapy in terms of "the operation of primitive defense mechanisms" (p. 168) such as splitting, projection, and projective identification.

Projective identification is not synonymous with the defense mechanism of projection. When patients project unwanted parts of themselves onto the therapist, usually the therapist is aware of the process and experiences the projections as ego alien. The therapist experiences projections as the patient's distortions of the therapist, that is, as a distortion of who the therapist really is. However, when projective identification is successfully employed by the patient, the therapist feels as if the patient's projections, which are distortions, are actually a part of him- or herself. It is as if the patient wraps a cloak of badness around the therapist which the therapist unknowingly accepts and wears as if the "badness" actually belongs to him or her. Overall, when projective identification is employed by the patient, the therapist has a diminished awareness of the distortion that is taking place.

We know that the group can become a maternal object for its members. The group can function as both a good mother and a bad mother. In fact, its bad mother functions, when analyzed, are especially healing and pave the way for the healing of splitting and the further development of object constancy. Libidinal object constancy is a developmental achievement that "consists of (1) the ability to develop and maintain a constant, predominantly libidinal (positive, object-related) attachment to a specific other; (2) the capacity for firmly established affective evocative memory; and (3) the resolution of factors such as defensive splitting which interfere with the functional use of this memory" (Wells & Glickauf-Hughes, 1986, p. 461). More simply stated, libidinal object constancy addresses the capacity of the self to sustain positive feelings about a good-enough mother when the self is feeling frustrated or deprived; and the capacity to function as a good-enough mother by providing self-soothing functions for the self. In my work with patients, development of libidinal object constancy is a primary goal with patients whose primary defenses are splitting and projection. The bad mother group phenomenon can pose special challenges for the group clinician. The concept of the bad mother reflects a dynamic process and a way of understanding group work in general. It is not limited to use with an all-Black women group. The good and bad mother is a metaphor used to describe the process of identifying the mother role of the group. Failure to explore and work through this defensive phenomenon may be disruptive to the group and could possibly lead to its dissolution.

Ganzarain (1989) observed that exploring "bad mother" group images can prevent the stereotyping of an idealized "good mother" group, while the therapist or others are rigidly cast in " bad" roles:

> The mother group functions, good and bad, should become instead interchangeable in psychotherapy groups, fluctuating within the group as an entity, the therapists, one member or another, or another group. Achieving this fluidity of roles provides varied opportunities for the patients to meet and to solve their individuation difficulties. The group can be especially suited to contain and to receive projective identifications from its members, for holding, modifying, and eventually returning them to the projectors, helping their selves to blossom and expand. (p. 84)

Certain treatment modifications and techniques have been found to be useful in healing the splitting that is evidenced by bad mother projections. They are as follows: (1) the placement of the individual session the day before group or the day after group (Youcha, 1984); (2) the use of brief phone contacts after the group session or the day following the group session for patients who may be experiencing themselves or the therapist in the all-bad state; (3) the therapist checking on the emotional pulse of the group; (4) the maintenance of the treatment plan—for example, patients may wish to drop individual or group treatment (special arrangements with fees may need to be developed).

1. *The placement of the individual session.* The placement of the individual session the day before the group or the day following group helps to minimize splitting. In this way, the patient is not left alone to deal with the experience of self or object as all bad. The patient's level of hostility that is associated with experiencing the self or object as all bad may be so intense that the group therapist may need to postpone dealing with the negative transference until the

individual session. This delay helps the patient's observing ego to regain its "reality assessment" (Ganzarain, 1989, p. 169). Repair to the narcissistic injury that may have been experienced in group can be worked on in the individual session. However, the therapist asks the patient to talk about her injury in group. Patients whose primary defenses are splitting and projection also have low frustration tolerance. Knowing that she will be able to meet with the therapist the day following group helps to minimize the anxiety that is stimulated by an injury in group. At times, patients may request to have the individual session the day before group. The patient may state that this allows her to address urgent concerns or concerns that she, as yet, does not feel free to share in group. Unconsciously, this may serve to minimize feelings of sibling rivalry that are stimulated in group. Or, more importantly, the placement of the individual session the day before group may serve to strengthen the attachment between the patient and the therapist. (See "The Bad Mother: Group Therapist" section, below, in which Andrea is discussed. Andrea requested that her individual session be held the day before group rather than the day after group.)

2. *Telephone contacts.* Telephone contacts after the group session or the day following may be used in a similar manner as the individual session. Telephone contacts can be used to minimize the patient's anxiety and/or rage so that she can function until her next individual session. The patient should always be encouraged to discuss her feelings in the next group session. Telephone contacts can be particularly helpful when therapy is being done in a clinic setting.

3. *Emotional pulse.* I have found it helpful, especially after a particularly emotionally charged session, to ask each member to state how she is feeling. Every group member who has a history of missing a group session following an intense group session is asked by the group therapist or by another member if she thinks it will be hard for her to come to the next group session. This technique is a way of taking an emotional pulse or reading of each member of the group before the group session ends. This technique is a way of encouraging members to be attuned to their feelings, to talk about their feelings, and to discourage acting out (by not attending sessions).

4. *Maintaining the treatment plan of combined individual and group therapy.* At times the patient's use of splitting may lead her to experience the group as all bad or the therapist as all bad or the self as all bad. This can create difficulties in maintaining both group and individual sessions. The patient may stop attending group and come only to individual sessions after feeling misunderstood or hurt in group. Or the patient may have more difficulty tolerating the individual session (as Andrea did at one time) and choose to only attend group and miss individual. The resistance must be explored and the treatment plan resumed.

## HOMOGENEOUS RACIAL GROUPS

When the group therapist is the same racial background as the group members, the group therapist may need to be alert to countertransference dynamics that may complicate the psychodynamic process. Identification of these countertransference aspects will then facilitate the group process. For example, during the planning stage of the all-Black female group, I maintained a preconscious fantasy that this group experience would be more positive than the interracial group. In effect, the fantasy was that it would be a more cohesive group because it was a homogeneous racial group and because I was a more experienced group leader. My fantasy contributed to a sense of surprise when there was an overwhelming outpouring of aggression from a subgroup of women during the initial phase of the all-Black group.

The aggression first of a member and then of a subgroup was manifested within the context of race.

> During the first two group meetings, Lee, an older woman of dark-brown coloring expressed hostility toward Roxie, a younger, light-skinned woman. In later group sessions Lee was able to discuss the meanings of the color difference within her family of origin. Lee came from a family with two distinct sibling groups: an older group of dark-skinned children and a younger group of light-skinned children. Lee was the oldest of the group of dark-skinned children. She experienced herself as unwanted and rejected by her mother. In fact, Lee's mother had not served as her caretaker for most of her childhood. Yet Lee's mother had served as the caretaker for her younger, lighter skinned offspring. Transferentially, Lee feared that her group mother would favor Roxie, a lighter skinned group member, who was symbolically her younger lighter sibling.
>
> After Lee's attack, Roxie felt very unsafe in the group. Roxie was not an identifiable African American woman by virtue of her color. In fact, people would often ask her to identify her racial group because her racial background was not discernible given her coloring and appearance. Roxie was very hurt by Lee's attack and threatened to leave the group. For Roxie, the group was all bad. Therapeutic work was directed toward helping her identify good aspects of the group experience so that she could remain in the group.

More of the African American women in the all-African American group than African American women in the interracial group had experienced actual separation from one or more parents during childhood. This factor may explain the greater propensity for expression of aggression in the all-African American female group than in the interracial group. It should be noted that all of the African American women in this group were functioning professional women with at least one college degree and most had some level of graduate education. Another factor is a cultural one. Some authors maintain that expression of anger is more acceptable in the African American community than in the dominant society (Grier & Cobbs, 1968).

As stated earlier, the intrapsychic goal for the patients highlighted in this chapter's case vignettes is to move each woman toward obtaining libidinal object constancy. After the establishment of libidinal object constancy, a patient will be able to function as her good-enough mother and will experience a stronger sense of self and object differentiation. Combined individual and group therapy is an effective treatment modality that helps patients minimize the defensive process of splitting and projection.

At this point I will offer three clinical examples to demonstrate how bad mother projections can be ascribed to the group-as-a-whole, to a group member, and to the group therapist.

## The Bad Mother: Group-as-a-Whole

This was the beginning phase of the African American women's group when members were expressing a lot of ambivalence about group or their displeasure about being in group. The leader wondered if group members' lateness and absences were related to their feelings about group. Barb said, "I like coming to individual and I get a lot from individual but I don't feel I am getting enough [attention, nurturance] here, especially when I have to come here at night." Roxie said, "I only agreed to come here because Judith felt it would be helpful; she knows I am not going to be here for years and years." Andrea said vehemently, "I think each week we should have a different topic to discuss and that someone needs to direct the discussion."

The members continued to discuss how hard it was to get nurturance from the group. These members were experiencing the group as a bad breast incapable of nurturing them. Yet they seemed to like being with one another. In fact, two of the women had paired. Alonso and Rutan (1979, p. 483) refer to this as "premature pairing in the dependency phase." The two members who paired were both lesbian women of similar dark coloring who split and projected their negative feelings onto a heterosexual woman of light coloring. Alonso and Rutan observe that the women in a group with men and women will often pair with other women and focus their negative feelings onto members who are male. Pairing in this group was expressed on the basis of the same sexual orientation and a similar dark coloring.

## The Bad Mother: A Group Member

This vignette is taken from an interracial all-female group in the middle phase of the group's history.

Diane, a group member, was the recipient of a lot of warm feelings from other group members who then became the bad mother. Diane, a white Jewish woman, was discussing her relationship with her lover, a married Christian man. She indicated that her involvement with him helped her feel worthwhile. The group members were very angry and attacking of Diane—unusually so.

This process happened over a number of sessions. The leader asked the group members to try to understand their intense anger and rejection of Diane's feelings and behavior. Initially, they maintained that their anger with Diane was related to their wish for her to end a relationship with a man who devalued her. But, as the group process unfolded, it became clear that what the group members most hated in Diane was what they most feared in themselves. These members had projected their unwanted aspects of themselves, their dependency needs, onto Diane. Their rage and insensitivity to Diane was a way of defending against their dependency needs and their devaluation of themselves as women.

## The Bad Mother: Group Therapist

When the group therapist is experienced as the bad mother by the group or by a very vocal subgroup, the group therapist is particularly challenged to understand and work through countertransference reactions that may be harmful to the group.

Andrea, an African American lesbian woman in her late 20s, is the youngest of four children from a working-class family. She came to therapy to work on her relationship with her father. Andrea had been her father's favorite child. He would not discipline her and he related to her more as his "wife" than as his daughter. He would seek her counsel, take her out on "dates," and at times leave her mother home. When her father learned she was gay, he disowned her, stopped paying her college tuition, and made it difficult for her to continue living in the family home. Andrea then decided to leave the family home. After being disowned by her father, Andrea maintained minimal contact with her mother and siblings.

Andrea—who proudly identifies herself as a graduate of a prestigious women's college—began to question her devaluation of her mother as weak and childlike in contrast to her idealization of her father as intelligent and creative. It was her experience in both individual and group therapy that disrupted her identifications.

In individual she maintained an idealizing transference. When group was added, she began to devalue the group leader. She observed that the group therapist should provide the group with more direction—for example, choose a topical theme that they could discuss each week.

When the group therapist failed to be more "directive," Andrea became the "chairperson" of the group. She had become the alternative leader of the group as Bion (1961) described in the dependency phase of group.

The group was used to help Andrea become more aware of how members responded to her "chairperson" behavior. Given her strong desire to be liked by the group, she tried to work on learning to listen. During this period, in individual therapy, the therapist confronted Andrea's devaluation of her mother and her idealization of her father. Over time, she began to wonder who had actually held the family together when her father was hospitalized for an unknown psychiatric disorder and who had supported the family when her father impulsively quit his job. She began to express some feelings of admiration for her mother's role in consistently supporting the family.

In group, she alternated between experiencing the group therapist as good-enough and being the bad mother. For Andrea, the therapist was the wicked witch who refused to bail her out when she was threatened with being evicted from her apartment for failing to pay the rent. For a few group sessions Andrea was the leader of a subgroup that experienced the group therapist as the depriving punitive parent. Andrea also led the group in having postgroup sessions in front of the therapist's office building.

During the fight/flight phase of group (Bion, 1961), Andrea consciously hated the therapist for being the powerful mother/leader but unconsciously admired the leader for asking her to respect the norms of the group and individual treatment. Several months later Andrea joked in group with another group member about how persistently the therapist pursued her when she would take a "hiatus" from individual or group. It was curative for Andrea to feel wanted despite her "rejecting" behavior.

One of Andrea's concerns was that she had not been able to maintain a friendship with a woman without the friendship becoming a sexual relationship. Her participation in group would give her the opportunity to do so. Yet she was afraid of developing erotic transferences toward group members. Her most intense negative transference toward Roxie, another group member, became less toxic after Andrea said that she was often attracted to women who looked like Roxie, who were similar in coloring and hair texture to her mother. Andrea was also able to own her projections and accept aspects of her bad self in Roxie.

What helped the therapist manage her countertransference response? We had developed a positive working alliance before group was added to individual therapy. Continuing individual sessions while Andrea was in group helped to modulate the bad mother transference that would intensify in group. In fact, after a brief hiatus from group, Andrea asked if we could move her individual session to the day before group because she felt that it would be easier for her to come to group if we did so. This arrangement may have helped to minimize the splitting so that Andrea could maintain more of the positive transference. Andrea's estrangement from her family because of her sexual orientation strengthened her wish/fear dilemma for a new family, the group.

## The Bad Mother: A Male Group Member

Men were integrated into the all-female interracial group in the seventh year of the group. A few women specifically requested that new group members be men rather than women. But a number of women were opposed to the addition of men. The case below demonstrates how a male member was initially experienced as the bad mother by a subgroup of women. It also describes how the working through of this projection moved the women in this subgroup to greater self-awareness.

> Matt was a man who grew up on the West Coast of the United States, and who had recently relocated to the East Coast after being promoted by his corporation. Matt was a good-looking professional African American man. In individual therapy, Paula, a very attractive overweight African American woman, informed her therapist that she found Matt very attractive. He was in fact the kind of man she would like to marry but she feared that such a man would reject her. Work in individual therapy was directed toward exploring Paula's fantasy and her fear of rejection. Finally, in one group session, Paula was able to directly communicate her interest to Matt. It was truly significant for Paula to be able to openly share her attraction to Matt and to explore the meaning of the attraction with the group. Matt was able to talk openly of the qualities he admired in Paula. However, in a subsequent group session Matt suggested that he was more attracted to another female African American member. Although currently married to his second wife, Matt had informed the group that his first wife was White. In the midst of an angry exchange with Matt, Paula asked Matt to identify the race of his current wife. The therapist interrupted the group process and told Matt not to answer the question and then asked Paula to state what motivated her to ask Matt this question. Paula was furious with the group therapist for being interrupted and for being asked to consider what feelings or thoughts prompted the question. The group therapist then asked group members to consider the question as one they would be asking and then to think of what feelings or thoughts might give rise to this question. A subgroup of women talked about their annoyance with successful African

American men or men of color who marry White women. Group members stated that Paula's question was surely related to her expressed attraction to Matt. The group process was able to help Paula withdraw her projections from Matt and talk more openly about her desire to find a man with Matt's qualities given her intense fear of being rejected.

In summary, it was clear to me that it was important to make interventions that interpreted members' wish/fear for a powerful preoedipal mother. I understood their defensive splitting as a way of protecting themselves from mother's powers. However, I think that it would have been helpful to have been more attuned to the positive transferences that were in the latent communication of the group process.

With both groups I fantasize that I am trying to create a uterine environment, a group matrix, to facilitate the emotional growth of its members and to "hold" them when they feel bad or when the badness is projected onto the group therapist, and to accept their loving and erotic longings.

## SUMMARY

I have discussed the use of combined psychoanalytically oriented individual and group therapy with all-female groups, an interracial one and a homogeneous racial group comprised of all African American women. This chapter has reviewed the impact of race/ethnicity on transference and countertransference in an interracial group and in a homogeneous racial group. An object relations theoretical perspective with the focus on the defensive use of splitting has been discussed to understand the bad mother transferences that are stimulated in doing combined work. Treatment modifications and techniques that have been found helpful in healing the splitting evidenced by the bad mother projections have been proposed.

As our country becomes more racially and ethnically diverse, and as more African American people and people of color become more economically stable, clinicians will be faced with the need to integrate the powerful forces of race, ethnicity, and gender with psychoanalytically psychodynamic theory.

## ACKNOWLEDGMENTS

I wish to thank Dr. Beverly Greene for her consistent encouragement in preparing this chapter and Dr. Mary F. Hall for her support and critical commentary. Earlier versions of this chapter were presented in 1996 and 1998 at the Group Colloquium, Analytic Group Department, Postgraduate Center for Mental Health, New York City.

## REFERENCES

Akhtar, S., & Byrne, J. (1983). The concept of splitting and its clinical relevance. *American Journal of Psychiatry, 140*(8), 1013–1016.

Alonso, A. (1987). Discussion of women's groups led by women. *International Journal of Group Psychotherapy, 37*(2), 159–162.

Alonso, A., & Rutan, S. J. (1979). Women in group therapy. *International Journal of Group Psychotherapy, 29*(4), 481–491.

Bion, W. R. (1961). *Experience in groups.* New York: Basic Books.

Caligor, J., Fieldsteel, N., & Brok, A. (1984). *Individual and group therapy combining psychoanalytic treatments.* New York: Basic Books.

Durkin, H. E. (1954). *Group therapy for mothers of disturbed children.* Springfield, IL: Thomas.

Edwards, N. (1984). The preoedipal development of the critical superego and its manifestations in psychoanalytic group psychotherapy. *This Journal, 34,* 47–66.

Ganzarain, R. C. (1989). The "bad mother" group. In R. C. Ganzarain, *Object relations group psychotherapy: The group as an object, a tool, and a training base* (pp. 67–103). Madison, CT: International Universities Press.

Glatzer, H. T. (1959). Some clinical aspects of adult therapy: The pre oedipal fantasy. *American Journal of Orthopsychiatry, 29,* 383–390.

Glatzer, H. T. (1965). Aspects of transference in group psychotherapy. *This Journal, 15,* 167–176.

Glatzer, H. T. (1987). Critique of women's groups led by women. *International Journal of Group Psychotherapy, 37*(2) 155–158.

Greene, B. (1996). African-American women: Considering diverse identities and societal barriers in psychotherapy. *Annals of the New York Academy of Sciences: Women and Mental Health, 789,* 191–210.

Grier, W. H., & Cobbs, P. M. (1968). *Black rage.* New York: Basic Books.

Helms, J. (Ed.). (1990). *Black and White racial identity: Theory, research, and practice.* Westport, CT: Greenwood Press.

Karon, B. P., & Widener, A. J. (1995). Psychodynamic therapies in historical perspective: Nothing human do I consider alien to me. In B. Bongar & L. Beutler (Eds.), *Comprehensive textbook of psychotherapy: Theory and practice* (pp. 24–47). New York: Oxford University Press.

Kibel, H. (1993). Object relations theory and group psychotherapy In H. Kaplan & B. Sadock (Eds.), *Comprehensive group psychotherapy* (pp. 165–176). Baltimore: Williams & Wilkins.

Klein, M. (1930). The psychotherapy of the psychoses. *British Journal of Medical Psychology, 10,* 242–244.

Klein, M. (1948). *Contributions to psychoanalysis, 1931–1945.* London: Hogarth Press.

McWilliams, N., & Stein, J. (1987). Women's groups led by women: The management of devaluing transferences. *International Journal of Group Psychotherapy, 37*(2), 139–153.

Segal, H. (1973). *Introduction to the work of Melanie Klein* (2nd ed.). New York: Basic Books.

Smith, C. E. (1976, May). *Race and ethnicity in psychotherapy.* Lecture given at the Postgraduate Center for Mental Health, New York.

Wells, M., & Glickauf-Hughes, C. (1986). Techniques to develop object constancy with borderline clients. *Psychotherapy, 23*(3), 460–468.

White, J. (1994). The impact of race and ethnicity on transference and countertransference in combined individual/group therapy. *Group, 18*(2), 89–98.

Youcha, I. (1983, March). *Treatment of borderlines in group.* Lecture given at the Group Colloquium, Group Psychoanalytic Training Program, Postgraduate Center for Mental Health, New York.

## CHAPTER 11

# The Icon of the Strong Black Woman

## *The Paradox of Strength*

### REGINA E. ROMERO

She wears it like a suit of armor, a badge of courage. While it helps her to remain tenacious against the dual oppressions of racism and sexism, it is also an albatross around her neck. It keeps her from falling victim to her own despair, but it also masks her vulnerabilities. It is the substance around which folklore and legends, fact and fiction, have been written. "Strong Black woman" (SBW) is a mantra so much a part of U.S. culture that it is seldom realized how great a toll it has taken on the emotional well-being of the African American woman. As much as it may give her the illusion of control, it keeps her from identifying what she needs and reaching out for help.

While the historical antecedents of SBW are obvious, what is less clear are the effects of maintaining this self-definition in such an uncritical fashion. From a clinical perspective, African American women entering therapy must often struggle to get beyond some of the messages of SBW simply to join with the therapist in a journey of exploration. So threatening is it to redefine the basic tenets of SBW that many African American women present with and work hard at maintaining the facade. Some leave therapy prematurely without resolving the conflicts inherent in the SBW messages they have internalized. While many SBWs present with symptoms of depression, anxiety, and sleep and eating disturbances, the therapist must be cautioned against a symptom-only treatment plan or simply delving into family dynamics. Without addressing the cultural issues associated with the presenting symptoms, it is very likely the symptoms will persist.

Two primary themes of the SBW are explored in this chapter. The first suggests that African American women are strong, self-reliant, and self-contained. The second suggests that it is the African American woman's role to nurture and preserve family.

This chapter examines these themes, explores the messages associated with each, and clarifies what maintains SBWs and their psychological defenses. Through clinical vignettes, I explore the impact of SBW on the therapeutic relationship and, by inference, how it affects the African American woman's relationships with others. Finally, I propose methods of intervening that are culturally competent.

## THEME ONE: AFRICAN AMERICAN WOMEN ARE STRONG

Perhaps the single most consistent term African American women use to describe themselves is *strong*. I have heard clients refer to their "strength" numerous times in therapy sessions and I have often explored its meaning with them. Its full significance became even more apparent to me, however, when I attended a luncheon hosted by a group of African American women who had an "adopt a school" relationship with a majority Black, inner-city, junior high school. They geared their programs toward high-achieving females at the school. At the luncheon intended to honor them, they asked each young lady to come forward and introduce herself. The youth were quite creative in their self-descriptions, many comparing themselves to different animals. What was most intriguing to me was the fact that the vast majority of these young women used the term "strong" as a self-reference. As I listened to one youth after another use this term, I wondered how these self-descriptions might sound if the speakers were of a different ethnic or racial background. I also wondered what it meant that the identification with strength seemed so complete at such a young age.

In their study of identity development in young African American women, Shorter-Gooden and Washington (1996) found that the term "strong" was consistently used as a self-reference or to refer to those who had most impacted the respondents. In some cases, "strength," "strong," and "stronger" were used more than a dozen or more times throughout the interviews. Strength had two definitions for the respondents: it referred either to the determination and capacity to deal with the adversity associated with being African American, or to having such a strong sense of self that one's identity could not be obscured by others. The young women in the study either felt they already possessed strength or they were striving to achieve it. In either case, strength was a central component of their identity.

No doubt, women of other racial and ethnic groups have experiences that would lead them to self-identify as strong and nurturing. However, the basic difference for African American women is rooted in the historical context and social construction of her images as they developed through slavery and beyond. The image of the strong, self-sacrificing Mammy, for instance, has been institutionalized through books, movies, and folktales. West (1995) noted that "mental representations or images are difficult to alter and can occur without conscious intent or awareness" (p. 458). She also observed that "culturally imposed images may influence Black women in ways quite different than for women of other racial groups" (p. 463–464).

It appears that early in their development many African American women internalize the message that they should not expect to be able to rely on anyone else for their needs, and that they must become fully self-sufficient, first emotionally, and then economically. As one client pointed out to me, "You just have to do it [be strong]. I was raised that way. Society doesn't give you a choice. When you want to get off the merry-go-round, you can't."

"Strong" refers less to its physical strength than to emotional resilience. Ironically, it is often the physical kind of strength and caring for one's body that is neglected by those who try to live up to the SBW paradigm. Society expects the African American woman to handle losses, traumas, failed relationships, and the dual oppressions of racism and sexism. Falling short of this expectation is viewed by many African American women as a personal failure. This may bring about intense feelings of shame that they work hard to contain. Unconsciously, they learn to defend themselves against such onslaughts to their sense of self.

The external world may see the SBW as needing to be in control. Depending on how well she has developed coping skills, she may present as either inflexible and close-minded or as poised and competent. Others may perceive her as always handling things well. The African American woman herself, on the other hand, may not understand why others see her as "so together" when internally she feels anxious and depressed. She often does not make the connection between her own behavior and how others perceive her. To protect herself from feelings of vulnerability, she is inclined to utilize such rationalizations as "They really don't know me" or "They don't want to know me because then they would have to act differently." Showing vulnerability is unacceptable to an SBW. Crying, for instance, is a secret act shared only with the closest few—if with anyone. Exaggerated terms are often used to describe the simple act of crying. "Falling apart" or "breaking down" are common references. This is not a matter of being dramatic or using colorful language. Rather, the SBW actually experiences crying as "falling apart." One of my clients who was particularly well practiced in masking her vulnerabilities noted: "I even cry quietly!"

The SBW facade is an especially significant challenge in therapy. A therapist may easily underestimate the degree of distress the client is experiencing because the SBW client is just as likely to present herself as composed and collected in therapy as she would do in other situations. African American women have learned to mask their true feelings for self-protection. It is almost as if there are two separate beings: one she shows to the world and one she hides. In the course of therapy, the therapist must work to gently coax the SBW's hidden feelings out into the open. Exploring such issues as (1) *why* she needs to hide her feelings, (2) *where* she picked up the message that she should not share her feelings, and (3) *what* purpose hiding and not sharing feelings has for her now may prove revealing for the SBW.

One difficulty inherent in presenting a strong face to the world is that the SBW often inherits other people's problems. She may appear to be quite relational. Family and friends, colleagues and associates, seek her out for counsel. It is very hard for her to say No. Yet she isolates herself when she is feeling particularly vulnerable. She is unlikely to initiate phone calls, to get together with friends, or otherwise reach out to others. Because she so rarely presents herself as needy, others in her life do not know how to respond when she does. For instance, I had one client who was a member of a Black women's support group. As I explored her role in that group, I learned that she was the embodiment of emotional strength for all of its members. She was a few years older than most of the members and was more professionally accomplished. Looking up to her was easy for other members. They could not imagine that they had much counsel to offer her. When she did expose herself and seek their support, their apparent lack of appreciation for her struggle profoundly disappointed her. Her perception was that they listened to what she had to say, made a few cursory remarks, then moved onto someone else they felt they could help. Their apparent lack of concern devastated her. Recognizing that the other women in the group had come to rely on her as the wise sage and would unconsciously work to keep her in that position was difficult for her. She would have to examine how important it was to her to maintain this role and whether she was willing to reestablish herself in the group in a new status more consistent with her real needs.

This position of needing help but having difficulty asking for it is a common manifestation of the SBW theme. Secondary gain is derived from self-protection, which keeps her from confronting her more fragile self. It is also achieved by maintaining a position of some authority, control, and power in what otherwise may feel like a powerless, out-of-control existence.

Many feelings hide just below the surface of the SBW facade. Anger, fear, shame, pride, and loneliness are some more common ones. These are all particularly difficult emotions to express. Anger, for example, is often experienced as something physical or harsh, a sense of lashing out. It is an emotion that places the SBW very close to a sense of feeling out of control. The intense difficulty with the expression of anger that the SBW experiences may be related to her internalization of historical and racial representations. One image of African American women as overtly hostile and contemptuous, particularly of African

American men, is discussed by West (1995). It is difficult for the SBW to accept anger as a legitimate feeling, one that if expressed appropriately would not create the devastation to herself or others she often imagines. As a result, the SBW may accept responsibility for others' discomfort (Greene, 1994). She may strive to appear passive and nonthreatening, or she may unwittingly misdirect her anger against those she may perceive as safe targets for it. Depending upon the nature of her relationships, there are several common "safe" targets for her anger. Four safe targets are (1) male partners she may perceive as being emotionally unavailable or being verbally or physically abusive or irresponsible; (2) children, for acting in demanding and entitled ways; (3) parents, for placing unrealistic expectations on her shoulders at a very early age, or for not protecting or loving her enough; and (4) God. One client noted, "He [God] wants you to come to him broken. I have no idea why he would want that." Acknowledging painful feelings is particularly difficult for the SBW because they connect the SBW to her sense of neediness, which is unacceptable to her. She has never learned to say "I need," and those around her fail to take her seriously when she does have needs. This ensures a vicious cycle which ultimately becomes maladaptive to her physical, emotional, and spiritual well-being.

Taking on much more than she can realistically handle both professionally and personally is typical, for example, for the SBW. On the job, bosses and colleagues view her as a high achiever, someone on whom others may depend. The more they expect of her, the more she will strive to prove herself. Externally, she will appear undaunted by these challenges. Her message to herself is that she is just doing what she is expected to do, and that doing anything less is unacceptable. Pride ensures her that she will "never miss a beat." While she may be quite accomplished, she does not seem to relish her successes. She will take responsibility for her mistakes and is likely to highlight and remember them far more than her successes. While she will often acknowledge that she is in a "rat race" and may even admit to her part in maintaining it, she cannot acknowledge the impact it is having on her physical, emotional, and spiritual well-being. She is likely to see working as the "real" world, and to regard leisure time, having fun, and pampering herself as the "fantasy" world, a place to be engaged in only sporadically.

## THEME TWO: TO NURTURE AND PRESERVE FAMILY

The role of caregiver is perhaps the most clearly defined and accepted role of the African American woman. A common saying in the African American community is "African American women love their sons and raise their daughters." While this is an oversimplification of some very complicated relationships, it does raise ideas worth considering. One translation is that we expect African American women to be responsible caregivers in the community, while we provide men with a firmer sense of unconditional love. For the African American woman, then, being perceived as loveable becomes intricately tied to her ability to take care of others. Such caretaking requires a level of selflessness that involves suppressing one's own needs. The contradiction, of course, is that the search for unconditional love is a human condition requiring the acknowledgment of needs.

Because they have learned to feel that asking directly for their needs to be addressed is unacceptable, some African American women unconsciously employ indirect means. Some of these means are quite self-devaluing and disruptive of equitable, intimate relationships. One SBW client had tremendous difficulty getting her needs met with her spouse of 12 years. This was her second marriage and she was most ambivalent about her feelings toward him. She had grown increasingly angry and depressed. She fantasized about having an affair, but knew that would only create further complications. However, she found herself withdrawing from her spouse. When they were together, she badgered him about things she wanted done around the house. It was as if his level of willingness to complete such tasks was the closest approximation she could expect of his desire to care for her. It was much easier for her to assert her wishes for the household than it was to express her wishes for their relationship. Her true needs remained unspoken. Meanwhile, she experienced herself as hostile and controlling, which further impacted her level of self-esteem and left her questioning whether she even deserved the love she sought.

During her formative years society gave the SBW messages that love was associated with what she did and how she looked, not who she was. It is very common in therapy sessions as African American women explore their past for them to lament these messages to camouflage their dark skin, thick lips, large posteriors, and kinky hair. Harvey (1995) observed that skin color issues, for instance, have been observed to be a central variable in many issues impacting the psyche of African American men and women. For many women, the "Black is beautiful" consciousness raising of the 1960s and 1970s did little to counter negative internalized views of their physical appearance. As she is not imaged as beautiful, her behavior (i.e., her willingness to give of herself) becomes the condition for love.

As an adult, she searches for unconditional love, yet unconsciously she tends to avoid relationships with kind, gentle men who are emotionally mature. Fear of intimacy may be the primary obstacle. For it is in the context of intimacy that vulnerabilities such as fear, self-doubt, shame, and hurt run the risk of being exposed. I have worked with several women, for instance, who at some point in their lives were involved with a nurturing, supportive man quite capable of providing the love they were seeking. However, over time, these women discovered some "fatal flaw" that overshadowed the man's loving nature. Limited power and financial security are two very common flaws. The inability to work together on these issues generally lead to the demise of the relationship.

The SBW is more likely to be attracted to someone who either has difficulty working out his own problems or whose personal or professional growth has somehow been curtailed. She will gradually take on the task of "fixing" him. Believing that it is better to absorb and take on another's problems, she has difficulty listening to her partner without exercising her compelling need to problem-solve for him. The unwitting message she conveys is that she is the only competent person in the relationship. Over time, incidents will occur to support and preserve this view. For instance, I have worked with several female clients who took over the financial management responsibilities in their households because of past money management and credit difficulties their partners experienced. The pair colluded in a unilateral financial takeover by the female. They were unable to sort through their financial issues as partners and learn to view money matters as joint problems to which they could both bring their unique views and problem-solving abilities. The male, often struggling with his inability to express feelings, eventually comes to resent the SBW's control and acts out his anger in passive–aggressive forms, ultimately creating additional financial problems.

One woman described the entrepreneurial dreams she and her husband had shared early in their relationship. Both worked for large corporations and were quite financially successful. Their plan was to save enough money to support a start-up business within a few years. As time went on, however, she saw her husband forging out on his own and making unilateral decisions regarding the business. He left his corporate position but was ill-prepared to follow through on the details of a business plan. His drinking accelerated, further exacerbating his depression and withdrawal. The increased financial burden was left to the wife to handle, who sought to carry it for some time prior to both of them seeking treatment.

Intimacy and finances are not the only arenas in which the SBW finds herself in untenable situations. Parenting is a particularly difficult challenge. She vacillates between doing everything for her children and treating them like miniature adults capable of making mature decisions and demonstrating responsible behavior in any situation. For example, one client expressed her frustration that her very bright, capable adolescent daughter did not want to attend a high school with high academic standards, but insisted on enrolling in a school with a very mediocre record. The daughter's reason for this choice was that she did not want to be stereotyped as a "nerd," which would surely happen if she attended the superior program. She also threatened to pay little attention to her studies if her mother insisted on her choice of school. The mother presented in therapy as exasperated, disgusted with her daughter's thinking, and fearful for her future. She felt ashamed of her daughter and powerless to do anything. As we explored this dilemma, many issues surfaced for the mother. First, she was viewing this as solely her daughter's decision. She remembered numerous situations in which her mother had imposed her will on her, thus leaving her feeling invisible and without a voice. While she had come to see the wisdom in many of her mother's decisions, she continued to struggle with the way she issued them. She had consciously determined that she would be different from her mother, that she would be a friend to her child. Having turned over the power to make decisions to her daughter, she felt depleted. She was unable to state emphatically that her daughter did not have the final decision. Rather than letting her daughter know that she was willing to hear her concerns and try to help her with them, the mother engaged in manipulative, bargaining approaches in an attempt to get her daughter to do her bidding.

Striking a balance between her own needs and those of her children is very difficult for the SBW. This struggle appears to intensify for single mothers and for women who have taken on all the responsibility for parenting to the exclusion of the fathers. The SBW's view that she should be able to "do it all" leaves her feeling guilty when her child's behavior, attitudes, or accomplishments fall short of parental expectations. This guilt creates further obstacles in her capacity and willingness to take care of herself. That is, if her child is having difficulties, how can she focus any attention on herself? Rather, a self-sacrificing posture develops that may predispose her not only to feeling resentful but to a variety of health problems as well.

## THE THERAPEUTIC RELATIONSHIP

The therapeutic alliance provides one avenue for a relationship that only requires the client to bring some level of motivation to participate in the process of self-exploration. Greenson (1986) defines this working alliance as a relatively rational transference phenomenon that requires the client "to work purposefully in the treatment situation" (p. 192). It has been my experience that African American women often seek out an African American female therapist. Their reasons typically center around the belief that another African American woman can relate to them better and more adequately understand how they feel. Many African American women I have seen have previously been in therapy, often with a White therapist (male or female). While this may have been helpful at the time, they often felt limits in mutual understanding, and believed that they did not receive the feedback they sought.

Researchers and clinicians have already written much about cross-racial therapy (Abramowitz & Murray, 1983; Atkinson, 1985; Sue, 1988). While it is not my intention here to take a position on the efficacy of cross-racial therapy, I would like to suggest, that for many African American women, the choice of another African American female as therapist may serve as the basis for the development of positive self-regard. In other words, what an African American woman client seeks in the therapeutic relationship is a reflection back to her, whether in words, feelings, or nonverbal messages, of a picture that looks more like herself and that conveys a healthy appreciation for her struggle. Even in choosing an African American female therapist, however, there is always the risk that the SBW will not get what she seeks. There is so much heterogeneity among African American women that the selection of an African American female therapist by no means guarantees the success of the therapeutic alliance. Yet for many African American female clients, racial congruity provides a level of comfort that helps them get beyond some of their initial resistance to seeking a therapist.

Traditional models of psychotherapy often neglect significant facets of racial and ethnic material, relegating them to defense and resistance against the exploration of underlying conflicts (Evans, 1985). By inviting the examination of this material, the client may experience a more balanced and complete understanding of herself and better resolve conflicts associated with her racial and ethnic heritage (Evans, 1985).

I have worked with many African American women in therapy who would describe their own mothers as SBWs who expected nothing less from their daughters. Many of these women came from stable households with one or two parents and extended family members living in the home. They experienced many opportunities in their formative years and felt a reasonable level of familial support. At the same time, many other SBW clients came from very chaotic families, from mothers who were depressed, drug- or alcohol-addicted, or otherwise unable to provide for them emotionally. These women learned to be the primary caretakers for their mothers, in an emotional and tangible reversal of roles. In either situation, the African American female client's capacity to identify with another African American woman as her therapist may suggest an unconscious desire to be loved and nurtured for herself as she is and for whom she would like to be. In the early stage of therapy, however, the SBW client may try to nurture the therapist, thus making it difficult to assert her own needs. Similarly, because the SBW tends to be quite self-critical, she may project those feelings onto the therapist and experience the therapist as a source of criticism.

## Countertransference and the African American Female Therapist

The African American female therapist must struggle with countertransference issues related to the SBW image. Already in a helping profession, the therapist may be particularly vulnerable to presenting herself (consciously and unconsciously) to her clients as a resourceful, dependable, emotionally self-reliant, intellectually competent SBW. The therapist becomes an easy repository for the projected fantasies of the client, who both needs the image of a SBW in front of her, and may feel too vulnerable and envious of such an image, believing that her therapist "has it all together." Comas-Díaz and Jacobsen (1991) observe some of the issues involved in intraethnic transference phenomena. The "omniscient–omnipotent therapist" is one such manifestation that is particularly relevant. Because of the ethnic and racial similarity between client and therapist, the client views the therapist as a savior or folk heroine. In the former instance, the therapist's perceived capacity to manage in mainstream society creates the fantasy that the therapist will be able to reach out and "rescue" the client. In the latter case, the therapist is viewed as one who has "made it." Conversely, the therapist may become the object of envy and resentment. Here the therapist is viewed as a traitor who betrayed her culture in order to achieve personally. Thus, the transference may be one of idealization or devaluation. Comas-Díaz and Jacobsen observe that "ethnocultural transference and countertransference reactions may emerge at various times during therapy. They can act as catalysts for the acceptance of disparate parts of the self. Monitoring and properly addressing such reactions can advance the therapeutic process and promote growth" (p. 400).

The African American female therapist is also of a particular hue, and has a particular hair texture, body type, and the like. How thoroughly she has explored these issues in her own life may determine her comfort in raising them with clients who may have a similar or very different look from her own. The therapist's unacknowledged issues with historically volatile physical characteristics may also impact her capacity to empathize with her client without overidentifying. Such overidentification may lead the therapist to make excuses for her client for any maladaptive patterns that have developed around these issues. Further, the therapist may make assumptions about the impact of these issues on her client. For example, I am a light-skinned person with green eyes and relatively straight hair. Such characteristics are familiar in my family of origin, and, in my recollection, were neither coveted nor rejected. A more significant struggle I internalized was coming of age in the late 1960s and questioning "if I were Black enough." While I could not do anything about my skin color (short of an occasional tan), I went through much effort to create the largest, bushiest "Afro" I could to display my political ideology, my commitment to "the cause," to protect my identity from being called into question. Many years later as a therapist I was working with a woman whose physical attributes and age were close to my own. Unconsciously, I made the error of assuming that her experience around these issues would be similar. Later in the therapy I realized that my client was the only light-skinned child in a large family, and that several family members had ridiculed her and singled her out negatively because of her light skin. She held a great deal of pain and mistrust as a result. Fortunately we could examine these matters quite fully and to a good degree of resolution. Had I been more open to her experiences from the beginning, we would most likely have gotten to them much sooner.

## Developing the Therapeutic Alliance

Entering therapy for the SBW holds all of the ambivalence it would for anyone else. However, the SBW must also wrestle with issues particular to the Black world. In the African American community therapy is still a relatively misunderstood and unaccepted phenomenon (Boyd-Franklin, 1989). It is not at all uncommon for African American clients, female or male, to acknowledge that they had a very difficult time making that first appointment. Coming to therapy was proof that they "had lost it" (their minds). Others noted that they were ashamed of "airing dirty laundry in public." They should, after all, "be able to handle [their] own problems." Moreover, many African American women experience spiritual conflicts because they have been taught that therapy is inherently conflictual with religious beliefs and their relationship with God (Boyd-Franklin, 1991). They may perceive the need for therapy as a sign that their faith is not strong enough and that they need to pray more. In the early phase of therapy, even in short-term models, getting a sense of the client's view of being in treatment is critical. Such discussion will help diminish the impact of cultural and religious negative images of therapy.

The therapeutic relationship poses a major dilemma for the SBW. On the one hand, she has sought out treatment and recognizes a need for help. She may quickly come to see therapy as a safe place where she is free to unburden herself. On the other hand, she may struggle with whether doing something personal for herself is acceptable. She may perceive therapy as a narcissistic luxury. That is, she may experience taking time for herself to reflect, explore, unburden herself, and plan as excessively self-indulgent in a world where African American people, overall, have so little.

As the relationship between client and therapist develops, the SBW's struggles with acknowledging her needs and accepting support will usually become quite apparent. For instance, she may try to be the "perfect patient" by pleasing the therapist and achieving in treatment. "Achieving" means that she continues to look competent and successful in her attempts to resolve issues. Even after an especially vulnerable moment in therapy, she might well return to the next session as if everything were just fine. Indeed, she will likely report on her many accomplishments and positive interactions that occurred between sessions. At times, her attempts to hide her pain is an effort to protect her therapist from it. Again, she may take on the role of the caretaker with her therapist.

Compartmentalizing is another method of managing the needs/support conflict. For instance, African American women who are very spiritual may be reluctant to raise spiritual issues in therapy. Boyd-Franklin (1991) notes that this may be due to a perceived lack of interest by the therapist in spiritual matters. Also, therapy may cause inner conflict with their religious beliefs and what they have heard from the pulpit. For the SBW, these are especially salient issues that if unexplored may create considerable conflict in the relationship with the therapist. For instance, the notion that "God will never give you more than you can handle" is a common message that can be a very affirming reminder as a client deals with the day-to-day challenges and responsibilities in her life. However, she may also interpret this belief as suggesting she should be able to handle all that God (and life) give her, and then some, by herself. Helping the client to reframe such an interpretation may be an important step in her capacity to disengage from the negative expectations of the SBW image while simultaneously valuing her spirituality and that which exists between client and therapist.

The client may also be afraid of disappointing her therapist because she does not "get it" readily enough. If the therapy lasts longer than she initially anticipated, for example, she may view that as an indication that she is not doing something right. Since her validation comes from what she does, she will attempt to rectify this situation by presenting as much less depressed or anxious than she actually feels. She may even bring up termination prematurely to assure herself and her therapist that she is fine.

The SBW client experiences strength and vulnerability as polar opposites. It is extremely difficult for her to accept the idea that it takes strength to expose vulnerabilities and conflicts and to understand defenses and other unconscious phenomenon, and that such exposure is a key aspect of the work of therapy. As we discussed this concept of vulnerability as strength, one client observed to me: "I'm so afraid to let go . . . I'll just crack up and crumble." She viewed her SBW face to the world as something that had carried her through many difficult times. Indeed, there was much truth to this. However, she had considerable difficulty hearing my suggestion that she may want to work through the SBW messages she had internalized to achieve a more balanced view that was more consistent with her current reality.

This balance is one indication of successful resolution. Initially, many clients report no sense of how to change or even that they could be different. As the client becomes more experienced with observing her own behavior and assessing her motives, as she becomes increasingly intrigued by unconscious processes and patterns in her relationships, the path to change begins to unfold. By creating simple boundaries with others, she is less likely to feel consumed by their needs. She may begin to do some very simple things for herself, such as pampering, submitting bills to get reimbursed from her insurance company, or making clear choices when requests for sexual intimacy are made. Because she is more comfortable with herself, she will experience increased comfort when alone. As she becomes more comfortable being with and giving to herself, she will come to relish moments of quiet, reflective time.

The task is not to become less strong. One SBW client observed toward the end of her therapy that she had truly come to appreciate her strength. Others had always remarked on it and had come to have very high expectations of her ability to deliver no matter what the situation. However, she had been afraid to really embrace her strength, particularly when boundaries with family members and others were so loose. She was afraid she would be engulfed by them. As she gradually learned in therapy to establish more balanced relationships, she felt much freer to accept her strength as a blessing to be nurtured rather than as an expectation to be exploited by self and others.

## STRONG BLACK WOMAN: ASSET OR LIABILITY?

Any overused asset that develops uncritically, that is, without ongoing evaluation and attention to changing needs and demands, runs the risk of becoming a liability. This may be the case with the SBW paradigm that has become a central theme for so many African American women. Unraveling the messages, limitations, and contradictions inherent in this culturally internalized image will have very significant meaning for many African American women in therapy.

The therapist's ability to enhance the therapeutic alliance and invite a nonjudgmental exploration of these issues can make a significant difference in the therapeutic outcome. It is critical for the therapist to appreciate that despite racial and cultural images, each African American woman has a unique story and an individual worldview.

For many African American women, challenging the messages inherent in the SBW paradigm is quite threatening. One client noted to me that reframing some of her beliefs associated with the SBW image was tantamount to "getting rid of myself." She recognized that many externally and internally imposed demands overwhelmed her. Yet she worried that if she let go of even a few of her deeply internalized beliefs, a loss of control would ensue. Thus, for most clients, this process proceeds slowly.

As the client grows in her understanding of the influences of this paradigm, she is likely to experience much more freedom in the way she images herself, in accepting the parts of her that are resilient, and in forming more meaningful, mutually supportive relationships with family, partners, colleagues, and other significant people in her life. She will become more comfortable sharing her vulnerabilities with trusted companions, and will be able to accept support from her therapist and others. Just how emotionally available others, particularly men, have become often surprises her. She learns to be more flexible in her approach toward others. She is better able to differentiate how and when to use her strength such that it can be much more the asset we project it to be in our cultural folklore.

# REFERENCES

Abramowitz, S. I., & Murray, J. (1983). Race effects in psychotherapy. In J. Murray & P. Abramson (Eds.), *Bias in psychotherapy* (pp. 215–255). New York: Praeger.

Atkinson, D. R. (1985). A meta-review of research on cross-cultural counseling and psychotherapy. *Journal of Multicultural Counseling and Development, 1,* 138–153.

Boyd-Franklin, N. (1989). *Black families in therapy: A multisystems approach.* New York: Guilford Press.

Boyd-Franklin, N. (1991). Recurrent themes in the treatment of African-American women in group psychotherapy. *Women and Therapy, 11*(2), 25–38.

Comas-Díaz, L., & Jacobsen, F. M. (1991). Ethnocultural transference and counter-transference in the therapeutic dyad. *American Journal of Orthopsychiatry, 61*(3), 392–402.

Evans, D. (1985). Psychotherapy and Black patients: Problems of training, trainees, and trainers. *Psychotherapy, 22S,* 457–460.

Greene, B. (1994). African-American women. In L. Comas-Díaz & B. Greene (Eds.), *Women of color: Integrating ethnic and gender identities in psychotherapy* (pp. 10–29). New York: Guilford Press.

Greenson, R. R. (1967). *The technique and practice of psychoanalysis* (Vol. 1). New York: International Universities Press.

Harvey, A. (1995). The issue of skin color in psychotherapy with African Americans. *Families in Society: The Journal of Contemporary Human Service, 76*(1), 3–10.

Shorter-Gooden, K., & Washington, C. (1996). Young, Black, and female: The challenge of weaving an identity. *Journal of Adolescence, 19,* 465–475.

Sue, S. (1988). Psychotherapeutic services for ethnic minorities: Two decades of research findings. *American Psychologist, 43*(4), 301–308.

West, C. M. (1995). Mammy, Sapphire, and Jezebel: Historical images of Black women and their implications for psychotherapy. *Psychotherapy, 32*(3), 458–466.

## CHAPTER 12

# African American Women and Moral Masochism
## *When There Is Too Much of a Good Thing*

### CHERYL L. THOMPSON

One of the challenges for many African American women—whether they seek treatment or not—is to determine how to have their own needs met while those for whom they are caretakers are provided for. When an appropriate balance is not established, the result is often role strain. West (2000) and Lerner (1988) observe that regardless of their ethnicity, many women face the potential for role strain. Attempts to manage the multiple roles of mother, worker, intimate partner, daughter, sister, extended family member, and more put many women at risk. However, this problem appears to be heightened in African American women. African American women often earn less, are less formally educated, have lower job status, and are more likely to be single or single heads of households than their White female counterparts (West, 2000). Because of the extended rather than nuclear structures of African American families, African American women may be more likely to be called upon to provide support or to function as caretakers to people outside of their immediate family. West (2000) and Greene (1994, 1997) observe that the "Mammy" stereotype of African American women, when internalized by them and by male African Americans, contributes to the perception of African American women as infinite resources for others, always strong in the face of adversity and having no need for caretaking themselves. Women who believe this stereotype often confuse the behavior that leads to role strain with African cultural derivatives or mandates. While this is a problem for poor African American women, it also appears to increase in proportion to the occupational, financial, or material success experienced by these women. The experiences of achievement often result in an even greater conflict between the right to meet individual needs and a sense of responsibility for loved ones (Comas-Díaz & Greene, 1994). These factors exist in a dynamic tension that can often serve to inhibit or limit success. While these issues are not unique to African American women, they unfold in treatment with such a high degree of consistency that one must speculate that something in African American women's experience predisposes them to this form of symptom expression. A historical perspective is needed in order to create a framework for understanding this phenomenon.

A significant source of the difficulty seems to be the result of an extended family structure that may or may not be limited to blood relatives and a sense of self that is more tied to family structure than to the individual (Boyd-Franklin, 1991). I hasten to add that extended family structures per se are not the problem. When family systems of obligation operate in a reciprocal and balanced manner, the result can be greater resources for all members without creating undue burdens for any single individual (Boyd-Franklin, 1991; Hill, 1971). Put simply, the burdens are shared. The real problem arises when the burden to carry the family's needs is placed on the shoulders of one person, rather than being shared among many. While it is clear that an individual cannot be the sole matrix of health or the sole individual who sustains the entire family, it should be equally clear that the sacrifice of an individual cannot sustain an entire family system either. Many of my patients are left feeling that they alone are responsible for the well-being of other family members. Psychodynamic psychotherapy is uniquely positioned to address these issues within the dynamic complex in which they exist.

In this chapter I discuss a way of being in the world that is often accepted as nonsymptomatic. Indeed, this way of being in the world is often accepted by African Americans as the way things have to be or should be, because they are culturally mandated. The strength and self-sacrifice observed in African American women has served an adaptive purpose in that it has been an important survival mechanism. African American women have a tradition of bearing their suffering as if it is inevitable and sometimes as if it is a manifestation of their ethnic identity (Greene, 1994). Often, the perception these women have of themselves is not that they are suffering, but that they are strong, autonomous beings who can survive anything without help, despite any and all difficulties they confront. In fact, many perceive the need to ask for and accept help from anyone as an intolerable expression of weakness. Seeking psychotherapy is often seen as a sign of weakness for many African American women, a problem that can delay their obtaining much-needed help.

The history of African American women is one of struggle to overcome many obstacles and to keep families intact as much as possible. Because of racism, African American women were not accorded the courtesies of femininity that were available to White women (Greene, 1994, 1996). Slavery did not recognize African Americans as human beings and the status of slave superseded the status of woman. Hence, African American women worked outside the home in many forms of labor that were considered unsuitable for White women. Because the women's liberation movement initially viewed working outside the home as the key to women's liberation, many African American women felt that they were already liberated because since the days of slavery Black women had been defined as workers (Greene, 1994, 1997). Hence many African American women felt they had no need for a women's movement. Their ability to endure hardship and take on many of the roles that their White counterparts did not have to manage contributed to the myth of the ubiquitously strong woman who can take care of everyone, often with no consideration for herself. In many cases, stoicism is taken to such an extreme that the behavior begins to look masochistic (Marcus, 1981).

The definition of masochism, like many psychoanalytic concepts, has changed over time as the result of acquisition of increased knowledge and experience. Initially the term was used to describe people, typically women, who derived erotic pleasure from sexual pain. This earlier definition is a part of drive theory. Mattei (1996) observes that drive theory has been criticized for its androcentric and "ethnocentric reductionism" in which social and psychological dynamics are universally attributed to the sexual conflicts that were particular to 19th-century Europe. My use of the term *masochism* in this chapter refers to moral masochism. *Moral masochism* is a level of excessive personal sacrifice that assumes pathological proportions. The moral masochist derives a sense of well-being or nonerotic pleasure from excessive sacrifice despite the pain of giving too much or giving to the point of personal depletion. This later definition is more consistent with interpersonal psychodynamic theories.

Hence, African American women may often have an inability to appropriately define and acknowledge their own suffering. They may also feel that seeking help is a sign of weakness, a critical flaw. This concept, and the idea that true mental health is based on the American ideal of autonomy (prioritizing your own needs first and the needs of others second) are two constructs that I have struggled with as an African American woman and as a psychoanalyst. Each represents an extreme, rather than a balanced, position. The object relation theorists such as Fairbairn (1954) and Winnicott (1965) have been tremendously useful in helping me to understand the construct of autonomy (Hartmann, 1951). All (Fairbairn, 1954; Hartmann, 1951; Winnicott, 1965) have helped me understand that a construct of "mature dependency" is a more meaningful idea. It is also an idea that is more consistent with my own understanding of human beings as social animals and a need that I believe I share with other women to feel successfully related to people who are important to me.

External variables are a significant source of the difficulty that many of my patients face (Boyd-Franklin, 1989; Greene, 1994; Hill, 1971; Thompson,

1987, 1995). Success for many Black people often comes as a result of great sacrifice. One person in a family may have stood out as capable, and other family members may have worked in order to assist that person's move along an educational or career path. The individual who has benefitted from the family's help and is now successful is expected to share the fruits of that success with those who made sacrifices on her behalf (Boyd-Franklin, 1991; Comas-Díaz & Greene, 1994). The expectation is sometimes stated openly, but most of the time it is unspoken. The successful individual may also find herself on the receiving end of a double message regarding her success. Family members and peers may idealize the degree to which material success minimizes or entirely removes other struggles, particularly struggles with racism. But family members and peers may also view the successful individual's transition across educational and/or class boundaries as a betrayal of those left behind. Such feelings may be communicated in subtle or overt ways, even while families continue to exhort the successful individual to do well. These individuals may find themselves the target of the jealousy of other family members and may be treated as if they are now undeserving of care, because of their success (Comas-Díaz & Greene, 1994).

The result for the successful person is often a feeling of not deserving her success or of feeling guilty for having achieved it, resulting in an experience best described as survivor's guilt (Comas-Díaz & Greene, 1994; Spurlock, 1985). Others, especially those who are sensitive to experiences of deprivation, may sabotage their own success. They may do this to avoid feeling responsible for those who may expect a significant return for their assistance. An example of this may be observed in professional women who after lengthy struggles to obtain advanced degrees either delay, avoid, or sabotage themselves around completing dissertations or theses, or taking licensing, certification, or professional exams. Such things often symbolize the last hurdle to success, without which the forward progression of their careers is halted. If they have internalized racism and sexism they may doubt that their success is an accurate reflection of their efforts. Such women may feel like frauds and expect that the next challenge will reveal the "truth" of their incompetence or undeservedness. Hence, they avoid that last step. For a variety of reasons, many Black women manifest clear feelings of ambivalence about their success and may undermine themselves in both conscious and unconscious ways.

Therapists who work with African American patients often neglect to monitor interpersonal and intrapsychic issues simultaneously and in the context of external or reality pressures. The need to monitor the salience of external, societal barriers in this population is often greater because the external realities of isolation and tokenism in corporate or professional life often serve to exacerbate the sense of guilt and responsibility toward loved ones. These realities stand in stark contrast to most people's association with success and to the kinds of experiences these patients really have. Because inner and outer reality can so easily serve to confirm neurotic ideation, such as a belief that success is undeserved or that it occurred purely by accident, the analyst must offer a working model of health that includes as much reality as possible. Thus the analyst needs to have a clear working model for what it means to be a psychologically healthy functioning person of color.

The issues of obligation, responsibility, guilt, and deprivation often work together to defeat the aspirations of many of my patients. Further, this constellation has often served to reduce their pleasure about their accomplishments. The external pressure that exacerbates the conviction that this level of taking care of others is appropriate comes from the stereotype shared by African Americans, specifically those from the middle class, that they are the moral barometer of the society. Thus, many successful African Americans feel obligated to exhaust their limited resources without an adequate assessment of their realistic limits. When these issues are explored from all necessary vantage points, patients experience significant growth.

The cases that follow reflect a number of traditionally successful African American women who have entered treatment because of concerns or symptoms that were not the issues that became most compelling to me as their therapist. I hope that my experiences with them are helpful to other therapists. Identifying details have been disguised to protect the confidentiality of patients.

## CASE EXAMPLES

### Case One

Ms. A began psychotherapy with me 7 years ago. At that time, she was depressed, had suffered significant weight loss, and was unable to get through the day without crying. Her depression was precipitated by her knowledge that her husband was involved in an extramarital affair. Ms. A was dimly aware that this affair had been long-standing but managed to ignore it until the husband's behavior had become widely known and the topic of gossip in her small community. Ms. A did not want to leave her husband because she believed that she could not survive without him. When we began psychotherapy, antianxiety medication was prescribed for Ms. A. She used it very sparingly; she did not want to take the medication because she was concerned about its addictive possibilities. In addition to her concern about medication, she wanted to understand how "she got herself" into this predicament.

At the onset of treatment, Ms. A was in her early 40s, was employed full time in a professional career, and had one daughter, who was 14 at the time, with whom she had a good relationship. She was worried about the lessons her daughter might learn based on the bad marriage she was in but wanted to maintain. Ms. A felt that being married was a privileged status for a Black woman.

Most of her close female friends had never been married. As we began to probe and discuss her need to be married despite the pain and frequent humiliation she endured as a result of her husband's behavior, Ms. A recalled her childhood experiences with her parents (her father was now deceased but her mother was alive and in good health).

Ms. A experienced her mother as demanding and complaining. She frequently tried to avoid being with her mother because she felt belittled by her. The mother presented herself as someone worthy of her daughter's attention and care because she had sacrificed her safety and comfort in order to provide a financially secure environment for her daughter. This constellation is described by Menaker (1979) and Panken (1993) as a frequent source of masochistic development. Ms. A's mother had lived in an abusive marriage and looked to her daughter for recognition and appreciation. Ms. A remembered many times when her father would beat her mother. Ms. A would hide in her room when they were fighting. When the house fell silent, Ms. A would walk around the house looking for her mother, fully expecting to find her dead. Ms. A's mother never allowed herself to know the pain her daughter endured as she watched her parents' marriage. In therapy Ms. A came to believe that her mother was often so difficult that her father could only confront her after drinking too much. However, his substance abuse resulted in his loss of control and subsequent extremely violent outbursts. Ms. A recalled being confused by her mother's behavior with her father, because Ms. A could tell when her father had had too much to drink and subsequently left him alone. She wondered why her mother wouldn't do the same thing. She passed through a period of deep resentment regarding her mother because she felt it was unfair that she should have been subjected to the repeated fear that her mother would be killed by her father.

Ms. A did not hold her father responsible for his behavior, which she attributed to his alcoholism. Moreover, she believed that her mother was in greater control in the relationship. Ms. A's father died prior to her beginning treatment and she believed that she had made peace with him. There was a period before he died in which he stopped drinking and they had an opportunity to repair some aspects of their relationship. We explored my patient's belief that her mother held the upper hand in her parents' marital relationship and connected it to her belief that she too had caused her husband to be unfaithful. Ms. A believed that she had committed some unspoken crime that resulted in her need to be punished by her unfaithful husband. As we addressed these issues, Ms. A began to see that she was so fearful of marrying a husband who would be violent like her father that she settled for a man who was not openly abusive but who was psychologically abusive and who left her filled with self-doubt. He was often silent and used my patient's meal preparation or household activities as excuses to leave the house in order to be with his mistress. Ms. A was very resistant to the idea that her husband's behavior was self-motivated rather than reactive. Several years of work were required before Ms. A would accept this reality. Ms. A did come to understand that her husband was abusive but different from her father and that her relationship with him represented an attempt on her part to avoid the problems she observed in her parents' relationship. When she came to understand that her relationship with her husband reflected her desire to avoid physical abuse, she felt relieved enough to truly explore the reality of her marriage. When she accepted that her marriage was painful and that there was no hope that she could change the quality of that relationship, she divorced her husband. When the divorce was final, Ms. A felt relieved. She found support in her friends and slowly began to make a life for herself. She now has a circle of good and loyal friends and has a hobby that gives her great pleasure.

A crisis in her treatment erupted when her daughter became pregnant. Both my patient and her daughter are religious people so that her daughter felt that her only option was to have the baby. Ms. A was devastated. She felt wounded and betrayed. Ms. A stated that her daughter negated all her sacrifices and had forsaken all of her dreams for her by choosing a path that Ms. A had never considered. Ms. A was so ashamed of her daughter's decision that she threatened to abandon her daughter. As we worked on this problem, my patient could see that she was behaving like her own mother. When she accepted her daughter as a young adult who had made a life choice, Ms. A was better equipped to assess the situation differently. She now feels that her daughter has moved forward in the family history of male–female relationships. Ms. A's daughter has been able to establish a strong, mutual relationship with her own husband, which allows Ms. A to feel good about her daughter's choices.

Ms. A is no longer depressed and has resolved many of the problems that were part of her treatment. At this point, we are working on termination. This treatment has been essentially successful. Ms. A has been able to reestablish a relationship with her mother, and is pleased with her ability to relate to her mother. The construct that followed Ms. A throughout her treatment was her confusion about dependency, appropriate neediness, and masochism. Ms. A never wanted to have a relationship with anyone that involved acknowledgment of her own needs. For her, to be in need of someone was to be vulnerable to possibilities of abuse and humiliation. Ms. A had arranged her life so that no one knew of her dependency needs. She never allowed her husband to provide for the family. All expenses were divided 50-50. She came to understand that this was a means of defending herself from the awful dependency she believed occurred between her parents. Ms. A now understands that her fear of letting people know what her needs are allowed people to ignore her, to believe that she needed nothing, or to think that she was capable of taking care of herself regardless of what others did to her.

At this point, as we are ending treatment, I am concerned that Ms. A does not have enough personally meaningful interests or activities to insulate her from the possibility of becoming involved with someone who has no awareness of her needs or concerns. She has a group of friends, but she struggles with letting them know what she needs or allowing them to be supportive of her. Allowing herself to be dependent is not natural for her, but fortunately her friends are accepting of her. She has now surrounded herself with people who see mutuality as a core aspect of relationships. Ms. A has found that as she has opened herself to other women, she has not been alone in denying her own needs or in having family expectations that exceed one's own ability to provide and still meet appropriate personal demands.

Ms. A has committed herself to her treatment until we can discover her resistance to allowing herself more private pleasure.

## Case Two

Ms. B is a professional African American woman who, like Ms. A, entered treatment 7 years ago. She was in her early 40s at the time we began our work. She entered treatment because of her difficulty adjusting to her husband's disfiguring surgery. For the first year of her treatment we talked only about her husband and her daughter. Ms. B has only one child, which is fairly common for professional African American women. She, like many patients, devoted her life to providing for her husband and her child. Ms. B was deeply saddened when her daughter became a drug user and barely finished high school. Ms. B stopped talking to her colleagues and social acquaintances when her daughter had a child who was born with a handicapping condition. When I began working with her, my patient and her daughter had a close but antagonistic relationship. Ms. B was an extremely reluctant grandmother. In her treatment, she often talked about her friends and their daughters' weddings or college graduations and how hurt she was that her daughter could not see how important these experiences were for both of them. She felt that her daughter made different life choices in order to cause her pain.

Ms. B has not been able to find support or understanding within her extended family. The family perceives her as the strong successful one who should be and has always been available to meet the family's needs for advice, direction, or financial support. My patient reinforced her family's perception of herself by always agreeing to drop any activity of her own to address family problems and by her willingness to provide financial support to her less successful family members.

Ms. B had become an extravagant gift giver. She had excessive financial obligations and was often very worried that she would not be able to meet her expenses. Initially she saw her financial situation as a reflection of her husband's need to keep his resources for himself. She was never able to talk with him about her feeling that he did not contribute enough to the maintenance of their home. Over time, she became able to give less, but whenever a person in the family fell upon hard times she was convinced that it was her obligation to assist that person because she had the best job in the family.

Ms. B would not heed my suggestions that maybe she was exhausting herself and that she was giving to others in excess of her ability. Ms. B was angry with me and felt that I had no understanding of her plight. Instead of seeing me as helping her, she twisted my advice and claimed that I was telling her that she should ignore her family's needs and just think about herself. This is not an uncommon reaction from such clients when the therapist raises this issue or suggests that the patient is overextending herself. She believed that I was encouraging her to be selfish, which created marked anxiety for her. According to Ms. B, she had no right to think about herself, for to do so would result in the loss of her family (Panken, 1993).

I was getting nowhere on this issue. In each session, Ms. B began by complaining about how little money or time she had for herself. It took a health crisis to alter her perception of our work with each other. Her husband fell seriously ill and required major life-threatening surgery. Ms. B accompanied her husband to many medical consultations and translated the medical information that he received from the doctors into plain English so that he could understand what he was being told. Her husband went through the surgery and experienced multiple organ collapse during recovery. After one postsurgical week, her husband died. My patient felt that she had contributed to his death. It was through this crisis that I was able to help her see that she was not responsible for her husband's decision to have the surgery. We were able to look at her role in the management of his illness and to talk through the seriousness of his health problems. Ms. B recalled that her husband told her that he didn't think he would be around for Christmas that year.

In reconstructing their marriage, and the choices that led her to this marriage, we began to understand her need to give to others to the point of giving excessively and depleting herself. My patient always felt excessive guilt because of her parents' bad marriage, her own success, and her previously unspoken demand for caretaking of her daughter by her own mother when she was a single parent. Ms. B finally was able to acknowledge that she wanted her mother to make up for her failure as her mother by caring for Ms. B's daughter. She wonders at this point if her daughter's drug use could be related to the intermittent care she provided. She continues to have doubt about this idea, especially since there is some support for a biological explanation of drug use. Ms. B observes that her daughter's behavior became uncontrollable when she (Ms. B) married her daughter's father. The daughter was 13 at the time of the marriage.

My patient came to see that she hoped through her giving not only to make reparation for her need of significant others but also to show them that despite their failure to meet her needs, she could "turn the other cheek" and give to them. She also secretly believed that the reason her family let her down was because her need was excessive. When she came to understand that her needs were ordinary, both in the family and in the Black community, we made progress. She needed to know that she was not responsible for other people in her family or in the community who had not been as successful as she. It was her need to expiate her own sense of guilt that propelled her to give to the point of self-destruction.

We are continuing to work on this and other issues. Ms. B is not ready to end therapy. Indeed, she has allowed herself to become dependent in the treatment. However, to date she has not allowed herself any tears. She is afraid that if she starts to cry she will never be able to stop. My patient continues to be seen by her friends and colleagues as a strong woman who needs very little. She is less willing to maintain the facade of unlimited supplies and now tells people what she is willing or unwilling to do when others ask for her help. She has become able to express pride in saying no to people when she does not want to give too much.

## DISCUSSION

African American women often accept the myth of the strong Black woman who nurtures all and needs no one or nothing for herself. This is a myth that is supported by cultural interdependence among family and community members, as well as by the adaptability of African American women as a survival mechanism against racism. African American women are seen as successful inside and outside of their communities. They are often portrayed as successful and without needs. It is not surprising that many African American women would have no awareness of their suffering because they are doing what they think is expected of them. My concern is that as the social milieu becomes increasingly less supportive of the vulnerable and the weak members of our society, the resources of often fragile middle-class Black family members will become exhausted as they attempt to care for family members when it is beyond their means. This burden falls particularly heavily on women in the family, as they are presumed to be the ubiquitous caregivers with little thought to their own care.

My patients have found it extremely difficult to consider that their own personal needs are valid and are not excessive. When they consider their personal needs, many of my patients have become terrified that disaster will result. Menaker's (1979) concept suggests that moral masochism removes the suffering emanating from a loved one and places it in a depersonalized domain. This means that the suffering is caused by impersonal powers or circumstances. This concept has been extremely helpful in assisting me to understand the phenomenon and then discuss it in ways that proved to be helpful to my patients. We have been able to look at external demands and conditions and address them in ways that liberated my patients from their bondage. Even though these patients have major issues with their families of origin that need to be explored and reconstructed, I have found that exploration of the social milieu needs to precede that exploration in order for my patients to feel able to explore their issues with the family.

For these patients, the additional variable of race presents as a factor that must be explicitly explored because there is a cultural worldview that supports the idea that African American women have very little need, and that loss, rejection, and abandonment do not result in a need for social or family support for them. Professional African American women are often psychological orphans. Their suffering is denied because their success is all that is acknowledged. Their success in the larger world has often come at the expense of rejection by the family and the community with no real acceptance or inclusion in the world of the dominant culture that would be more consistent with their success.

In order for these women to alter their self-definitions, an exploration of their experiences in their workplaces and in their nonfamilial relationships was an essential part of their treatment. These women need to be encouraged to think about themselves as children who once needed care, and as women who deserve some degree of mutual dependence in their adult relationships. They need to learn not to feel responsible for the lack of success of extended family members or others in their community. The failures of others have to be understood as something independent of, that is, not tied to, their own success.

In these women masochism shifts from symptom to defense. Their masochism defended them against dependency that aroused more anxiety than they could contain. The denial of their own appropriate dependency was a significant factor in their relationships with their own mothers (Panken, 1993), as well as in their relationships to money, marriage, sexuality, and work.

One difficulty in working with the suffering of these women is the very limited social support they have for the expression and acceptance of mutuality of need. Their behavior is not seen as symptomatic in their families or other relationships so that sometimes the excesses to which these women go in their relationships are not even discussed in treatment. Many of these women have unconsciously selected peers, mates, and other relationships with people who are comfortable with their tendency to deny their personal needs. Such individuals may not support the patient if she rejects the role of the ubiquitous caregiver, begins to change, and expects greater mutuality. We need to be aware that this situation exists and listen for it in our work with professional African American women. The sorrow of these women exceeds individual psychopathology. There are no easy solutions to such problems, but we need to be aware that conflicts like those presented in the patients discussed in this chapter often reflect a larger context of external reality as well as the internal demands of the specific woman.

## REFERENCES

Boyd-Franklin, N. (1991). Recurrent themes in the treatment of African-American woman in group psychotherapy. *Women and Therapy, 11*, 25–40.

Comas-Díaz, L., & Greene, B. (1994). Women of color with professional status. In L. Comas-Díaz & B. Greene (Eds.), *Women of color: Integrating ethnic and gender identities in psychotherapy* (pp. 347–388). New York: Guilford Press.

Fairbairn, R. (1954). *An object relations theory of the personality.* New York: Basic Books.

Greene, B. (1994). African-American Women. In L. Comas-Díaz & B. Greene (Eds.), *Women of color: Integrating ethnic and gender identities in psychotherapy* (pp. 10–29). New York: Guilford Press.

Greene, B. (1997). Psychotherapy with African American women: Integrating feminist and psychodynamic models. *Journal of Smith College Studies in Social Work: Theoretical, Research, Practice, and Educational Perspectives for Understanding and Working with African American Clients, 67*(3), 299–322.

Hartmann, H. (1951). *Ego psychology and the problem of adaptation* (D. Rapaport, Trans.). New York: International Universities Press.

Hill, R. (1971). *The strength of Black families.* New York: National Urban League.

Lerner, H. (1988). *Women in therapy.* Northvale, NJ: Jason Aronson.

Marcus, M. (1981). *A taste for pain,* New York: St. Martin's Press.

Mattei, L. (1996). Coloring development: Race and culture in psychodynamic theories. In J. Berzoff, L. M. Flanagan, & P. Hertz (Eds.), *Inside out and outside in: Psychodynamic clinical theory and practice in contemporary multicultural contexts* (pp. 221–245). Northvale, NJ: Jason Aronson.

Menaker, E. (1979). *Masochism and the emergent ego.* New York: Human Sciences Press.

Panken, S. (1993). *The joy of suffering.* Northvale, NJ: Jason Aronson.

Spurlock, J. (1985). Survival guilt and Afro American achievement. *Journal of the National Medical Association, 77*(1), 29–32.

Thompson, C. (1987). Racism or neuroticism? An entangled dilemma for the Black middle-class patient. *Journal of the American Academy of Psychoanalysis, 15*(3), 395–405.

Thompson, C. (1995). Self-definition by opposition: A consequence of minority status. *Psychoanalytic Psychology, 12*(4), 533–545.

West, C. M. (2000). Developing an "oppositional gaze" toward the images of Black women. In J. C. Chrisler, C. Golden, & P. D. Rozee (Eds.), *Lectures on the psychology of women* (2nd ed., pp. 220–233). Boston: McGraw-Hill.

Winnicott, D. W. (1965). *The maturational processes and the facilitating environment, studies in the theory of emotional development.* New York: International Universities Press.

## CHAPTER 13

# Feminist and Psychodynamic Psychotherapy with African American Women
## Some Differences

### FRANCES K. TROTMAN

I am an African American woman. I have served as founder, director, and supervisor of a large, predominantly White psychotherapy institute in a socioeconomically and ethnically heterogeneous area of suburban New Jersey for the past 20 years. In my capacity as director of the center, I perform all the initial client interviews and then assign clients to the therapist whom I believe is most appropriate and therapeutic for the presenting problem and personality. Of the male and female social workers, psychologists, and psychiatrists whom I supervise, 80 to 90% are European American, yet we still have the largest number of licensed African American psychologists of any center in the state.

Originally as the first African American woman to be licensed as a psychologist in New Jersey, and now as one of only a few African American psychologists in the state, I see a disproportionately large number of African American women who present themselves for psychotherapy at the center. There are few other African American therapists. I cannot personally treat all of the African American women clients, nor is that desirable. Therefore, I must often assign African American women to European American therapists. It is my responsibility to decide which approaches and personalities, and what knowledge embodied in a European American therapist can be most therapeutic for the African American client. Underlying this task is an assumption of some differences, social, cultural, emotional, historical, relational, and ancestral, between African American and European American women.

Since I supervise each therapist of the diverse group weekly, I am well aware of each of their approaches, styles, and personalities. The therapists are licensed clinicians who are trained in various theoretical approaches and techniques. Many are psychoanalytically trained. As their supervisor, I must be well versed in a wide range of psychotherapeutic theories and approaches. I attempt strategically to encourage selective use of various and varying parts of the approaches to effect the maximum growth and well-being of the clients under the institute's charge. I have been trained in and practice psychodynamic psychotherapy with African American women, yet I have been guilty of hesitating to espouse it when supervising European American therapists who are treating African American women. I have in fact been reluctant to assign psychoanalytically trained European American therapists to African American clients at all.

In my capacity as an educator and director of a graduate program in psychological counseling at a small, overwhelmingly White, private university, I am responsible for educating and training students in the science and art of psychotherapy. In my teaching and supervision of future therapists, my inclination has been subtly to indoctrinate students with the more existential/ humanistic and feminist approaches. I deem these approaches less potentially harmful to African American clients in the hands of European American therapists than psychodynamic approaches. Though I teach students all the major theories of counseling and psychotherapy, from Freud and Adler through Ellis and Lazarus, I have always conveyed a feminist perspective in my lessons. I have claimed to want students to choose the theoretical framework that is most appropriate to their individual histories, personalities, and inclinations. As an African American woman, the contradiction between what I practice and what I teach can be explained by my belief that a psychoanalytic approach lends itself to being used in an authoritarian manner. It is my fear that students, often fearful and inexperienced, who are armed with a psychoanalytic approach might use it to conceal their anxiety behind the veil of the all-knowing therapist. Given the reality of racism and race relations in the United States, countertransference that is a function of White privilege (Wildman, 1995), and the lack of expertise associated with managing this form of countertransference is very difficult to escape. By sharing their interpretations and insights too soon or too knowingly, White therapists can and often do mirror the racism in American culture. They may behave in ways that indicate that it is the White therapist who knows the Black client better than she knows herself.

Despite my stated apprehensions, I am aware that psychodynamic psychotherapy has many important, and, in the right hands, therapeutic aspects. Childhood events do influence who and what we become and how we behave. A skilled therapist who can understand and interpret the nuances and subtleties of African American childhoods and parental influences can unlock the secrets of pathologies and perhaps improve lives and well-being. This may, however, be less possible to effect for the European American therapist trained in a psychological environment that does not adequately consider and understand the important differences that can differentially influence significant aspects of the lives of Black and White women.

## SOME DIFFERENCES BETWEEN SOME AFRICAN AMERICAN WOMEN AND WHITE WOMEN

Do African American women have special therapeutic needs? Often there is a well-meaning assumption, sometimes explicit but often implicit, that African American women are like all other women and can therefore be treated as such. There are, however, factors that contribute uniquely to the development of African American women that have implications for therapy. The notion that the needs of African American women are just like the needs of women of other ethnic groups is problematic. The history of African American women differs from that of European American women. It is not surprising, therefore, that the present-day behavioral patterns of African American women have evolved out of their historical experiences. Mays (1985) concurs that "the process of slavery and its debilitating effects on the development of a self-identity imposed on the African American present a unique psychological development that is not comparable with any other group lacking such an experience" (p. 385).

Looking at differences between African American and European American women, Williams and Trotman (1984) examined four areas that contribute to the uniqueness of the African American female experience: (1) physical characteristics; (2) historical/social/cultural dynamics; (3) emotional/intellectual characteristics; and (4) sex roles and male–female relationships.

### Physical Characteristics

Gunnar Myrdal (1944), in *An American Dilemma* over half a century ago, attributed skin color and identifiability as the basis of racism and discrimination against African Americans in the United States. In addition to skin color, there are a number of other characteristic physical features (nose, lips, hair texture, etc.) that distinguish the African American person. Physical differences are the basis of initial and ongoing differences in the treatment of all African Americans by both European Americans (male and female) and other African Americans (male and female). The general perception of an African American person is often based on stereotypes associated with physical characteristics, resulting in discrimination in all institutions (educational, social, legal, political, religious, business, etc). The physical characteristics that distinguish African American women are also often the basis of adverse treatment by other members of her own family and by the greater African American community. Intragroup verbal, social, and physical rejection is often based on such factors as skin color, facial features, and hair texture. These factors and the dynamics that accompany them are discussed in greater detail in Chapter 8 of this volume. The physical characteristics that distinguish some African American women from White women stimulate an association with negative stereotypes and deficits in American society. The presence of such negative stereotypes can result in a need to respond to being treated as if one is the embodiment of the negative stereotype. The presence of these negative stereotypes results in psychologically destructive behavior by others.

A therapist will need to know, first of all, that this phenomenon exists. It must not be ubiquitously misunderstood as the client's abdication of personal responsibility. Second, therapists will need to know how a particular African American woman understands, experiences, and copes with this phenomenon. Many women will enter therapy in part because they have not learned how to successfully cope with this ever present stressor. The danger is that the therapist, regardless of ethnicity, will not understand that process or seek to understand it. When this occurs, the client is at risk for having this stressful phenomenon repeated in the therapy process itself. Negative treatment based on the perception of negative stereotypes associated with race is a routine feature of most African American women's experience and psychological life. Therefore, it must be considered in the organization, composition, and direction of therapeutic interventions that address African American women.

## Historical/Social/Cultural Dynamics

The African origins of African American women contribute a cultural framework as well as physical characteristics to her experience. An oral rather than a literary tradition, polyrhythmic musical influences, Black English, an extended family, the central role of religion, and a variety of nonmainstream (i.e., White) values, priorities, and attitudes are the legacy of African and slavery influences perpetuated across centuries in the United States by racism and isolation. The major impact of culture on personality relates to the behavior of others toward an individual and the individual's observations and resulting patterns of behavior and responses toward people and objects (Barber, 1998; Linton, 1945; Manstead, 1997; Molloy & Herzberger, 1998; Nigel, 1976; Stack, 1986). Because of these factors, African American women's perceptions of self may depend on the degree to which they have experienced segregated neighborhoods, schools, and colleges, or whether they have had the opportunity to experience acceptance and rejection by both African and European Americans. All the cultural influences brought to bear on Black women, rural versus urban, northern versus southern, West Indian versus Caribbean, African versus American, and so on, cannot begin to be addressed in this chapter. A knowledge of these differences and how their profound effects distinguish the psychological life of African

American women is, however, crucial to the successful psychotherapeutic conduct of therapy for African American women. Bulhan (1985) examined the ethnocentric basis of the history of psychological assessment, theories, and research findings central to the teachings of psychotherapy, and concurs that "mental health professionals who seek to work with blacks must learn their history, culture, communication patterns, hurts, strengths and aspirations as they experience and define them not as professionals assume them to be" (p. 176).

## Emotional/Intellectual Characteristics

The professional who works with African American women in therapy must also consider the emotional and intellectual characteristics that distinguish her from White women and other women of color. Differences in the incidence of female-headed households, poverty, extended family traditions, and the experience of strong female role models have facilitated the development of the mythical "Black superwoman" image with its concomitant expectation that African American women must "do all" and "be all," often ignoring her individual needs. Regina Romero and Cheryl Thompson (Chapters 11 and 12, this volume) provide an extensive discussion of this phenomenon and some of its frequently ignored but potentially self-destructive consequences. Alice Walker, reporting to Bradley (1984), underscores this subtle difference in emotional and intellectual outlook by pointing out that "white feminism teaches white women that they are capable, whereas my [Black] tradition assumes I'm capable" (p. 36). Staples (1981) goes on to say that because of their history, Black women are "more aggressive and independent than white women" (p. 31), and Ladner (1971) posits that adaptive Black female strength has been confused with dominance. Staples (1981) asserts that any inordinate powers that Black women possess are owed to White racist employment barriers in the United States. The net effect of this phenomenon, he believes, is not Black female dominance but greater economic deprivation for families deprived of the father's income. Smith (1982) found that "whereas black young women formulated their work commitments on a socialized sense of family economic responsibility, white women more often indicated that they desired to work for self-fulfillment" (p. 282). All these views point out the often subtle but important differences that distinguish African American women's experiences. The therapist's awareness of these different realities facilitates the potential for optimum growth for African American women in therapy.

## Gender Roles and Intimate Relationships

Another difference between heterosexual African American and European American women whose understanding is relevant to the optimum conduct of African American women's psychotherapy is that of male–female relationships and roles. Thomas and Dansby (1985) argue that "black professional women with advanced degrees have competently balanced the work role (with its racial and sexual discrimination) and the home role." The authors go on to state that "with the increased participation of white married women in the labor force, there is much they can learn from the experience of well-educated black women" (p. 405). Implications of this finding for the conduct of therapists must be understood (Bethea, 1998; Essed, 1994; Ferguson & King, 1996; Letlaka, Kedibone, Helms, & Zea, 1997; Nkomo & Cox, 1989). African American heterosexual couples' interactions are much more egalitarian than those of European American couples (Bethea, 1998; James, Tucker, & Mitchell-Kernan, 1996; Thomas & Neal, 1978). This does not mean, however, that sexism is not a problem in the African American community.

Proportionately more African American women have always worked outside the home than European American women. Historically, the slave woman was first a piece of property /full-time worker for her owner and only incidentally a wife, mother, and homemaker. As slaves, Black women learned that their ability to work was much the same as Black men's abilities because they were forced to work alongside their men. They were not exempt from harsh forms of labor deemed inappropriate for White women (Greene, 1996, 1997). Ironically, this lack of protection of her "femininity" gave her the experiences in the workplace needed to debunk the mythology that only males could perform certain tasks. She developed the qualities of hard work, perseverance, self-reliance, tenacity, resistance, and sexual equality (hooks, 1982). As popular depictions portray them (Burton, 1996a, 1996b; Mitchell, 1993), most African American women have not been raised with the expectation that a man would take care of them or that marriage would relieve them of the need to work outside the home. Yet many "black women view their familial responsibilities in a very stereotypically female manner" (Helms, 1979, p. 40).

Simultaneously, African American women outnumber African American men to such an extent that many heterosexual African American women who wish to marry may never have the opportunity (Jarrett, 1994). Of those who wish to have children, many will become mothers only if they are willing to be single heads of household, while still others of this group may live out their lives with neither husband nor children (Jackson, 1976; Jarrett, 1994). It is important, however, that therapists understand that not all African American women are heterosexual and that not all heterosexual African American women are seeking a husband and family. The bonds of the African American community do not automatically include or protect women who are lesbians from heterosexism within the African American community. This complicates relationships for African American lesbians. Greene (Chapter 5, this volume) provides a more extensive discussion of relationship issues among African American lesbians. It is also important to note that all heterosexual African American women are not seeking a male life partner or a traditional marriage, and still others may not have children because of their own personal choice rather than by default. Still other single African American women, both lesbian and heterosexual, may make a decision to have or adopt children that is independent of their choices in relationships. Other African American women who may be single or who do not have natural children of their own are actively involved in the raising of the children of siblings or other family members. They may provide critical and not simply casual childcare and financial support, particularly if they are more economically successful family members. As African American women constitute a heterogeneous group, the absence of a traditional lifestyle should not automatically be seen as a problem for that person. A wide range of potential choices in relationships and family structures should be entertained.

White feminists are often puzzled by what is perceived to be a lack of formal acknowledgment or commitment on the part of African American women to the feminist political movement. They may not realize that African American women's experience of racism may result in her perception of whiteness, not gender, as the major factor preventing equity. Indeed, hooks (1982) reports that "in the 19th and early 20th century America few if any similarities could be found between the life experiences" (p. 122) of African American and European American women. Wright (1991) notes that "although they were both subjected to sexist victimization, as victims of racism, black women were subjected to oppression no white woman was forced to endure" (p. 122). In fact, "white racial imperialism granted all white women, however victimized by sexist oppression they might be, the right to assume the role of oppressor in relationship to black women and black men" (Wright, 1991, p. 123). In her award-winning one-woman play, *Pretty Fire*, author Charlayne Woodard writes:

> When the women's lib movement came about, we were all very anxious to hear grandmama's views on that subject. She said, "Generations and generations of Woodard women have always had . . . the opportunity . . . to work like a man, at a man's job. . . . A woman must always be prepared to do whatever she has to do for the sake of her family and her loved ones. . . . But if any of you should find a nice young man . . . and this young man just happens to be offering you a pedestal I want you to climb up on it, and take a nap for me." (1995, p. 42)

The therapist must closely consider the physical, historical, and emotional context in which therapy takes place for all African American women. As the examples above suggest, there are often subtle but significant differences between African American and European American women that could affect the therapeutic experience. The therapist must also be "aware that all Black women are not alike and that the nature of the problems that they bring to counseling may differ depending upon such factors as socioeconomic status, family size, age, and marital or relationship status" (Helms, 1979, p. 41). Being born both a

Black person and a woman in 20th-century America represents double jeopardy, and for African American lesbians triple jeopardy, in terms of one's self-image. On the other hand, Black history and African cultural derivatives may have afforded African American women some degree of resilience that many White American women lack (Carey, 1979; Kuppersmith, 1987; Mahmoud, 1998).

Such things as skin color, hair texture, social class, sexual orientation, and environment have salient effects on African American women and their perception of who they are in America. This complex set of variables, including variations in living styles in different geographical regions, further reflects the complexity of African American identities and has implications for psychotherapeutic intervention in the life of African American women (Greene, 1996; Kuppersmith, 1987; see also Chapter 8, this volume).

## FEMINIST PSYCHOTHERAPY AND AFRICAN AMERICAN WOMEN

Given the differences between African American and European American women, issues in the psychotherapy of African American women are crucial, significant, and often controversial. As African American women increasingly seek professional consultation for emotional difficulties, it is imperative that we evaluate existing approaches for their relevance to the African American female experience. In examining the appropriateness of specific therapeutic interventions for African American women, several issues must be considered. Among the most salient are (1) the race of the therapist, (2) the importance of the culture and social class of the therapist, (3) the effect of therapists' attitudes, (4) the same-sex versus the different-sex therapist, and (5) the importance of role modeling.

### Race of the Therapist

As director of a psychotherapy institute in a socioeconomic and ethnically heterogeneous area, I have the responsibility of ensuring an appropriate match between therapist and client to maximize the therapeutic potential of the dyad. For the African American female client, an obvious consideration is the race of the therapist. It is understandable that the African American client will bring her preconceptions and perhaps strong feelings about race to the treatment situation. These feelings may be expressed in concerns about the race of her therapist. She might, for example, view the European American therapist as representative of a kind of authority figure who is more invested in defending and maintaining the status quo of racial hierarchies, because he or she benefits from them. The African American client in this situation may find it hard to believe that such a therapist is capable of empathically relating to her as a client. Usually, the African American therapist is less likely but not totally immune (if he or she has internalized racism, class guilt, or survivor guilt) to being seduced or manipulated by the particular African American female client who has learned to use her blackness as a weapon to maintain power or to punish others by eliciting compassion or guilt. Racial guilt may make the European American therapist reluctant to suggest that the African American client has to take responsibility for her own life.

Other behaviors that are more readily seen in the European American therapist–African American client relationship are the therapist acting as the self-appointed advocate, as the client controller, or as the self-effacing sympathizer. As the self-appointed advocate or as the client controller, the therapist assumes undue responsibility for the client; in his or her paternalism, the therapist subtly implies an inequality in their humanity and a disrespect for the client's judgment and abilities. Well-meaning, dedicated, and sympathetic European American therapists are often trapped by the symbolism of their white skin and the subtle pervasiveness of America's guilt. The self-effacing therapist is neither genuine nor completely available to the client.

In the relationship between the African American therapist and the African American women client, other potential dangers exist. One is the possibility that the African American therapist will become overidentified with the client as a "victim of the system" and aid her in denial of responsibility for her own life. Some of this behavior might enhance the relationship through a feeling of sisterhood. However, it is extremely important that the client develop a sense of responsibility for her own life despite any obstacles imposed by her ethnicity. Another danger for the African American therapist (and occasionally the European American therapist) is that he or she will attempt to raise the consciousness of any African American woman who is seemingly unaware of the circumstances, history, and implications of her blackness via intellectual discussion. Such interventions may be quite instructional and educational. They are not, however, always therapeutic and often lead to premature termination by a client who either may be uninterested in or defended against such information.

At the other end of the spectrum is the African American therapist who has dissociated his or her self from his or her own blackness, harboring a core of self-hatred, internalized racism, and rejection of anything reminiscent of African American culture. Such a therapist poses the danger of engendering feelings of rejection and self-hatred in the African American female client, thereby creating a relationship that not only fails to be therapeutic, but may in fact be detrimental.

On the other hand, the African American therapist–African American female clients' alliance has many advantages. Most African American therapists are aware of behaviors among African American women that are different from the European American norm and behaviors that are often pathologized by mental health. For example, African American women may harbor a distrust of police or authority figures. Such fears or distrust may be justified by the reality of corrupt ghetto police officers or other dominant-culture authority figures who have historically abused and continue to abuse their power in the African American community to the detriment of community members. Frequently African American patients are diagnosed as more severely disturbed by European American therapists than they would be by African American therapists (Bland & Kraft, 1998; Byington, Fischer, Walker, & Freedman, 1997; Lerner, 1972). Often, many nontraditional behaviors are appropriate and functional for African American women but less readily comprehensible to the European American therapist. For example, a therapist unfamiliar with African American culture may see belief in spiritualism or the seeking of "readers and advisers" as magical thinking and therefore pathological. Also the African American therapist is frequently more likely to realize that traditional interventions and the 50-minute hour are often less effective for the African American female, who may require active intervention and assistance with such things as housing or discrimination before she can begin to attend to her intrapsychic conflicts. Additionally, knowing what a client's words might mean symbolically in her experience obviously makes it easier for the therapist to translate her thoughts and feelings into a content that reveals more about herself. The ability to make these kinds of translations is essential to dynamic therapies (Altman, 1995; Edelson, 1975; Thompson, 1989).

There has been some interesting research about the salience of the therapist's race for the African American client in general that is likely to be applicable to African American women in particular. Turner and Armstrong (1981) found that European American therapists do not experience racial issues in psychotherapy with the same salience as African American therapists, yet they report higher levels of subjective distress in cross-cultural treatment. The European American therapists' distress focused on the "negative attitudes" of clients, therapists' feelings of not being able to help or to confront clients of a different race, or being oversolicitous or too distant with clients of a different race. Research on psychotherapy with African Americans suggests that "the nature and quality of therapist–patient interaction is a critical determinant in whether a black client continues psychotherapy" (Griffith & Jones, 1979, p. 229). Several studies indicate that African Americans drop out of therapy quite early at a high rate (Sue, 1977; Sue, McKinney, Allen, & Hall, 1974). Research has found that "depth of self-exploration" in African American clients was enhanced when those clients were seen by African American interviewers (Banks, 1972; Carkhuff & Pierce, 1967). Griffith and Jones (1979) report several other similar studies in which clients expressed preference for African American counselors or felt better understood by them. Sattler (1970) cites studies of assessment, interview, educational, and therapeutic situations to show an inhibiting effect on the African American client when the authority figure is European American.

## Culture and Class of the Therapist

Despite many of the challenges and complexities that I have discussed, African American patients from neurotic, middle-class populations have been shown to profit in cross-racial therapies (Jones, 1978). In the Jones studies outcomes and details of therapy processes in the four kinds of Black–White therapist–client matches were compared. No differences were found in an overall outcome as a group: clients in all the different possible permutations got better to about the same degree. There were differences by racial matchup, however, in the nature of the interpersonal dynamics that occurred between therapist and client.

Addressing the European American therapist–African American client relationship, Griffith and Jones (1979) note:

> The race difference appears to have its greatest impact early in treatment, particularly at the first encounter. If the white therapist can establish effective rapport at initial contact and build a therapeutic alliance in relatively rapid fashion, successful outcomes can be achieved with lower income black clients despite their initial sense of wariness and consequently slower movement in therapy. (p. 230)

I observe that African American women depend more on their initial affective assessment of the therapeutic situation than on any objective criteria over time. For African American women entering therapy, the therapeutic alliance may automatically conjure up the specter of an authoritarian institution operating on the potential client to her detriment. The history of psychiatric treatment of African Americans in America does not refute this (Bland & Kraft, 1998; Thomas & Sillen, 1972; Willie, Kramer, & Brown, 1973). Also, seeking professional consultation for psychological difficulties is not something that springs naturally from an African American woman's experience. She is understandably wary, and the cultural unfamiliarity may heighten her tendency to rely more on affective assessments as a way of judging whether or not this is going to be a useful experience. This may mean that a potential client may be particularly sensitive to the initial difficulties that are bound to occur between strangers, particularly those from different cultural backgrounds.

There are additional therapeutic considerations for African American women that are more specifically cultural or attitudinal than purely racial. Tomes (1976) cites various studies indicating differential attitudes toward African Americans who present themselves for treatment. The tendency to see African Americans as too sick or inappropriate for talking therapies or not really psychologically disturbed may be a way of "avoiding their own race and class attitudes on the part of the white professional" (Jenkins, 1982, p. 155). Jenkins (1982) also sees this as avoiding "exposure to the intense feelings that black clients may want to vent . . . concerning their social and racial as well as their personal concerns" (p. 155). Many African American women are very sensitive to any indication by the therapist that she may be masking or avoiding her own difficulties through quick preconceptions of African Americans and hasty inaccurate interpretations. This is obviously detrimental to the therapeutic process, particularly if it is kept undercover and unexpressed.

It is generally recognized now that the degree to which a person expresses herself verbally depends on the situation in which a person finds herself (Labov, 1972; Lerner, 1972). When lower class African Americans feel comfortable and understood, they are quite expressive and reflective. African American women may have traditional reservations concerning immediate trust and self-disclosure; the guilt feelings and anxiety of the therapist can cause the client to further strengthen her defenses against intimacy.

## Therapists' Attitudes

Dealing with Black anger and rage (Grier & Cobbs, 1968) is often both central and crucial to therapy with African Americans. The experiences of self-hatred and degradation imposed on Black people in America have left psychic wounds and scars that cannot be left unattended if psychological health is to be realized. Such experiences, which may include the subtle but perhaps devastating feelings among African Americans about variations of skin color and hair texture, or their childhood memories of being the scapegoated or idealized darkest or lightest member of the family or community, are often difficult or impossible for the African American client to express to her European American therapist. Yet these are often the very issues that cause the greatest pain and psychological destruction, particularly if left unexplored.

Along with the experience of anger and rage, a widespread feeling of sadness, a kind of "cultural depression," is part of many Black individuals' responses to historical and current conditions in America (Comer, 1972; Grier & Cobbs, 1968; Poussaint, 1972). It is essential for the therapist of African American women to understand and ideally to have felt these feelings to facilitate the therapeutic process for African American women clients. Black rage and "cultural depression" are certainly not the sole predispositions that are likely to be brought into therapy by African American women. Block (1981) suggests that "the black culture stresses early in life the ability to 'do it.' Emphasis is placed on actively managing difficult situations without showing stress" (p. 179). Many such cultural tendencies must be understood and preferably experienced by the therapist to create an authentic empathic connection with the African American female client. Whenever therapists have experienced situations and feelings similar to those of their clients, there is a greater likelihood of communicating empathy and understanding—not only mutual trust, but a deeper experience of kinship.

The gender of the therapist for African American women also has relevance to treatment. It would surely seem that by virtue of having a female body and the opportunity to have played the roles of girl baby, daughter, sister, lover, wife, pregnant woman, mother, divorcée, widow, and grandmother, a woman does have unique experiences different from those of men. These different understandings may prove especially useful in understanding her women patients, as well as in discerning which patients can benefit from specific therapist–patient arrangements (Goz, 1981, p. 516; see also Pikus & Heavey, 1996).

## Same-Sex versus Different-Sex Therapist

The superficial simplicity of these considerations is complicated, however, by Porché and Banikotes's (1982) findings that European American female counselors were perceived as more expert than their African American female counterparts, whereas the higher rating of male counselors was not influenced by the racial variable for African American adolescents. These findings are supported by recent research by Helms (1990), Helms and Carter (1991), and Nickerson, Helms, and Terrell (1994). This seems to suggest that the woman therapist in general and the African American female therapist in particular would have difficulty treating African American women because of their clients' low expectations and lack of respect for the "expertness" of the African American female therapist.

Given the view of African Americans and of women in the United States, these findings are quite understandable and do not, in fact, present the problems that they appear to. Chesler (1975) has noted that women in the past have preferred male therapists because they mistrusted women as both authorities and people. Similarly, many African American female adolescents have internalized society's view of African American women as not as "expert" as European American men. Despite these findings, anecdotal data suggest that African American women overwhelmingly request a female therapist and an African American female therapist specifically. This suggests that there is a difference between being recognized as a figure who has power and being regarded as one who has credibility. While European American therapists clearly enjoy a higher position in the hierarchy of social power when compared to African Americans, they are not necessarily more credible to African American women clients.

## Therapist as Role Model

Though her African American female client may not initially perceive her as "expert," the African American female therapist serves an important function as a role model for African American women in treatment. As she communicates honesty, sincerity, and love to her African American clients, the African American therapist subtly and simultaneously also identifies the details and mechanisms of her own success, thereby demystifying success and making it more accessible to the African American female client. In her authenticity, the therapist may relinquish the power and awe of her "expert" or "superwoman" status for the satisfaction of facilitating the possibility of duplication of her own success for her client.

This brings us to the actual conduct of the therapeutic relationship with African American women. A reduction of the traditional distance between therapist and client encourages African American women to take control of their lives rather than rely on the omniscient "master" who directs their behavior. A lifelong encouragement of African American dependency is subtly redirected by the "feminist" psychotherapeutic relationship and the embodiment of egalitarianism.

There are some obvious differences in the "feminist/psychodynamic" psychotherapy of African American women versus European American women. In raising the woman's consciousness about the impact of culture on her development, for example, both the culture and its impact will differ between the races. The cultures' view of what is "pretty," "sexy," "masculine," or "independent" may touch an African American woman's life very differently than it touches the lives of White women. African American women have historically been defined as "not" pretty, possibly "too" sexy, and "too" independent, perhaps to the point of being "castrating matriarchs" who took over her man's role when she was forced to support her family (Greene, 1994, 1996, 1997). These and other differences change the cultural context in which therapy must take place for African American women. It is imperative therefore, as I suggested above, that the therapist is intimately acquainted with African American women's culture.

A feminist psychotherapy approach that includes modeling an egalitarian relationship, authenticity, and encouraging the client to take responsibility for her own life are most likely to facilitate African American women's optimal development. Psychodynamic interventions can incorporate elements of feminist therapy as opposed to traditional authoritarian approaches. Such integrative models seem most effective in facilitating the therapy process.

If we attempt to offer the African American women client some of the added benefits of incorporating a psychodynamic approach, there is much to be considered. Many (Brown, 1990, 1995; Greene, 1994, 1995, 1996, 1997; Mays & Comas-Díaz, 1988) have lamented the failure of feminist formulations to reflect the full spectrum of diversity among women. Moreover, psychodynamic theory is notorious for its androcentric, heterocentric, and White, middle-class ethnocentric point of view.

## PSYCHODYNAMIC/FEMINIST PSYCHOTHERAPY
## WITH AFRICAN AMERICAN WOMEN

## The Role of African American Mothers, Foremothers, and Other Mothers

Much of psychodynamic practice, in general, and object relations theory, in particular, focus on maternal influences, with much gender, class, heterosexist, and cultural bias (Espin, 1995; Greene, 1996). If we are to attempt to incorporate psychodynamic psychotherapy into the feminist treatment of African American women, we must begin to examine the parental influences and significance of African American mothers, foremothers, and other mothers. The pervasiveness of therapists' White privilege (Wildman, 1995) and their roles in racial oppression have not been sufficiently considered as part of countertransferential reactions on the parts of European American psychotherapists (Altman, 1995). Much of adult personality, as well as problems that may arise from repressed emotions during childhood, are presumed to have their basis in conflictual relationships with significant caregivers. Yet the concepts of "mothers" and "mothering" are based on White middle-class constructs, leaving therapists with "a poor understanding of child care relationships in the many diverse contexts in which contemporary mental health clinicians encounter them" (Greene, 1997, p. 312). African American mothering is a process and a product of collective African and African American foremothers and African American community mothers. Given the isolating effects and peculiar nature of slavery, racism, discrimination, and oppression in America, many of the 17th-, 18th-, and 19th-century West African tribal customs, values, and attitudes brought here by our ancestors have been retained and passed on by our foremothers. The African American community has depended on itself and its foremothers for guidance in the most important areas of mothering. The language, concepts, and practice of African American mothering may be very different from those of the dominant White American culture. Psychologists may want to examine the words and stories of African American mothers and foremothers for a clearer sense of the meaning of motherhood and mothering for African American clients. The intensity of the African American mother–daughter connection was strengthened as stories were passed down through the foremothers. The role of the oral tradition and the history of storytelling is reflected by author Gayl Jones in *Corregidora* (1975): "My great-grandmama told my grandmama the part she lived through that my grandmama didn't live through and my grandmama told my mama what they both lived through and my mama told me what they all lived through and we suppose to pass it down like that from generation to generation so we'd never forget" (p. 9).

Recent feminist literature has begun to acknowledge the significant role of foremothers in the lives of women. They are now seen as "a model for autonomy and dependence existing side by side in a healthy interdependence" (Halperin, 1989, p. 160). The foremother is an "archetype which guides [us] . . . in our development, allowing us to unfold in harmony with our feminine selves and to experience the cyclical nature of life, not as a limitation but as a vehicle for individuation" (Lowinsky, 1990, p. 97). This linkage of foremothers has recently been acknowledged in feminist writings as a "motherline." Feminist psychologists are slowly beginning to honor the role and place of the foremother as more than symbiotic pathology or Electra-complex-inspired conflictual competition.

Understanding the roles of African American mothers, foremothers, and other mothers is important to the psychodynamic understanding and treatment of African American women. The cultural history of African American mothering is indeed crucial to the interpretation of transference and countertransference and the resolution of the transference neuroses—all significant concepts in psychodynamic treatment.

Among the significant differences to a psychodynamic understanding of the influences on African American women are the impact and import of African American mothers. Because the role of mother is one that is crucial to an analysis of a woman's intrapsychic forces in the psychodynamic framework, I now briefly discuss African American mothering. The difference from the eurocentric concept of "mother" and the practice of mothering is quite evident. Cooperation, a sense of community, interdependence, collective behavior, harmony, collectiveness, a sense of extended self, and "we"-ness often distinguishes African American women (Pack-Brown, Whittington-Clark, & Parker, 1998), in their mothering from European women. One of the tasks of psychodynamic psychotherapy is to help the client/patient to discover how her past influences her present. An underlying assumption in this endeavor is that both the therapist and the patient share or at least understand the same language of nuanced experiences. Complicating this endeavor is that the same word, spelled in exactly the same way in the English language, can mean very different things when spoken by the African American client and heard by the European American therapist, and vice versa. The result of this miscommunication can, at best, mean little discovery of how her actual past influenced the client's present and at worst a professional pathologizing of the client. This can lead to a concomitant lowering of the African American client's knowledge of self and self-esteem.

## The Voices of African American Mothering

In order to understand some of the differences in African American and European American maternal influences, it is important to view how the daughters, mothers, and foremothers of African America see each other. Some well-known African American women have spoken of their mothers. Their voices and thoughts on African American *grand*mothering must also be heard in order to give us an additional glimpse of African American life with which the psychotherapy session can be enriched.

African and slave ancestral legacies have always given great significance to the role and place of foremothers as a link to African American history and the future. African culture honors the ancestor as a significant guiding force. Eighteenth- and 19th-century African tribal customs and attitudes about the interdependence of the extended family and the role of the foremother are consistent with Lowinsky's (1990) description of the "motherline." Cattell (1994) reports that among grandmothers and granddaughters in Kenya, "[T]he most salient female relationships are . . . grandmothers and granddaughters. Age hierarchy is ever-present" (p. 163). "It is in the grandchildren that ancestral spirits are reborn" (Blacking, 1990, p. 120). This phenomenon may color or enhance the experience of aging for African American women. Typically, European American women are valued for their physical attractiveness. When this attractiveness begins to wane with age, they are viewed as less valuable. This phenomenon may be different for African American women who accrue a certain status as elders in their families.

In African American culture the grandmother often plays a central role in the parenting of her grandchildren. Kennedy (1991) found that, of all the groups studied, African American grandchildren were closest to their grandmothers. Today more African American children than ever—67% according to U.S. Bureau of the Census (1994) figures—are being born to single mothers. Often, it is the grandmother who has a major responsibility for mothering the African American child. African American grandmothers provide an important sense of historical continuity. They have usually been the family members who have directly experienced and can place in perspective important aspects of our history. Contemporary African American grandmothers were alive before the 1964 civil rights law was enacted and thus experienced life under U.S. racial apartheid.

While African American grandmothers are often the glue that holds the family together, this role can also be burdensome. Despite the presence of a natural mother in their households, many African American women were raised by their grandmothers. Many African American grandmothers provide necessary childcare and financial support to struggling mothers. Many work further into their later years than White women; indeed, some never really "retire" or feel a sense of retirement. Many experience significant stress when caring for very young children or for many children. The negative consequences of these practices must be considered in the stress-related health problems that many African American women develop that are associated with aging. Striking an appropriate balance between the grandmother's needs and those of her family is important.

Accordingly, Johnetta B. Cole, the first woman president of Spelman College, expressed some of the strength of the influences of the roles of grandmothers and ancestors in the lives of African American women. Speaking of "the nameless West African woman who represented all of our foremothers," Cole went on:

> Despite grueling work and ignominious abuse, she became both a student and teacher. She recognized her powerment. First she taught herself a new language. It certainly was not the standard American English of the time but it was enough to communicate with her slavekeepers and fellow slaves. And in this her motives were quite simple: Language would at least give her the power to name things in her captors' own words. This woman studied "white folks' ways" not in any grotesque desire to emulate them, but in order to recognize and anticipate the many faces of oppression, brutality, and cruelty. . . . (qtd. in Nikuradse, 1996, p. 118)

While feminists teach European American women that they are capable, it has always been *assumed* that African American women are both capable and proud. The attitudes of African American women concerning employment and their role in the family, as passed down from our foremothers, presents a subtle difference from those of her European American counterpart.

Psychotherapists must not underestimate the role and significance of African American mothers, extended families, community mothers, grandmothers, and ancestors in the lives of their African American clients. Boyd-Franklin (1989) has noted that strong kinship bonds are an enduring legacy of the African American heritage.

Many West African cultural traditions, attitudes, and behaviors were preserved by our foremothers directly in the lives of slaves in the United States. Jules-Rosette (1980, p. 275) identified six distinctive features of West African spirituality incorporated into the religious practices of African Americans:

1. The direct link between the natural and the supernatural.
2. The importance of human intervention in the supernatural world.
3. The significance of music to invoke the supernatural.
4. The strong tie between the world of the living and the world of the dead in defining the scope of the community.
5. The importance of participatory verbal performance, including the call–response pattern.
6. The primacy of both secular and verbal performance.

Even if African American families are not actively involved in a particular church, their religious heritage will probably shape their beliefs and values. In order to make well-informed intervention decisions, it is important that the therapist is aware that the "mother" church religious background and the influence of the foremothers may shape attitudes and practices.

Psychotherapists must not underestimate the role and significance of African American mothers, grandmothers, and ancestors in the lives of their African American clients. "The African American family structure evolved from African family structure, in which their strength has been the flexibility and adaptability of their family organization" (Sudarkasa, 1993, p. 89). It is often difficult for therapists unfamiliar with African American culture to truly understand and not pathologize the role of foremothers in African American families. They are often not only a source of comfort and pleasure, but of identification, strength, history, and inspiration. Therapists and counselors must understand not only the impact of specific mothers, but also the significance of African American *grand*mothering in general.

Feminist psychotherapists/counselors often speak of growth through feminine relationships. They might theoretical espouse Lowinsky's (1990) grandmother archetype that guides us "in our development, allowing us to unfold in harmony with our feminine selves and to experience the cyclical nature of life, not as a limitation but as a vehicle for individuation" (p. 97). Yet, in practice, these same therapists may mindlessly impose their own values, maternal struggles, and life experiences on clients as they see adult daughter–mother interdependence as pathological, and counsel their adult clients to "separate" from their mothers and grandmothers. As economic forces compel more adult children to stay at or to return home (Frankel, 1993) we might want to further investigate some of the positive aspects of African American *grand*mothering and the role of the extended family in fostering mental health and happiness.

## SUMMARY

Just as feminist psychology has been forced to develop a more inclusive discourse and has begun to recognize the full array of diversity among women, and the different shapes and effects of various types of oppression on women, psychodynamic psychotherapy will need to similarly evolve. When this evolution is complete, psychodynamic therapy may become more useful in assisting African American women at uncovering and interpreting their unconscious. Neither the early childhood nor the adult experiences, mothering relationships, and influences, or other developmental issues of African American women, can be accurately interpreted in White middle-class terms. Hence, there is much for the European American therapist to learn when conducting therapy with African American women.

## REFERENCES

Altman, N. (1995). *The analyst in the inner city: Race, class, and culture through a psychoanalytic lens.* New York: Analytic Press.

Banks, W. M. (1972). The differential effect of race and social class in helping. *Journal of Clinical Psychology, 28,* 90–92.

Barber, N. (1998). Sex differences in disposition towards kin, security of adult attachment, and sociosexuality as a function of parental divorce. *Evolution of Human Behavior, 19*(2), 125–132.

Bethea, P. (1998). African American women and the male–female relationship dilemma: A counseling perspective. In D. Atkinson, G. Morten, & D. W. Sue (Eds.), *Counseling American minorities* (pp. 87–94). Boston: McGraw-Hill.

Blacking, J. (1990). Growing old gracefully: Physical, social, and spiritual transformations in Venda society, 1956–66. In P. H. Spencer (Ed.), *Anthropology and the riddle of the Sphinx: Paradoxes of change in the life course* (pp. 112–130). New York: Routledge.

Bland, I., & Kraft, I. (1998). The therapeutic alliance across cultures. In S. O. Okpaku (Ed.), *Clinical methods in transcultural psychiatry* (pp. 266–278). Washington, DC: American Psychiatric Press.

Block, C. B. (1981). Black Americans and the cross-cultural counseling and psychotherapy experience. In A. J. Marsella & P. B. Pedersen (Eds.), *Cross-cultural counseling and psychotherapy* (pp. 177–194). Elmsford, NY: Pergamon Press.

Boyd-Franklin, N. (1989). *Black families in therapy: A multisystems approach.* New York: Guilford Press.

Bradley, D. (1984, January 8). Telling the Black woman's story. *New York Times Magazine,* pp. 24–37.

Brown, L. S. (1990). The meaning of a multicultural perspective for theory building in feminist therapy. In L. Brown & M. Roots (Eds.), *Diversity and complexity in feminist therapy* (pp. 1–21). New York: Haworth Press.

Brown, L. S. (1995). Antiracism as an ethical norm in feminist therapy practice. In G. Adleman & G. Enguidanos-Clark (Eds.), *Racism in the lives of women: Testimony, theory, and guides to antiracist practice* (pp. 137–148). New York: Haworth Press.

Bulhan, H. A. (1985). Black Americans and psychotherapy: An overview of research and theory. *Psychotherapy, 22*(2), 370–378.

Burton, L. (1996a). The timing of childbearing, family structure, and the role responsibilities of aging Black women. In E. Hetherington & E. Blechman (Eds.), *Stress, coping, and resiliency in children and families* (pp. 155–172). Mahwah, NJ: Erlbaum.

Burton, L. (1996b). Age norms, the timing of family role transitions, and intergenerational caregiving among African American women. *Gerontologist, 36*(2), 199–208.

Byington, K., Fischer, J., Walker, L., & Freedman, E. (1997). Evaluating the effectiveness of multicultural counseling ethics and assessment training. *Journal of Applied Rehabilitation Counseling, 28*(4), 15–19.

Carey, P. M. (1979). Black women: A perspective. *Tenth-Year Anniversary Commemorative Monograph Series, 1*(3). New York University, Institute for Afro-American Affairs.

Carkhuff, R. R., & Pierce, R. (1967). Differential effects of therapist, race, and social class upon patient depths of self-exploration in the initial clinical interview. *Journal of Consulting Psychology, 31,* 632–634.

Cattell, M. G. (1994). "Nowadays it isn't easy to advise the young": Grandmothers and granddaughters among the Abaluya of Kenya. *Journal of Cross-Cultural Gerontology, 9*(2), 157–178.

Chesler, P. (1975). Women as psychiatric and psychotherapeutic patients. In R. K. Unger & F. L. Denmark (Eds.), *Woman: Dependent or independent variable?* (pp. 137–162). New York: Psychological Dimensions.

Comer, J. P. (1972). *Beyond black and white.* New York: Quadrangle.

Edelson, M. (1975). *Language and interpretation in psychoanalysis.* New Haven, CT: Yale University Press.

Espin, O. (1995). On knowing you are the unknown: Women of color constructing psychology. In J. Adleman & G. Enguidanos (Eds.), *Racism in the lives of women* (pp. 127–135). New York: Haworth Press.

Essed, P. (1994). Contradictory positions, ambivalent perceptions: A case study of a Black woman entrepreneur. *Feminism and Psychology, 4*(1), 99–118.

Ferguson, S., & King, T. (1996). Bringing organizational behavior therapy together: Counseling the African American female on "job socialization failure." *Women and Therapy, 18*(1), 47–58.

Frankel, J. (1993). *The employed mother and the family context.* New York: Springer.

Goz, R. (1981). Women patients and women therapists: Some issues that come up in psychotherapy. In E. Howell & M. Bayes (Eds.), *Women and mental health* (pp. 514–533). New York: Basic Books.

Greene, B. (1994). Diversity and difference: The issue of race in feminist therapy. In M. Pravder-Mirkin (Ed.), *Women in context: Toward a feminist reconstruction of psychotherapy* (pp. 333–351). New York: Guilford Press.

Greene, B. (1995). An African American perspective on racism and anti-Semitism within feminist organizations. In J. Adleman & G. Enguidanos (Eds.), *Racism in the lives of women* (pp. 303–313). New York: Haworth Press.

Greene, B. (1996). Psychotherapy with African American women: Considering diverse identities and societal barriers. In J. A. Sechzer, S. M. Pfafflin, F. L. Denmark, A. Griffin, & S. Blumenthal (Eds.), *Annals of the New York Academy of Sciences: Women and Mental Health, 798,* 191–209.

Greene, B. (1997). Psychotherapy with African American women: Integrating feminist and psychodynamic models. *Smith College Studies in Social Work, 67*(3), 299–322.

Grier, W. H., & Cobbs, P. M. (1968). *Black rage.* New York: Basic Books.

Griffith, M. S., & Jones, E. E. (1979). Race and psychotherapy: Changing perspectives. In J. H. Masserman (Ed.), *Current psychiatric therapies* (Vol. 18). New York: Grune & Stratton.

Halperin, S. M. (1989). A neglected triangle: Grandmother, mother, and daughter. *Contemporary Family Therapy, 11*(3), 151–168.

Helms, J. E. (1979). Black women. *Counseling Psychologist, 8*(1), 40–41.

Helms, J. E. (1990). Three perspectives on counseling and psychotherapy with visible racial/ethnic group clients. In F. Serafica (Ed.), *Mental health of ethnic minorities* (pp. 171–201). New York: Praeger.

Helms, J. E., & Carter, R. T. (1991). Relationships of White and Black racial identity attitudes and demographic similarity to counselor preference. *Journal of Counseling Psychology, 38*(4), 446–457.

hooks, b. (1982). *Ain't I a woman? Black women and feminism.* Boston: South End Press.

Jackson, A. M. (1976). Mental health delivery systems and the Black client. *Journal of Afro-American Issues, 4,* 28–34.

James, A., Tucker, M., & Mitchell-Kernan, C. (1996). Marital attitudes, perceived mate availability, and subjective well-being among partnered African American men and women. *Journal of Black Psychology, 22*(1), 20–36.

Jarrett, R. (1994). Living poor: Family life among single-partner African American women. *Social Problems, 41*(1), 30–49.

Jenkins, A. H. (1982). *The psychology of the Afro-American: A humanistic approach.* New York: Pergamon Press.

Jones, E. E. (1978). Effects of race on psychotherapy process and outcome: An exploratory investigation. *Psychotherapy: Theory, Research, and Practice, 15,* 226–236.

Jones, G. (1975). *Corregidora.* New York: Random House.

Jules-Rosette, B. (1980). Creative spirituality from Africa to America: Cross-cultural influences in contemporary religious forms. *Western Journal of Black Studies, 4,* 273–285.

Kennedy, G. E. (1991). Grandchildren's reasons for closeness with grandparents. *Journal of Social Behavior and Personality, 6*(4), 697–712.

Kuppersmith, J. (1987). The double bind of personal striving: Ethnic working class women in psychotherapy. *Journal of Contemporary Psychotherapy, 17*(3), 203–216.

Labov, W. (1972). *Language in the inner city: Studies in the Black English vernacular.* Philadelphia: University of Pennsylvania Press.

Lerner, B. (1972). *Therapy in the ghetto: Political impotence and personal disintegration.* Baltimore: Johns Hopkins University Press.

Letlaka, R., Kedibone, L., Helms, J., & Zea, M. (1997). Does the womanist identity model predict aspects of psychological functioning in South African women? *South African Journal of Psychology, 27*(4), 236–243.

Linton, R. (1945). *The cultural background of personality.* New York: Appleton-Century-Crofts.

Lowinsky, N. R. (1990). Mother of mothers: The power of grandmother in the female psyche. In C. Zweig (Ed.), *To be a woman: The birth of the conscious feminine* (pp. 86–97). Los Angeles: Tarcher.

Mahmoud, V. (1998). The double binds of racism. In M. McGoldrick (Ed.), *Re-visioning family therapy: Race, culture, and gender in clinical practice* (pp. 255–267). New York: Guilford Press.

Manstead, A. (1997). Situations, belongingness, attitudes, and culture: Four lessons learned from social psychology. In G. McGarty & A. Haslam (Eds.), *The message of social psychology: Perspectives on mind in society* (pp. 238–251). Oxford, U.K.: Blackwell.

Mays, V. M. (1985). The Black American and psychotherapy: The dilemma. *Psychotherapy, 22*(2), 379–388.

Mays, V. M., & Comas-Díaz, L. (1988). Feminist therapy with ethnic minority populations: A closer look at Blacks and Hispanics. In M. Dutton-Douglas & L. Walker (Eds.), *Feminist psychotherapies: Integration of therapeutic and feminist systems* (pp. 228–251). Norwood, NJ: Ablex.

Mitchell, A. (1993). Signifying women: Visions and revisons of slavery in Octavia Butler's *Kindred*, Shirley Anne William's *Dessa Rose*, and Toni Morrison's *Beloved*. *Dissertation Abstracts International, 53*, 8-A.

Molloy, B., & Herzberger, S. (1998). Body image and self-esteem: A comparison of African American and Caucasian women. *Sex Roles, 38* (7–8), 631–643.

Myrdal, G. (1944). *An American dilemma: The Negro problem and modern democracy.* New York: Harper.

Nickerson, K., Helms, J., & Terrell, F. (1994). Cultural mistrust, opinions about mental illness, and Black students' attitudes toward seeking psychological help from White counselors. *Journal of Counseling Psychology, 41*(3), 378–385.

Nigel, C. (1976). *The human conspiracy.* New York: Viking Press.

Nikuradse, T. (1996). *My mother had a dream: African-American women share their mother's words.* New York: Dutton Books.

Nkomo, S., & Cox, T. (1989). Gender differences in the upward mobility of Black managers: Double whammy or double advantage? *Sex Roles, 21*(11–12), 825–839.

Pack-Brown, S. P., Whittington-Clark, L. E., & Parker, W. M. (1998). *Images of me: A guide to group work with African-American women.* Boston: Allyn & Bacon.

Pikus, C., & Heavey, C. (1996). Client preferences for therapist gender. *Journal of College Student Psychotherapy, 10*(4), 35–43.

Porché, L. M., & Banikotes, P. G. (1982). Racial and attitudinal factors affecting the perceptions of counselors of Black adolescents. *Journal of Counseling Psychology, 29*(2), 169–174.

Poussaint, A. F. (1972). *Why Blacks kill Blacks.* New York: Emerson Hall.

Sattler, J. (1970). Racial "experimenter effects" in experimentation, testing, interviewing, and psychotherapy. *Psychological Bulletin, 73*, 137–160.

Smith, E. J. (1982). The Black female adolescent: A review of the educational, career, and psychological literature. *Psychology of Women Quarterly, 7*(3), 261–287.

Stack, C. (1986). The culture of gender: Women and men of color. *Signs, 11*(2), 321–324.

Staples, R. (1981). The myth of the Black matriarchy. *Black Scholar, 12*(6), 26–34.

Sudarkasa, N. (1993). Female-headed African American households: Some neglected dimensions. In H. P. McAdoo (Ed.), *Family ethnicity: Strength in diversity* (pp. 81–89). Newbury Park, CA: Sage.

Sue, S. (1977). Community mental health services to minority groups: Some optimism, some pessimism. *American Psychologist, 32*, 616–624.

Sue, S., McKinney, H., Allen, D., & Hall, J. (1974). Delivery of community mental health services to Black and White clients. *Journal of Consulting and Clinical Psychology, 42*, 794–801.

Thomas, A., & Sillen, S. (1972). *Racism and psychiatry.* New York: Brunner/Mazel.

Thomas, M. B., & Dansby, P. G. (1985). Black clients: Family structures, therapeutic issues, and strengths. *Psychotherapy, 22*(2), 398–407.

Thomas, M. B., & Neal, P. A. (1978). Collaborating careers: The differential effects of race. *Journal of Vocational Behavior, 12*(1), 33–42.

Thompson, C. (1989). Psychoanalytic psychotherapy with inner-city patients. *Journal of Contemporary Psychotherapy, 19*(2), 137–148.

Tomes, H. (1976). The impact of cultural influences on psychotherapy. In J. L. Claghom (Ed.), *Successful psychotherapy* (pp. 197–203). New York: Brunner /Mazel.

Turner, S., & Armstrong, S. A. (1981). Cross-racial psychotherapy: What the therapists say. *Psychotherapy: Theory, Research, and Practice, 18*(3), 375–378.

U.S. Bureau of the Census. (1994). *Statistical Abstract of the United States: 1994.* Washington, DC: U.S. Government Printing Office.

Wildman, S. (1995). *Privilege revealed: How invisible preference undermines America.* New York: New York University Press.

Williams, B., & Trotman, F. K. (1984, April). *Black women: The original superwomen.* Paper presented at the annual meeting of the New York State Psychological Association, New York.

Willie, C. V., Kramer, B. M., & Brown, B. S. (Eds.). (1973). *Racism and mental health.* Pittsburgh: University of Pittsburgh Press.

Woodard, C. (1995). *Pretty fire.* New York: Penguin.

Wright, M. (1991). African American sisterhood: The impact of the female slave population on American political movements. *Western Journal of Black Studies, 15*(1), 32–45.

## CHAPTER 14

# African American and American Jew
## A Tale of Two Women Searching for Home

### CHERYL L. THOMPSON

African Americans and American Jews share unique aspects of their respective histories. Both groups have suffered extensive histories of institutional and personal oppression and rejection that have included horrendous loss of life. It would seem that this shared history of oppression based on group membership might reinforce the bonds between the two groups. Paradoxically, we often observe hostility and tension between members of these groups despite their shared experiences as targets of genocide. At this time, a tragic gulf exists between African Americans and American Jews in general. Such a gulf not only results in the presence of bad feelings but may have more dire implications. Each group is significantly weakened politically because the contemporary forces of bigotry benefit from their division and flourish.

In this chapter I discuss two psychotherapy patients, both women, one African American and one Jewish American, whose personal struggles metaphorically exemplify the struggles of their respective people. In my analysis I hope to offer a means of reconciliation.

It is important to note that both of these individuals are patients who reflect the neurotic pursuit of a "home" that may be observed in individuals in both cultures. They do not, however, represent the wide range of diversity or a healthy psychological adjustment in either group. Rather, they represent examples of neurotic adjustments. For each of these patients, something in her development has gone awry. Both have been rejected by their parents. When pathology of this sort or any other serious pathology occurs in the person or in the family, the ordinary avenues and opportunities for appropriate identification may be unavailable. Pathology interferes with an individual's ability to take in appropriate objects of identification, even when they are present. It is infinitely more difficult when appropriate objects are not readily available. Specifically, parental rejection makes the process of identity formation fraught with difficulty, and its presence may be seen as a precursor to the development of problems in establishing a healthy sense of self and identity.

One may ask why an exploration of these issues in a Jewish woman in therapy would be relevant to the treatment or understanding of an African American woman. Justifiably or not, African Americans and Jewish Americans have been compared to one another. Both have endured parallel histories of genocide and both find themselves in an "adopted" land where they have been treated as unwelcome and suspect intruders. Understanding the varied survival mechanisms employed by any one group can help us in our attempts to understand those mechanisms or their absence in other groups.

Both patients and their respective groups have ambivalently sought a place to call "home," with all the complexities of feelings experienced when the longing for home is met with rejection. Both struggle to manage the rage and shame resulting from repeated experiences of prejudice. Both may be seen as siblings cheated of their rightful places within their birth and national families. Both of these patients and the groups they represent are experienced by their parents and their nation as unwanted, ungrateful, and unworthy children. Metaphorically, the problems encountered by these patients mirror some of the challenges that African Americans and Jewish Americans face in developing a cohesive ethnic or cultural identity in their "adoptive" motherland, the United States, when that motherland is rejecting as well. I would contend that these challenges are intensified for people of color because their skin color heightens their visibility and in some ways their vulnerability.

My conceptualization of these issues and my treatment of both patients is rooted in my work as a psychodynamically trained clinical psychologist and a formally trained psychoanalyst. Psychodynamic theory and techniques are often the object of scathing criticism when they are applied to the treatment of African Americans and women. They are assailed for their perceived failure to incorporate the national and cultural context in which human development and behavior is embedded, one that includes institutional oppression, in their developmental paradigms and their therapeutic practice. Psychodynamic theory is viewed by its critics as a theoretical framework that focuses exclusively on intrapsychic mechanisms and presumes they should and do develop in a universal fashion, independent of social or cultural influences.

In a previous work (Thompson, 1996) I observed that African Americans are not well represented in the development of psychoanalytic theory or the psychoanalytic movement. Some writers have even suggested that African

Americans were not analyzable (Cohen, 1974; Kardiner & Ovesey, 1951). My view is that pejorative references to African Americans as "primitive" in fact represent the disapproved wishes that all human beings—and thus our society—have, for example, those expressing sexuality, aggression, or emotionality. These are feelings that people are ambivalent about, deny in themselves, and often project onto African Americans. I am also aware of psychoanalytic literature that views women as damaged creatures who wish to be men and who satisfy that need by giving birth to males (Thompson, 1996). However, other psycho-analytic writers (Chodorow, 1978; Gilligan, 1982; Klein, 1975), not coincidentally women, have made contributions to psychoanalytic theory that contradict views of women as "castrated men." African Americans, American Jews, and all women constitute groups who step outside of their place when they advocate or move toward autonomy and social equality in the United States. Often, the response to this has been to pathologize members of these groups as self-hating (if they do not accept the subservient societal roles that are imposed on them), unworthy, and—like the patients discussed in this chapter—ungrateful for what little they have been given (Thompson, 1996).

In my view, the failure to appropriately frame the patient's developmental history and current dilemma in a social context, the failure to consider society's role in promoting and condoning institutional discrimination and its effects on a patient's development and adjustment, is the failure or unwillingness of the analyst or therapist to do so. It represents the therapist's countertransference resistance and is not the result of an absolute mandate of the theory itself (Thompson, 1987, 1989, 1996). When Freud (1914, 1917, 1923, 1938) grappled with the conceptualization of the superego, he viewed it as the internalization of cultural values and prohibitions. This conceptualization, one that explicitly included a consideration of the role of culture, pointed to the role of the family as a major translator or mediator in the transmission of cultural values (Blatt & Lerner, 1983). The superego as an intrapsychic structure was not considered something that developed in isolation from cultural variables; rather, it reflected them as they were communicated by the family. Intrapsychic structures were believed to represent the result of complex interactions between a child's biological endowments, temperament, and predispositions and the interpersonal matrix of the family and the culture. No appropriate analysis of a patient can take place without understanding these contextual variables (Thompson, 1996).

My personal affinity for this orientation is based on the fact that as a technique it elicits a narrative from the patient that is uniquely personal. Therapy proceeds by allowing the patient to tell his or her own story. It is the therapist's responsibility to help provide a safe, by definition, nonattacking environment in which the patient's story may be told. The therapist must then help organize and facilitate an understanding of the patient's story or narrative using the patient's own words and the patient's conceptualization of the problem.

This occurs as the therapist attempts to understand how the experiences contained in the patient's narrative have contributed to the development of the patient's unconscious psychic mechanisms. It is also the therapist's responsibility to facilitate an understanding of the nature of the therapist and patient's interaction in the treatment, and to use that understanding as a model for understanding how the patient negotiates other relationships in his or her world. Developing an understanding of the patient and therapist's interaction is referred to as *the analysis of the transference*. Ultimately the task is to help the patient to connect his or her feelings about aspects of his or her life to the actual experiences contained in his or her own personal narrative. Establishing a connection between the two must take place for authentic insight into the experience to take place. When insight takes place, the patient is no longer relegated to feeling shame about these experiences and feelings (what was unknown or misunderstood), nor is he or she doomed to repeat the same problematic behaviors.

Although I am trained to conduct psychoanalysis, my work with the patients discussed in this chapter does not constitute a formal analysis; rather, it was guided by an object relations psychodynamic theoretical approach. A common element in both approaches is their explicit assumption that unconscious processes and their understanding are important. In the object relations framework, we understand that people come to be who and what they are because of what occurs both inside and outside of them (Fairbairn, 1954; Greenberg & Mitchell, 1983). Winnicott's (1965) and Kohut's (1971) work is useful in describing how we come to be social beings in the many cultural contexts in which we live.

Winnicott (1971) discusses how people come to relate to the culture and describes the "bridges" to culture as *transitional phenomena*, or spaces. Some of these "bridges," such as religion and art, are considered to be shared illusions. Other illusions are individual, and still others are deemed idiosyncratic. The latter may be viewed as neurotic. The hallmark of group membership is the presence of a collection of shared illusions. Kohut (1971) helps us to understand how we come to develop a self as an outgrowth of our biological selves as we move from our family of origin out into the world. Family relations are the template that we carry into the broader culture. The culture may then help to sustain the family template, to challenge it, to destroy it, or leave the individual confused and/or conflicted about a sense of self. One role of the family is to help individuals develop a healthy sense of self and teach its young members how to negotiate the world, or culture. An inherent difficulty in executing these tasks is that the cultural template is always broader than the family and changes from generation to generation. Hence the cultural world is never exactly like the family template. The contemporary world will contain challenges to individuals that their parental figures did not encounter and for which they cannot necessarily prepare their offspring (Greene, 1998). Thus, it is important that the family support the development of a self that has a cohesive core but that is also flexible and as such able to negotiate a wider range of societal demands.

Encouraging the development of a self based on dichotomous, rather than multiple, conceptions of identity leaves family members at risk. If the family boundaries are too rigid and do not permit the self of members to be flexible or "different enough" from family, such individuals may be rendered unable to comfortably function in a wide range of cultural contexts lest they risk the loss of family (or nation) support (Greene, 1997, 1998, 2000; Thompson, 1996).

The distinctions between psychoanalysis and psychodynamic therapy are important and therefore deserve description. Psychoanalysis with these patients would have focused more intensely on developing and analyzing the transference in the treatment. While an analysis of transference constituted a part of their therapy, it was not the major focus of treatment. Another distinction between analysis and psychodynamic therapy as applied in these cases is that the inquiry in the latter is more connected to reality rather than to fantasy, and there is less waiting for material to unfold because the therapist asks more direct questions. In my experience, this approach is more conducive to work with African American patients. If the therapist is too "quiet," African American patients tend to feel that they are not getting anything from the therapist (Thompson, 1996). Conversely, too much or premature interpretations can leave these patients feeling attacked. By definition, unconscious material is unconscious because it is painful to acknowledge. If the therapist uncovers material through interpretation before the patient is ready to be exposed to it and its meaning, such exposure can be experienced as the therapist inflicting pain on or attacking the patient. Because of their history of discrimination and ongoing painful encounters with it in their day-to-day life, many African Americans enter therapy already feeling attacked (Thompson, 1996). When the therapist interprets or moves too quickly to painful material, this behavior may intensify the experience of being attacked or found wanting. An approach in which the therapist's inquiries are framed as questions is effective with African American patients. Such questions are experienced as interest in the patient's narrative and what it means to the patient. I find it particularly helpful to end each session with a meaningful probe that combines a question and an interpretation for the patient to consider.

Using concepts from object relations theory, I assume that social beings replicate previously ingrained early childhood notions of authority, nurturance, and community, and project those early experiences onto all aspects of adult life (Fairbairn, 1954; Klein, 1975). Comparing the nation to a family is a useful way to metaphorically understand and explore the experience of African Americans and American Jews. This notion also includes the projection of an individual's early life experiences and dynamics in his or her relationships onto the national political scene. In this manner, the political landscape becomes a symbol of or exemplar for what is expected within the family. Thus, at some level, every individual is in the midst of a scenario in which he or she is reenacting his or her roles in his or her family in the larger, fantasy-based context of the nation as an imaginary extended family.

The national family, for people born and raised in the United States, is the broader American culture as well as any subcultures the patient belongs to. The United States as a national family has been selectively welcoming and rejecting to different ethnic immigrant groups. It is fair to say that this national family has been hostile and rejecting to both African Americans and American Jews, albeit in different ways and at different points in history. These are only two of many groups who have been treated this way. Despite the differences in the specific legacies of rejection, the existence of legal discrimination against both groups leaves both groups in the position of being treated metaphorically like unwanted children/siblings in a family, competing for what they are told are meager resources that are ultimately begrudged them.

Unfortunately, our national "family" appears to have a need to set the jealous siblings at war. When siblings maintain a hostile position toward one another, the parents can both conceal and continue their own narcissistic involvement with themselves, and define the family problem as the hostility between the "children," taking no responsibility for their role in these damaged relationships.

## CASE EXAMPLES

### Case One

Carol, a 16-year-old, African American, high school senior, entered psychotherapy at the request of her mother and stepfather. Carol's mother believed that Carol was involved in a relationship with a boyfriend that was too intense.

Carol was happy to enter therapy because she believed that her parents did not understand her and would not listen whenever she tried to explain her behavior to them. Carol presented as a solemn young woman who was mature beyond her years. Sometimes her depression was palpable. I viewed her as someone who was neurotically depressed because she was able to continue to work quite successfully. Even though she was not doing well in high school, she had passing grades and had been promoted on two occasions because of her intellectual competence.

Carol began her therapy by talking about the poor relationship she had with her mother. Carol felt that her mother did not care for her or her older sister because the mother's relationship with their father had failed. The parents met while they were in college. They quickly became lovers and Carol's mother became pregnant. Neither she nor her family believed abortion to be an option, so the couple married when the mother was 4 months' pregnant. Carol's mother was 19 years old at the time of the marriage and the father was 20 years old. The mother dropped out of college after the birth of Carol's older sister. The father stayed in college and graduated. After graduation, he was able to work very successfully in banking. Carol was born when her mother was 21 years old. Carol's mother and father were in continuous conflict, and the marriage finally ended when Carol was 6 years old.

The mother expressed deep concern and anger that Carol was in danger of repeating her mistake. She wanted Carol to "date around" and not focus on one boy so early in her life. The mother repeatedly told Carol to look at her, to consider how hard she had worked, and to remember the many years that she had floundered before meeting her current husband. The mother and step-father met when Carol was 13 years old. The mother would often tell Carol that she didn't want her to have to wait until she was 34 years old to have a life she was not ashamed of.

Carol was able to work successfully and to save money. She saw this ability as something that would help her live independently the following year. It was her plan to leave her parents and set up her own living arrangements as soon as she graduated from high school. In the course of her treatment, Carol revealed that she was sexually active and had been for 2 years. She defended her sexual activity by stating that she loved her boyfriend and used contraception. She felt that she was in no danger of repeating her mother's experience. Her sexuality resulted in a further rift in the family when it was discovered that her boyfriend had sneaked into the house and spent the night in Carol's bedroom. As a result of this discovery, Carol was banned from her own house for several days. During this period of banishment, Carol slept in the garage. Carol was willing to remain in the garage because she saw this as a form of confrontation with her parents. She hoped that the neighbors would question them, and that they would be embarrassed by the harshness of their punishment of her. Carol could have moved in with her sister but did not believe that it would affect her parent's treatment of her. She was allowed back in the house following a day of heavy rain in which she became soaked. Her parents stated that she was allowed to return to the house because they were afraid she would get sick.

Throughout her treatment, Carol's parents remained convinced that they had provided all they could for her. They expressed a desire for her to remain in treatment in order to encourage separation from them so that they could move on with their own lives. The parents intended to leave the state and begin a new life with a family of their own.

Thus Carol's belief that her parents no longer wanted to be burdened by her or her sister was confirmed. Carol believed that her parents' bitter divorce was only partially responsible for her mother's intense desire to close this chapter in her life. She believed that her mother wanted to separate herself from her girls because they knew all about her life before her second marriage. Carol described her mother as a woman who had frequently used marijuana and who had many sexual encounters with different partners for several years before settling down and presenting herself as a stable middle-class person. Carol often made a hostile joke about her mother "finding her virginity" after years of "whoring around."

Carol would often say that she did not want to feel sorry for herself but she could not help but wonder what would have happened to her if her parents had cared about her at all. Carol experienced the parental relationship as so bad that she was relieved when they decided to divorce. She did not realize at the time that her father would leave the area and have no further contact with her. Carol's mother believed that her father left the state in order to avoid paying child support. As a result of not having child support, the mother had to work both a full-time job and a part-time job. Consequently, the girls rarely saw their mother while they were growing up. There was no extended family to provide any caretaking because Carol's mother was estranged from her own family. The extended family believed Carol's mother to be the source of the discord in her marriage and blamed her for the divorce. Carol's grandparents were very pleased that their son-in-law was as successful as he was. The grandparents are deeply religious people who firmly believe that all marriages have difficulty and divorce should be avoided. As a result, the grandparents were unavailable to Carol and her sister.

The sisters were close and shared their perceptions of rejection by their mother. When the mother met the man she would eventually marry, the girls felt further rejection. Carol described her mother during this courtship as like a giggly teenager who spent time on the telephone with her boyfriend. When the parents came together as a couple, it was clear to Carol that there was no space in this new relationship for the girls. Carol explained that the relationship was very good for her mother, for it enabled her to quit one of her jobs and finish college. She was then able to resume work with a much better salary and to have a position that she felt was more in keeping with her ability.

Carol saw her mother as a much younger person, basically as a sibling, so that Carol was often left with a deep longing for a maternal figure. Sometimes this longing would get her into deep trouble because she would borrow items of her mother's clothing and wear them. On one occasion she took a very expensive pair of shoes that the mother was particularly attached to and ruined them by wearing them in bad weather. Her mother was furious, so unforgiving that this episode severed their relationship. Carol moved out of the house and thereafter lived with her sister. She had only one semester left to graduation from high school.

As she became more estranged from her mother, Carol began demanding more and more of her boyfriend's attention and time. He found these demands excessive and eventually left her. Carol was quickly able to understand that her demands on her boyfriend were the result of her feeling isolated from her family and her need to find a sense of belonging elsewhere. However, she still felt betrayed by her boyfriend as he too had marked difficulties in his family relationships and depended upon her to support him. She believed that he wanted more from her than he was willing to give to her. Carol did come to understand that both she and her boyfriend were using each other to address the deep feelings of rejection and hurt they experienced in their family relations (Willis, 1990).

Some of the problems that brought Carol to treatment are common to many adolescents today. Divorce is common and children of divorced parents are often exposed to parental sexuality in ways that might not have occurred if the parents had stayed in a long-term marriage. The feeling of rejection is also a common experience in psychotherapy patients. Carol's rejection was not just a feeling: she was rejected in fact. While it is not rare to hear young parents say that they will not sacrifice their lives for their children, this attitude appears to be most intense in those parents who have not experienced themselves as accepted as unique individuals in their birth families (Miller, 1981). The inability to sacrifice for a child appears to be a result of believing that the sacrifice has already occurred. It requires no great leap of logic to see that Carol's mother believed that she had tried to please her own parents but was rejected when her real-life, unexpected problems interfered with their expectations. Furthermore, there is a strong force in American society that compels one to think primarily of oneself and not to be concerned about the needs of the group, even the family group. Carol found herself struggling to take care of herself at a very early age. While she could be proud of her ability to do so, this very ability took her out of synchrony with most middle-class children who now experience a very protracted adolescence.

This case almost represents a stereotype of the "strong independent African American woman." However, what becomes apparent in the patient is that the facade of independent functioning and strength is extremely fragile. This young woman is on a path of loneliness and vulnerability that has the potential to destroy her. I selected Carol for this discussion because she highlights a struggle often observed within the African American community and her personal survival symbolically represents the group as surviving despite many real and fantasied obstacles. However, in the African American community, when there is a struggle for identity or the need for a sense of belonging, there is no concrete or clear place to begin such a process. Whether we believe such a place is necessary or not, such a place does not exist for African Americans. Instead, what tends to happen is that significant relationships bear the brunt of the early pain and rejection that is never mediated. Thus, we see marked difficulty in male–female relationships because the relationship cannot withstand the excessive demands aimed at compensating for the history of deprivation (Willis, 1990).

## Case Two

Sarah entered psychotherapy at age 19 years. She was about to begin her junior year in college and found herself unsure of her major, her future, and her identity. Sarah came to treatment with me after a brief visit to Israel. She had decided that she was going to return to Israel, live on a kibbutz, and study Hebrew. Her parents were in a panic about her decision. They had never considered the possibility that any of their children would not complete college. Sarah was the older of two siblings. The parents hoped that since I was not Jewish I would be able to quickly convince Sarah that a trip to Israel at this time was not in her best interest.

Sarah was anxious and depressed. She felt that her parents did not understand her and were only concerned about what others would think of them if one of their children did not complete college. Sarah wondered whether I could help her since I did not have a Jewish identity and could not understand her quest for self-knowledge. Sarah left treatment after 5 months and returned to Israel. Her parents accepted her choice even though they were upset about it. She remained in Israel for many months. However, she eventually returned to the United States and renewed her therapy with me.

Sarah decided to move to a religious community and became involved in an ultraorthodox group, which she found warm and inviting. As Sarah became more overtly religious, she also became more estranged from her family because she could not eat their food and would not travel on the Sabbath. She had different families with whom she could spend the Sabbath and she always felt accepted. The religious community's rules about life and relationships helped Sarah feel more secure in the world. Sarah presented as intensely worried about doing or saying the right thing. Her religious community helped her address her anxiety. As we worked together, we found that Sarah grew up in a family that did not allow her to develop sound judgment. Her mother was critical and disapproving. Her father, in an apparent attempt to compensate for her mother's critical posture, was completely accepting. He praised his daughter for every effort, but Sarah experienced his approval as false. She described her father as a person who never grew up and as someone who always received the mother's disapproval because of his immaturity. Sarah perceived her father as her mother did: he was a silly, perpetual adolescent. Sarah found substitute parents in the structured religious community. For example, her dating life was somewhat supervised in that she met men who were chosen for her. She was able to discuss her dating life with her rabbi, who would often advise her about whether to leave someone or to remain in the relationship.

Sarah's increasing involvement in this ultraorthodox community further pushed her estrangement from her parents. They worried that she was being seduced into a cult. Her parents were minimally practicing Jews whose families emigrated to the United States in the early 1900s. By the time Sarah was an adult, the parents attended a temple led by a woman rabbi, but only for high holy days. They saw themselves as progressives and could not understand what appeared to them to be a regressive pull in their daughter's return to stricter religious practices. They felt ashamed of their daughter.

Sarah remained depressed but became increasingly aware that she was really trying to find a home. Sarah described herself as someone who had no idea about herself or her work, and had no sense of direction. Sarah understood that it was her mother's recurrent rejection of her that was at the core of her struggle. However, she remained unable to explore that relationship in order to gain enough understanding to become less incapacitated by the rejection. She continued to blame herself. Sarah believed that the external structure supplied primarily by religion would alter her internal structure. As Sarah's understanding about herself and her family increased, she became able to speak to her mother about her deep feeling of rejection. While this did not change their relationship, it did allow Sarah to experience a sense of self. As of today, she has found no one with whom she can make a permanent attachment.

## DISCUSSION

Neither of these cases was experienced by the therapist as a treatment success. Both young women have gone on to claim their lives as their own and to live them with some happiness and the conviction that they have made choices that fit their needs. I think every therapist hopes that their patients will succeed in all of life's challenges. Knowing that each of these women has experienced such profound rejection that each harbored a deep fear of intimacy, I hoped they would remain in treatment until they could feel safe in an intimate relationship. However, each ended treatment before these changes could take place. Both women left their therapist as a defense against rejection by the therapist that they were convinced would inevitably happen. Because their departure from treatment was defensive, rather than marking the end of their work, I do not feel the treatment could be considered wholly successful.

These cases highlight some of the differences between African Americans and American Jews. Some of the differences are represented in individual psychopathology and some represent the larger cultural differences that often result in African Americans and American Jews appearing competitive about their histories of oppression (Terkel, 1992).

The first case was selected because she highlights the difficulty often seen within the African American community around the struggle for identity, the struggle for intimacy, and the experience of community. Many African Americans have attempted on an individual or small-group basis to select a specific African country as a source of identification (West, 1993). The changes in the American community of people of African descent about how they wish to be addressed reflect a quest for a place to describe as "home." However, "African American" is probably too vague a term to be curative. Africa is a large continent. The fact that Africans were all "Black" has never meant that Africans regard themselves as one unified and homogeneous people or nation. Indeed, Africa has always consisted of many different nations and tribes with many different languages, customs, and values. Many of these nations and tribes do not now and never have considered themselves "brothers and sisters"—even if they may be idealistically viewed in this manner by people of African descent who live in countries where they are by far numerical minorities, or by White Americans who see all Black people and all people of color as if they are the same, because they are not White. However, romanticized depictions of the Africa that existed during slavery suggested the opposite, despite a litany of pejorative information from the dominant culture about Africa and African people. Over time, more accurate depictions of the African continent that contradict the prevailing view have become available. During the 1960s and 1970s when more affirmative models of Black identity were asserted, they were accompanied by positive identifications with being a person of African descent. Africa, like the birth mother from whom one was stolen, given up, or both, and hence never really known, is to some extent idealized. It is for many African Americans akin to the fantasy of the birth mother who was never known. The relationship to her is based on an illusion, not on the history of a realistic relationship. Despite the ambivalence that is always a part of such relationships, the fantasy that is created is always better than the reality.

There is probably some unconscious awareness that some of our African brethren actively contributed to our slave status. The decisions about who would go and who would remain have never been clarified and are virtually taboo to discuss openly. It is clearly more comfortable to view White oppressors as the solitary and absolute enemy with a conspicuous omission of some consideration of the circumstances that permitted our sale and trade by other Africans. This phenomenon can be likened to the defensive operation of *splitting* (Kernberg, 1975), in which there is a failure to integrate the good and bad elements of an object, person, or relationship, with the result that it is either idealized or devalued. Since no person or relationship is "all good" or "all bad," engaging in this kind of defense does not allow for the integration of all elements of an object nor does it facilitate changing the experience. Considering the role of Africans in the selling of Africans does not relieve the dominant culture in the United States of the responsibility for the cruel and harsh nature of slavery nor the more than a century of legal racial discrimination and disenfranchisement that followed. It is, however, an essential piece of this historical conundrum that requires discussion if our dilemma is to be fully contextualized. Thus, we as African Americans have been rejected by our birth mother (Africa) as well as by our cruel and rejecting foster or adoptive mother (America).

A well developed Black or African American identity is one that leaves the individual feeling secure about who he or she is but also flexible. African American identity was initially deliberately stripped and hidden from us. Because this history was distorted, it was often rejected. However, in the 1960s and 1970s, the civil rights movement served as a catalyst for the development of a more affirmative and accurate African American identity. However, for some African Americans, a sense of African heritage and African identity is still elusive. When the insecure individual experiences this elusiveness, it may be a source of anxiety for him or her. The response may be to become rigid about how one's ethnic identity is defined and to experience people who defy those definitions as a source of anxiety and something to be defended against. Using the authenticity of one's "blackness" to exclude or minimize other aspects of a person's identity is an example of such rigidity. Group boundaries are used to control the behavior of group members who might step outside the acceptable realm. What is threatened in the individual who is insecure about his or her own identity is the fantasy of a Black or African American identity that is clearly and absolutely defined for all African Americans, for all time.

For Jewish people who also struggle with issues of identity, the situation is different, for they have a real place they can call "home": Israel. Yet most American Jews were not born in Israel. They are the descendants of Jews who were born in different European countries in which they were ill-treated and from which they were often banished. In addition, Israel has been a Jewish state for merely 50 years, and thus does not constitute a birth mother per se. Israel cannot satisfy the need for a home that is a birth mother. Israel can be seen dynamically as a devouring stepmother because it requires the bloodshed and lives of its young to maintain the security of its borders. This is not a criticism of the need to defend those borders or its people, nor is it intended as a criticism of the importance of the existence of the state of Israel. It is simply a statement of the high cost of doing so. In psychodynamic thinking, Israel is a cause for ambivalence. Ironically, this dream of the historical home brings with it the reality of war and endless cycles of terror and violence to defend its borders. Israel may never be able to offer a truly safe territory or home because of the long-standing political and military contentiousness regarding its borders and its right to exist. It is noteworthy that some of the most belligerent and zealous young Israelis are American-born Jews. Their anger appears to reflect the ease they may find in expressions of rage to the stranger rather than to the familiar. That is, for many American Jews it is easier to fight the Palestinians than to fight against American anti-Semites for acceptance in the land of their birth, the United States.

The dilemmas of these young women can be seen as metaphor for the oppressed and rejected populations they represent. Their mothers are homelands who offer no succor. Each patient stepped out of her proverbial place and violated the family's expectations. Neither of them lived up to the parents' fantasy of achievement or interpersonal relationships. Neither chose people or life paths that would enhance the family status, as their parents hoped. In both

cases, the parents would or could not see what their child really was and accept her for what she was. Both sets of parents could only relate to their child
in response to the ways that the child had disappointed them. Both young
women are left with the issue of what to do with this profound experience of
rejection. Hence both are left to look for a home someplace else. When there
is no home, the search becomes intense and often futile, because there is no
clarity about what constitutes such a place. Each of the women is looking for
a place of comfort based on fantasy, just as the two oppressed groups they represent are looking for a place of acceptance and appreciation based on a fantasy of a place and not a realistic relationship with that place.

Neither Africa nor Israel can be a true home for those who struggle with
their identity in this manner because one can never return to that which only
exists as metaphor or as a fantasy representation of what one wishes were home.
In the fantasy, home can be anything wished for; however, the reality never
lives up to the fantasy creation. As a result of their mutual struggle to find a
connection with a nonrejecting mother, the groups can be seen as competitive
siblings, vying for acknowledgment of whose suffering is worse. The reality is
that both have suffered; both experiences are real; and the consequences for
both are devastating.

The sources of envy between the groups rests in some of the developments
that are unique to their experiences in America. The Jewish experience in
Europe uniquely positioned them for success in the United States (Sowell,
1994). Jews were for the most part urban dwellers, and they possessed a strong
intellectual tradition in which formal academic and scholastic achievement was
accorded a high priority. The presence of an intellectual tradition is not synonymous with simply being smart or intellectually cogent. I am not suggesting that African Americans were intellectually lacking or disinterested in learning. An intellectual tradition, however, is defined by a long history of learning
in a formal, often hierarchical, institutional setting. The Jewish culture is highly
verbalized, where the expression of words (particularly in writing), the ability
to verbally express thoughts, and to actively engage in debate and argue ideas
are highly prized (Langman, 1997).

In contrast, African Americans were stripped of their languages as a part
of their cultural genocide. They were not only forbidden to attend formal
schools but until 1865 laws forbid African Americans to learn to read and write.
Violating such laws warranted punishment by death or banishment for both
the teacher (even if White) and the pupil. Thus, learning had to take place in
secret. It is instructive that African Americans routinely put their lives in peril
by learning to read and write and seeing to it that their children did so too.
Often, the Bible was the only book available to use. This is a different experience than one in which the intellectual tradition in one's own language or other
language continues uninterrupted. African Americans did not have the resources
to "learn" in American insititutions and were often banished from them. Hence

they were forced to value other ways of "knowing" such as entrepreneurship and alternative forums of leadership (via offices in churches, masonic lodges and other community-based "corporations").

The presence of the intellectual tradition among emigrating Jews and the importance of the written word was also more consistent with Western educational traditions and learning styles than those in Africa. The way that education and learning were framed in Jewish culture is similar to the way it is framed in Western society. This factor positioned American Jews for success in the broader American society in ways that African Americans were not similarly positioned.

African Americans have been uniquely positioned not to succeed in their unchosen land. Blackness, the distinction of skin color in and of itself, denies people the option to assimilate or to become fully acculturated. Furthermore, African Americans were denied access to the country's intellectual institutions. This made it easier for White society to block their access to opportunities that required institutional credentials. It also made formal intellectual achievement more difficult, despite the later emergence of Black educational institutions. African Americans are left to struggle with the United States, an angry and ungiving adoptive mother, with a full awareness that there is no place else to find a safe and secure haven.

American Jews had also learned to seek employment in professional or portable forms of employment as a result of needing occupations that could survive banishment from a country. Arrival in the United States with its short history and a style of life that allowed a subculture to flourish has fostered the development of Jewish Americans as an intellectual and economically powerful minority. Again, the strength of the group, that is, its identification as a cohesive group that depends on group members more than on the broader American culture and the subsequent failure to fully assimilate, is also its vulnerability. These strengths in the group make it a target that remains an identifiable entity, often feared for its economic and intellectual power. Their power and influence is often exaggerated because of that fear.

A source of a lack of empathy among African Americans for American Jews is the perception that in America, American Jews need only renounce their Jewishness in order to become free to fully enjoy the privileges available to all who are White. African Americans are reluctant to acknowledge the depth of historical suffering that serves as the heritage of many American Jews, preferring to focus on their skin privilege as Whites. Conversely, many American Jews identify with their history of oppression and genocide but do not wish to examine the truth that they enjoy the privileges accorded people with white skin in America, even if those privileges are not equal to those accorded White Americans who are not Jewish. It is this perceived freedom of choice that often makes it difficult for African Americans to seriously sympathize with their more successful but oppressed sibling. If Jews were to acknowledge the power and privilege they have enjoyed in the United States, they would have to surrender the guilt they hold over some of mainstream America for their suffering. It is also likely that the harsher the oppression that any one group has suffered, in this case American Jews, the more group members may need to avoid identifying with members of other groups who currently suffer in ways that they have. To do so resonates too loudly emotionally. It elicits the need to deny and avoid reexperiencing the pain and fear in lieu of maintaining a sense of relief. The pain is a part of the ongoing pain that group members carry individually and collectively as survivors of oppression. The fear represents a rekindled fear, always lurking beneath the surface of consciousness, that the original horror could happen again, that one is never completely free of the threat of annihilation—hence one is never really safe. The relief that someone else and not you is the target of hostility makes it difficult to identify with those who are current targets.

Just as Carol and Sarah are clearly two lonely and hurt people, the two groups they represent are also lonely and hurt. The fragile alliance that once existed when discrimination was open and legal was an alliance that could not succeed because it was based on the superficial sameness of the groups. This phenomenon would occur in a family where one sibling is enormously successful, while another barely squeaks through, but the parents behave as if the children are indistinguishable. The less successful one may grudgingly accept help from the other, but neither believes that their position in the family allows for equal voice or equal respect from the rest of the family. Instead of being able to make sense of the success and the failure in the context of the demands of the family, it is acknowledgment of differences between the groups that could begin a dialogue about the forces that have resulted in their respective social positions. The awareness and acceptance of each other's pain would allow for the two groups to share more fully their strengths and become a source of empowerment probably sufficient to confront their mutual rejection. Jews have economic success and a formal intellectual tradition that can be helpful to African Americans who have numbers, perseverance, a historic desire to learn even at great risk, and a deep desire to also succeed in this, now their adopted motherland.

Both African Americans and Jewish Americans are aware at some level that their "adoptive mother" is consistently rejecting and that it is unlikely that any behavior on the part of these rejected "siblings" will result in the mother's approval. When both groups accept this idea individually, they are seen as hostile. When a rejected child accurately perceives his or her parents as hostile and deficient, the parents' defensive response to this truth, a truth they do not wish to acknowledge about themselves, is to redefine the child's accurate perception as if it were the child's deficiency or rejection of the parent. When a socially disadvantaged group correctly identifies the dominant, privileged group as hostile and rejecting, the dominant group's defensive response is to redefine the disadvantaged group's accurate perception as if it were unwarranted or hostile. The dominant group fails to acknowledge its role in the disadvantaged group's deprivation. The disadvantaged group's appropriate angry response to this redefinition and distortion of their perception is often interpreted as a rejecting desire for political separatism.

However, until there is willingness to understand that the rejection is real and permanent, no resolution or reconciliation can take place. Some African Americans view the position that American Jews hold, one just outside of the majority community, to be one born of their own choice. Even if this were a realistic and unambivalent choice, their pain is no less real. Rejection and banishment are no less painful whether one is banished to a gilded cage or to a concrete cell—neither one is of your own making. The rejection for each group is a result of its identity, whether by history and choice or by history and color. It is not a dialectic of choice or color but the shared reality of a history of rejection that can bring the groups together. Freedom, as in the case of the two rejected women and the two groups they represent, can only be gained when the rejection is fully acknowledged and the subsequent pain is experienced in its reality. Reconciliation occurs when one accepts the reality of a loss that cannot be changed, accepts the pain of that loss, and comes to terms with that reality in doing so. At that juncture, the individual can feel able to confront the stress of life and to manage it in accordance with the resources he or she has, to be aware of the resources he or she needs, and to make whatever changes are required to accomplish adapting to the demands of reality. This acknowledgment allows for the surrender of the bitter fantasy of pleasing and/or frustrating the rejecting parent. When African Americans and American Jews can acknowledge the shared experience of rejection, the possibility of repaired relationships can become a reality.

## ACKNOWLEDGEMENT

I would like to thank my husband, David Sard, PhD, for his editorial support and for being a person with whom ideas can be shared and explored. Without him this chapter would not have been possible.

## REFERENCES

Blatt, S., & Lerner, H. (1983). Psychodynamic perspectives on personality theory. In M. Hersen, A. E. Kazdin, & A. S. Bellack (Eds.), *Handbook of clinical psychology* (pp. 87–106). New York: Pergamon Press.

Chodorow, N. (1978). *The reproduction of mothering.* Berkeley and Los Angeles: University of California Press.

Cohen, A. I. (1974). Treating the Black patient: Transference questions. *American Journal of Psychiatry, 28,* 137–143.

Fairbairn, W. (1954). *An object relations theory of personality.* New York: Basic Books.

Freud, S. (1914). On narcissism. In J. Strachey (Ed. & Trans.), *The standard edition of the complete psychological works of Sigmund Freud* (Vol. 14, pp. 69–102). London: Hogarth Press.

Freud, S. (1917). Mourning and melancholia. In J. Strachey (Ed. & Trans.), *The standard edition of the complete psychological works of Sigmund Freud* (Vol. 14, pp. 239–258). London: Hogarth Press.

Freud, S. (1923). The ego and the id. In J. Strachey (Ed. & Trans.), *The standard edition of the complete psychological works of Sigmund Freud* (Vol. 19, pp. 12–63). London: Hogarth Press.

Freud, S. (1938). An outline of psychoanalysis. In J. Strachey (Ed. & Trans.), *The standard edition of the complete psychological works of Sigmund Freud* (Vol. 23, pp. 144–205). London: Hogarth Press.

Gilligan, C. (1982). *In a different voice.* Cambridge, MA: Harvard University Press.

Greenberg, J., & Mitchell, S. (1983). *Object relations in psychoanalytic theory.* Cambridge, MA: Harvard University Press.

Greene, B. (1997, June). Psychotherapy with African American women: Integrating feminist and psychodynamic models. *Journal of Smith College Studies in Social Work: Theoretical, Research, Practice, and Educational Perspectives for Understanding and Working with African American Clients, 67(3),* 299–322.

Greene, B. (1998). *Psychotherapy with African Americans: Ethnoracial transference and countertransference.* Unpublished manuscript.

Greene, B. (2000). Beyond heterosexism and across the cultural divide. In B. Greene & G. L. Croom (Eds.), *Education, research, and practice in lesbian, gay, bisexual, and transgendered psychology: A resource manual* (pp. 1-45). Thousand Oaks, CA: Sage.

Kardiner, A., & Ovesey, L. (1951). *The mark of oppression.* New York: World Publishing.

Kernberg, O. (1975). *Borderline conditions and pathological narcissism.* Northvale, NJ: Jason Aronson.

Klein, M. (1975). *Love, guilt, and reparation and other works: Vol. 1. 1921–1945.* London: Hogarth Press.

Kohut, H. (1971). *The analysis of the self.* New York: Basic Books.

Langman, P. F. (1997). White culture, Jewish culture, and the origins of psychotherapy. *Psychotherapy, 34(2),* 207–218.

Sowell, T. (1994). *Race and culture.* New York: Basic Books.

Terkel, S. (1992). *Race: How African Americans and Whites think and feel about the American obsession.* New York: New Press.

Thompson, C. (1987). Racism or neuroticism? An entangled dilemma for the Black middle-class patient. *Journal of the American Academy of Psychoanalysis, 15(3),* 395–405.

Thompson, C. (1989). Psychoanalytic psychotherapy with inner-city patients. *Journal of Contemporary Psychotherapy, 19(2),* 137–148.

Thompson, C. (1996). The African American patient in psychodynamic treatment. In R. Perez-Foster, M. Moskowitz, & R. A. Javier (Eds.), *Reaching across boundaries of culture and class: Widening the scope of psychotherapy* (pp. 115–142). Northvale, NJ: Jason Aronson.

West, C. (1993). *Race matters.* Boston: Beacon Press.

Willis, J. (1990). Some destructive elements in African American male–female relationships. *Family Therapy, 17,* 139–147.

Winnicott, D. W. (1965). *Maturational processes and the facilitating environment.* New York: International Universities Press.

# Index